Statistics for Biology and Health

Series Editors
M. Gail, K. Krickeberg, J. Sarmet, A. Tsiatis, W. Wong

Statistics for Biology and Health

Luc Duchateau
Paul Janssen

The Frailty Model

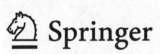 Springer

Luc Duchateau
Faculty of Veterinary Medicine
Ghent University
Salisburylaan 133
B-9820 Merelbeke
Belgium
luc.duchateau@ugent.be

Paul Janssen
Center for Statistics
Hasselt University
Agoralaan –Building D
B-3590 Diepenbeek
Belgium
paul.janssen@uhasselt.be

Series Editors

M. Gail
National Cancer Institute
Rockville, MD 20892
USA

K. Krickeberg
Le Chatelet
F-63270 Manglieu
France

J. Sarmet
Department of Epidemiology
School of Public Health
Johns Hopkins University
615 Wolfe Street
Baltimore, MD 21205-2103
USA

A. Tsiatis
Department of Statistics
North Carolina State
    University
Raleigh, NC 27695
USA

W. Wong
Department of Statistics
Stanford University
Stanford, CA 94305-4065
USA

ISBN 978-1-4419-2499-5   e-ISBN 978-0-387-72835-3

To Pascale, Veerle, and Katelijne (L.D.)

To Mia, Hans, and Marleen (P.J.)

Preface

Survival analysis techniques are used in a variety of disciplines including human and veterinary medicine, epidemiology, engineering, biology and economy. Proportional hazards models and accelerated failure time models are classical models that are frequently used for the analysis of univariate (censored) survival data.

In recent years a number of papers appeared, extending these models to models that are suitable to handle more complex survival data. In this context a lot of attention has been paid to frailty models and copula models. These models provide a powerful tool to analyse clustered survival data.

In this book the focus is on frailty models, but similarities as well as differences between frailty models and copula models are highlighted. Frailty models provide a nice way to capture and to describe the dependence of observations within a cluster and/or the heterogeneity between clusters. The specification of a frailty model is rather easy. Frailty models are hazard models having a multiplicative frailty factor. This factor specifies how frail subjects in a specific cluster are. The hazard factor in the model can depend on covariates and can be modelled in a parametric or a semiparametric way. Frailty models are conditional models. The frailty factor is random and therefore a frailty distribution needs to be specified in the frailty model. Different choices of frailty distributions are studied in detail in this book; attention is paid to the relation between the choice of the distribution and the type of dependence it generates between observations within a cluster.

Once the frailty model is specified we need to fit the model. This is often not an easy task and in many cases standard software to fit such models is missing. For particular choices of the frailty distribution, the frailties can be integrated out with respect to the frailty distribution from the conditional likelihood resulting in the marginal likelihood. For parametric frailty models, maximisation of the marginal likelihood then leads to estimates of the parameters in the model. However, for semiparametric frailty models, more complex estimation techniques are needed. These techniques include the EM algorithm, penalised likelihood techniques, and Gibbs sampling in a Bayesian context. This book does not give an exhaustive overview of all models and techniques that are available for the analysis of clustered survival data. We rather aim at an in-depth discussion of the most current techniques and we want to demonstrate, based on real data sets, how results obtained from the statistical analysis should be interpreted. By doing so, we hope to bring these important tools closer to the applied statisticians.

In the two final chapters of the book we consider more complex frailty models including hierarchical models with more than one level of clustering.

The data sets used in the book are taken from the different disciplines in which the authors worked during the last ten years. Three data sets are provided by the European Organisation for Research and Treatment of Cancer (EORTC, Brussels, Belgium): the periop data set (Example 1.5), the DCIS data set (Example 1.6), and the bladder cancer data set (Example 1.10). Another study in human medicine is a large asthma prevention trial that was run by Union Chimique Belge (UCB) to assess the effect of a new drug (Example 1.9). An infant mortality data set from Jimma (Ethiopia) resulted from a large longitudinal study run by the Public Health investigators at Jimma University (Example 1.11). The other data sets are from veterinary sciences. The first study (Example 1.1) deals with the epidemiology of East Coast Fever, an important disease of cattle in eastern and southern Africa. The data are provided by the Institute of Tropical Medicine (ITM, Antwerp, Belgium). The Department of Medical Imaging of Domestic Animals (Ghent University, Belgium) has provided data on time to diagnosis of fracture healing in dogs (Example 1.2). We further include two data sets from the Department of Physiology and Biometrics (Ghent University, Belgium) on mastitis and udder infection (Examples 1.3 and 1.4). Finally the Department of Reproduction, Obstetrics and Herd Health (Ghent University, Belgium) has kindly provided a culling data set (Example 1.7) and an insemination data set (Example 1.8).

This book is intended for students and for applied statisticians. It can be used as a graduate course for students who have had a course on survival analysis and a course on statistical inference. Applied statisticians will find a lot of examples in the book, which will help to get a better understanding of the theoretical ideas. The code of the programs used in the examples of the book is freely available from the Springer Verlag website. This gives the readers the opportunity to try the examples themselves and to adapt the code or write new code for their particular problems.

Selected parts of the book have been used as teaching material for a series of lectures at the Biometrics and Clinical Informatics Department of Johnson & Johnson Pharmaceutical Research and Development in Beerse, Belgium (October-November 2005) and for workshops in Nairobi (Kenya, 2004) and Addis Ababa (Ethiopia, 2005), sponsored by the Flemish Interuniversitary Council - University Development Cooperation. We also gratefully acknowledge the financial support from the IAP research network P6/03 of the Belgian Government (Belgian Science Policy).

We thank all those who provided in one way or another support to this book project: Bart Ampe, Sarne De Vliegher, Els Goetghebeur, Klara Goethals, Hans Laevens, Geert Opsomer, and Marije Risselada (Ghent University, Belgium), Tomasz Burzykowski, Goele Massonnet, and Noël Veraverbeke (Hasselt University, Belgium), Arnost Komárek (Catholic University Leuven, Belgium), Catherine Legrand and Ingrid Van Keilegom (Université Catholique de Louvain, Belgium), Dirk Berkvens (ITM, Belgium), Richard Sylvester (EORTC, Belgium), Catherine Fortpied (UCB, Belgium), Vincent Ducrocq (INRA, Jouy-en-Josas, France), Andreas Wienke (Martin-Luther-Universität Halle-Wittenberg, Germany), Samuli Ripatti (Karolinska Institute, Sweden), Virginie Rondeau (INSERM, Bordeaux, France), Elisa Molanes (University of La Coruña, Spain), Mekonnen Assefa and Fasil Tessema (Jimma University, Ethiopia), and Daan de Waal (University of the Free State, South Africa).

A word of special thanks from Paul Janssen goes to his next-door colleague for many years, Noël Veraverbeke, for many discussions on different issues in survival analysis and in statistics in general.

Luc Duchateau would like to thank Herman Ramon, Paul Darius, Bruno Goddeeris, Jef Vercruysse, and Christian Burvenich for their stimulating support in his different research undertakings.

Luc Duchateau
Paul Janssen
September 2007

Contents

Glossary of Definitions and Notation

Definitions are given for the case of the shared frailty model with one clustering level, with the first index i referring to the cluster and the second index j
referring to the jth observation within that cluster. For univariate frailty models or models without clustering, the first index i refers to the ith observation.
For hierarchical models with two clustering levels, the first index i refers to
the highest clustering level, the second index j to the second clustering level
and the third index k to the kth observation within cluster j which is nested
within cluster i.

The indexing for the conditional, joint and population density and survival
functions can be deduced from the corresponding hazard functions.

β	the fixed effects vector (of dimension p)
$\Gamma(.)$	the gamma function
δ_{ij}	censoring indicator with $\delta_{ij} = 1$ if the event time is observed, otherwise zero
ζ	(ξ, θ, β)
$\zeta(t_1, t_2)$	the cross ratio function
θ	the variance of a frailty density with mean one (except in the case of the positive stable frailty distribution)
ξ	vector containing the parameters of the baseline hazard $h_0(t)$
τ	Kendall's tau
Φ	the acceleration factor in the accelerated failure time model
$\phi(t_1, t_2)$	the ratio of the joint density function and the product of the two population density functions
$\psi(t_1, t_2)$	the ratio of the joint survival function and the product of the two population survival functions

c_{ij}	the censoring time
$C_{\boldsymbol{\theta}}(.)$	the copula function with parameter vector $\boldsymbol{\theta}$
d	the total number of events
d_i	the number of events in cluster i
$h_0(t)$	the baseline hazard function
$h_{0i}(t)$	the baseline hazard function for cluster i
$h_{ij}(t)$	the conditional hazard function
$h_{ij,c}(t)$	the conditional hazard function for observation j
	from cluster i with $u_i = 1$
$h_i(\mathbf{t}_{n_i})$	the joint conditional hazard function for cluster i
$h_{\mathbf{x},f}(\mathbf{t}_n)$	the joint hazard function for clusters of size n
	with covariate information $\mathbf{x}$ based on the frailty model
$h_{\mathbf{x},p}(\mathbf{t}_n)$	the joint hazard function for clusters of size n
	with covariate information $\mathbf{x}$ based on the marginal model
$h_{\mathbf{x},f}(t)$	the population hazard function for subjects
	with covariate information $\mathbf{x}$ based on the frailty model
$h_{\mathbf{x},p}(t)$	the population hazard function for subjects
	with covariate information $\mathbf{x}$ based on the marginal model
$H_0(t)$	the cumulative baseline hazard
$\mathbf{H}$	the Hessian matrix
$\mathcal{I}$	the Fisher information matrix
$\mathbf{I}$	the observed information matrix
$I(condition)$	the indicator function equal to one if the condition is true,
	zero otherwise
l_{ij}	the lowerbound of the interval that contains the event time
$l(.)$	the loglikelihood function
$L(.)$	the likelihood function
$L_{marg}(.)$	the marginal likelihood function
$L_{part}(.)$	the partial likelihood function
$\mathcal{L}(.)$	the Laplace transform
n_i	the number of observations in cluster i
p	the dimension of $\boldsymbol{\beta}$
r	the total number of distinct event times
r_{ij}	the upperbound of the interval that contains the event time
$R(y_{ij})$	the risk set for observation y_{ij}
	including all subjects at risk at time y_{ij}
$R_i(y_{ij})$	the risk set for observation y_{ij}
	including only subjects from cluster i at risk at time y_{ij}
s	the number of clusters
$\mathcal{S}$	the vector of scores
t_{ij}	the event time
u_i	the frailty term for cluster i
w_i	the random effect for cluster i
$W(\lambda, \rho)$	the Weibull density with scale parameter λ
	and shape parameter ρ

$\mathbf{x}_{ij}$ vector containing covariate information

$\mathbf{x}_{ij}\left(t_{ij1}\right),\ldots,\mathbf{x}_{ij}\left(t_{ijk_{ij}}\right)$ time-varying covariate vectors with k_{ij} timepoints

$\mathbf{x}$ $\left(\mathbf{x}_1^t,\ldots,\mathbf{x}_n^t\right)^t$

$\mathbf{x}_i$ $\left(\mathbf{x}_{i1}^t,\ldots,\mathbf{x}_{in_i}^t\right)^t$

y_{ij} the minimum of the event time and censoring time

$y_{(1)},\ldots,y_{(r)}$ the ordered event times

z_{ij} $\left(y_{ij},\delta_{ij}\right)$

1

Introduction

1.1 Goals

Survival analysis is an important statistical field that is required for data analysis in different disciplines. There are a large number of textbooks on the basic concepts of survival analysis, e.g., Collett (2003) and Machin et al. (2006). In recent years a number of papers have been published extending the classical survival models to models that are suitable for the analysis of clustered survival data: frailty models. A wide variety of frailty models and several numerical techniques to fit these models have been studied in these papers. Only a limited number of textbooks have chapters devoted to frailty models, all of them containing only some specific aspects on frailty models. Klein and Moeschberger (1997) have a chapter on the use of the EM algorithm in semiparametric frailty models. Ibrahim et al. (2001) discuss both parametric and semiparametric frailty models but only in a Bayesian context. Hougaard (2000) discusses, among other techniques to model multivariate survival data, the frailty model mainly assuming a parametric model. Finally, Therneau and Grambsch (2000) discuss inference for the semiparametric frailty model using penalised partial likelihood.

The main objective of this book is to study frailty models and the numerical techniques, needed to fit such models, in a unified and detailed way. Both proportional hazards models and accelerated failure time models are discussed; we consider parametric as well as semiparametric modelling. We fit models using both a frequentist and a Bayesian approach. Furthermore, different density functions for the frailty term are studied as each of them puts a different dependence structure on the data. We also discuss hierarchical models, i.e., models with more than one level of clustering. We do not attempt to give an exhaustive overview of the literature on frailty models as it is far too ambitious to do so; we rather prefer to explain the basic ideas and statistical techniques in detail. Some sections of the book are marked with an asterisk to indicate that they deal with more theoretical aspects. These sections can be skipped without losing the flow of the book.

1

A very important further objective is to make the frailty model techniques available to a wider audience. In spite of the amount of published material, the bottleneck is the lack of available public software. We will mainly use R, a freeware package, to fit the different models, and all the programs used are also freely available from the Springer Verlag website. Also software available in STATA and SAS is used to fit frailty models. WinBUGS, a freeware package, is used to perform most of the Bayesian analyses (Spiegelhalter et al., 2003).

1.2 Outline

In this first chapter, we introduce different data sets with time to event outcomes that will be used throughout the book to demonstrate the frailty model fitting techniques and the practical interpretation of the results. The introductory chapter further describes and explains some basic and general concepts in survival analysis to lay the foundation for the more advanced frailty models.

In Chapter 2, the simplest frailty model is introduced: the parametric model with clusters sharing the same gamma distributed frailty term. The simplicity is due to the fact that the frailties appearing in the conditional likelihood can be integrated out in a simple way to obtain the marginal likelihood that can then be maximised to obtain parameter estimates. Both the frequentist and the Bayesian approach are considered.

In Chapter 3, we consider models that, although different from frailty models, take the clustering of the data into account: the fixed effects model, the stratified model, the copula model, and the marginal model with robust variance estimators. We also demonstrate the relation between conditional and marginal models: given the hazard function and the hazard ratio in the conditional model and given the frailty distribution, the hazard function and the hazard ratio in the population can easily be obtained. These functions are important to understand how the population evolves over time.

In Chapter 4, different distributions for the frailty term are discussed and the type of dependence that they induce on the event times in the cluster is studied. The gamma distribution is most often used in practice. It belongs to the power variance function family proposed by Hougaard (1986a); other members of this family are also discussed: the inverse Gaussian and the positive stable distribution. The compound Poisson distribution is a further extension of the power variance function family. Characteristics of these distributions follow easily from their corresponding Laplace transforms. In practice also the lognormal distribution is often used for the frailty term. The use of the lognormal distribution mainly originates from work by McGilchrist and Aisbett (1991). They look at survival data from a mixed models viewpoint and therefore assume a normal distribution for the random effects which appear in the model formulation of the loghazard function. A drawback of the lognormal frailty distribution is that the Laplace transform does not take a simple form and hence the dependence imposed by the lognormal distribution is difficult to evaluate.

In Chapter 5, the semiparametric model is studied. Different numerical techniques have been proposed to fit semiparametric models, such as the EM algorithm (Klein, 1992), the penalised partial likelihood maximisation (Therneau et al., 2003), in a Bayesian context Laplacian integration (Ducrocq and Sölkner, 1994) or the MCMC algorithm (Clayton, 1991). The different techniques are studied in detail and the specific features of the different approaches will be compared.

Chapter 6 deals with frailty models with more than one frailty term. The chapter has two parts. First we discuss the case of two frailty terms within the same cluster, which occurs for instance if the objective in a multicentre trial consists of both looking at the heterogeneity between centres but also at the heterogeneity of the treatment effect between centres (Legrand et al., 2005). In the second part, nested or hierarchical models are discussed, with one clustering level nested within another clustering level.

In Chapter 7, further extensions of frailty models are discussed: frailty models for data with different censoring and truncation characteristics, correlated frailty models, joint modelling, and the accelerated failure time frailty model.

1.3 Examples

Different techniques to fit frailty models for clustered survival data are discussed in this book. All these techniques are applied to real data sets. We made a selection of examples so that we can demonstrate in later chapters how specific aspects of the data determine the appropriate inferential methodology used for the statistical analysis. A few important aspects that we will mention at this stage are (i) the cluster size, e.g., bivariate clusters versus clusters with large cluster sizes; (ii) the nesting or the hierarchy present in the design of the experiment; (iii) presence or absence of event ordering within a cluster, e.g., ordering is present in recurrent event data sets. Most of the examples do not have such ordering. If there exists an ordering, either in space or in time, we can still use techniques that do not take the ordering into account, although more specific models might be more relevant. We will therefore mention, whenever needed, that events in a cluster are ordered.

It is not our objective to give the complete analysis of the data sets; the data sets are rather used to illustrate how the different inferential techniques can be applied in practice.

We first consider data sets with one level of clustering. The simplest such data set consists of clusters of size one. Such a data set is given in Example 1.1. The models fitted to these data are called univariate frailty models. The simplest extension of this type of data set is to enlarge the cluster from one unit to two units. This type of data, called bivariate survival data, has received considerable attention. Typical examples include twin data (Wienke et al., 2003) and matched measurements on similar organs like eyes and kidneys (Mahé and Chevret, 1999a). We introduce two such data sets in Examples 1.2 and 1.3.

A data set with clusters of size four is presented in Example 1.4. In this example, we study time to infection in the four quarters of the udder of a dairy cow, the cow being the cluster. There is a certain ordering of the quarters, in the sense that front or rear udder quarters might have different characteristics.

In all the previous examples the cluster sizes are balanced, i.e., each cluster has the same number of units. However, many other examples exist where the cluster size differs from cluster to cluster and where it is often substantially larger than four. In fact this situation occurs most in practice. Four such data sets will be used. In Example 1.5 a breast cancer clinical trial data set is studied, with the hospital being the cluster and the patient the sampling or observational unit within the cluster. This data set has a restricted number of large clusters. In Example 1.6 a different breast cancer clinical trial is described. This particular breast cancer type, ductal carcinoma in situ, is a rather rare cancer, so that compared to the previous example, this study is characterised by the presence of many more hospitals with each of them having rather few patients. Examples 1.7 and 1.8 are based on studies in veterinary epidemiology; typical for these two examples is that we have a large number of rather small clusters. Example 1.9 is an asthma study: the patient is the cluster for which a varying number of event times are available. The event times clustered within the patient are now ordered in time and models taking this ordering into account will be the adequate ones.

In all the examples considered so far, one level of clustering is present. The clustering can be modelled by introducing a frailty term for each cluster inducing correlation between the units within the cluster. But for an appropriate analysis of the data it might be necessary to include more than one frailty term in the model, even for data sets having only one level of clustering. We will discuss such situation in Example 1.10. This data set is a collection of seven bladder cancer clinical trials. The data set is used to evaluate prognostic indices for bladder cancer. Apart from introducing a frailty term for the centre, an additional frailty term for the prognostic index is included for each cluster to study heterogeneity of the prognostic index effect. Therefore, although there is only one level of clustering, there are two frailty terms within each cluster. Finally, the data in Example 1.11 are hierarchical in the sense that there is more than one clustering level, in this example a collection of clusters is nested within a larger cluster.

The data sets could not be made publicly available, but data sets with exactly the same structure can be downloaded from the Springer Verlag website. The examples in the book are based on the real data sets.

Example 1.1 East Coast Fever data set: East Coast Fever transmission dynamics

Theileriosis or East Coast Fever (ECF) is a major cattle disease in eastern and southern Africa. The disease is caused by *Theileria parva* which is transmitted by the ticks *Rhipicephalus appendiculatus* and the closely related *Rhipicephalus zambeziensis* (Fandamu et al., 2005a). In order to study the transmission of the disease in southern Zambia, cows are followed up from birth until the time of first ECF contact in Nteme, a region in southern Zambia (Fandamu et al., 2005b). On a weekly basis, blood is collected and tested for the presence of antibodies to *Theileria parva* using the Indirect Fluorescent Antibody (IFA) test. After three consecutive positive IFA test results an animal is considered seroconverted. The time to first ECF contact is defined as the timespan from birth to one month before the first of the three consecutive positive test results (i.e., we set the date of contact with *Theileria parva* one month before the time of the first positive test result). Animals are followed up until one year after birth; if they do not seroconvert by that time, their time of seroconversion is right-censored. The data for a few animals are given in Table 1.1. We also consider the binary covariate breed. ∎

Table 1.1. East Coast Fever data set. The first column contains the cow identification number, the second column gives the time (in days) to ECF contact, the third column gives the censoring status taking value one (status=1) if seroconversion is observed and zero (status=0) otherwise. The last two columns give the breed and the month of birth.

Cowid	Time to ECF contact	Status	Breed	Month of birth
1	309	1	1	5
2	240	1	1	6
3	126	1	2	9
4	365	0	2	9
5	62	1	1	4
...				
232	365	0	1	3

Example 1.2 Diagnosis data set: Diagnosis of fracture healing

Medical imaging has become an important tool in the veterinary hospital to assess whether and when a fracture has healed. The standard technique in dogs is based on radiography (RX). Newer techniques based on ultrasound (US) are cheaper and do not require radioprotection. To investigate the performance of US for this purpose and to compare it to RX, Risselada et al. (2006) set up a trial in which fracture healing is evaluated by both US and RX. In total, 106 dogs, treated in the veterinary university hospital of Ghent, are included in the trial and evaluated for time to fracture healing with the two techniques. Only 7 dogs are censored for time to fracture healing evaluated by RX; no censoring occurs for time to fracture healing evaluated by US. The censoring is due to the fact that dog owners do not show up anymore. The data for a few dogs are given in Table 1.2. ■

Table 1.2. Diagnosis data set. The first column contains the dog identification number, the second column gives the time (in days) to diagnosis, the third column gives the censoring status taking value one (status=1) if healing is observed and zero (status=0) otherwise. The last column gives the diagnostic technique.

Dogid	Time to diagnosis	Status	Method
1	63	1	RX
1	30	1	US
2	83	1	RX
2	83	1	US
...			
106	35	0	RX
106	35	1	US

Example 1.3 Reconstitution data set: Reconstitution of blood–milk barrier after mastitis

When an udder quarter of a cow is infected (mastitis), the blood–milk barrier is partially destroyed and particular ions can flow freely from blood to milk and vice versa, leading to higher concentrations of, for instance, the sodium concentration Na^+.

The objective of this study is to demonstrate that the local application of a drug based on corticosteroids decreases the time to reconstitution of the blood–milk barrier in dairy cows. We therefore consider as outcome the time until the Na^+ concentration goes below a certain threshold (a concentration below the threshold value is considered to be normal again). Each udder quarter is separated from the three other quarters so that a quarter can be used as experimental unit to which a treatment is assigned. The Na^+ concentration in each of the experimental units is followed up. The rear udder quarters of 100 cows are experimentally infected with *Escherichia coli* (Vangroenweghe et al., 2005). After nine hours, one of the two infected udder quarters is treated locally with the active compound whereas the other is treated with placebo. Cows are followed up for 6.5 days, and are censored at that point in time if the Na^+ concentration is still above the threshold level. We further include

parity in the study as covariate. The parity of a cow is the number of calvings
(and therefore the number of lactation periods) that the cow has already experienced. Parity is often converted into a binary covariate, grouping all the
cows with more than one calving in the group of multiparous cows (heifer=0)
compared to the group of primiparous cows or heifers, cows with only one
calving (heifer=1). The data for a few cows are given in Table 1.3. ∎

Table 1.3. Reconstitution data set. The first column contains the cow identification number, the second column gives the time (in days) to reconstitution, the third
column gives the censoring status taking value one (status=1) if reconstitution is
observed and zero (status=0) otherwise. The last two columns give the drug application (active compound (drug=A) or placebo (drug=P)) and the heifer status
(multiparous cow (heifer=0) or primiparous cow (heifer=1)).

Cowid	Time to reconstitution	Status	Drug	Heifer
1	6.50	0	A	1
1	6.50	0	P	1
2	6.50	0	A	0
2	0.93	1	P	0
3	1.90	1	A	1
3	0.41	1	P	1
...				
99	3.80	1	A	1
99	6.50	0	P	1
100	4.93	1	A	1
100	6.50	0	P	1

Example 1.4 Mastitis data set: Correlated infection times in four cow udder quarters

Mastitis, the infection of the udder, is economically the most important disease
in the dairy sector of the western world. Mastitis can be caused by many organisms, most of them bacteria, such as *Escherichia coli*, *Streptococcus uberis*,
and *Staphylococcus aureus*. Since each udder quarter is separated from the
three other quarters, one quarter might be infected with the other quarters
free of infection. In an extensive study, 100 cows are followed up for infections.

The objective of this observational study is to estimate the incidence of the
different organisms causing mastitis in the dairy cattle population in Flanders.
Also the correlation between the infection times of the four udder quarters of a
cow is an important parameter to take preventive measures against mastitis.
With high correlation, a lot of attention should be given to the uninfected
udder quarters of a cow that has an infected quarter.

From each quarter, a milk sample is taken monthly and is screened for the presence of different bacteria. We model the time to infection with any bacteria, with the cow being the cluster and the quarter the experimental unit within the cluster.

Observations can be right-censored if no infection occurs before the end of the lactation period, which is roughly 300–350 days but different for every cow, or if the cow is lost to follow-up during the study, for example due to culling. Due to the periodic follow-up, udder quarters that experience an event are interval-censored with lowerbound the time of the last milk sample with a negative result and upperbound the time of the first milk sample with a positive result. In some examples, the midpoint (average of lowerbound and upperbound of the interval) is used for simplicity; in other examples the interval-censored nature of the data is taken into account.

In the analysis, two types of covariates are considered. Cow level covariates take the same value for every udder quarter of the cow (e.g., number of calvings or parity). Several studies have shown that prevalence as well as incidence of intramammary infections increase with parity (Weller et al., 1992). Several hypotheses have been suggested to explain these findings, e.g., teat end condition deteriorates with increasing parity (Neijenhuis et al., 2001). Because the teat end is a physical barrier that prevents organisms from invading the udder, impaired teat ends make the udder more vulnerable for intramammary infections. For simplicity, parity is dichotomised into primiparous cows (heifer=1) and multiparous cows (heifer=0).

Udder quarter level covariates change within the cow (e.g., position of the udder quarter, front or rear). The difference in teat end condition between front and rear quarters has also been put forward to explain the difference in infection status (Adkinson et al., 1993). In total, 317 out of 400 udder quarters are infected during the lactation period. A subset of the data is presented in Table 1.4. ∎

Example 1.5 Periop data set: Perioperative breast cancer clinical trial

Cancer clinical trials are often international multicentre trials due to the fact that quite a few patients are needed to have sufficient power to demonstrate a treatment effect. In survival analysis the power of a test used to study the treatment effect depends on the number of events rather than the number of patients within the study when the logrank test is used (Freedman, 1982). Therefore, especially trials with a low hazard rate such as early breast cancer trials are often large trials of a few thousand patients. Although the main interest is in showing a beneficial treatment effect, these data sets contain a lot of extra relevant information that is often not used. Indeed, in spite of the fact that all the patients in the trial are treated according to the same protocol, there still remains quite a lot of variability due to the fact that the trial is run in different cancer centres over the world. The scientific discipline that studies this type of heterogeneity is termed treatment outcome research (Legrand et al., 2002).

We investigate heterogeneity over centres for an early breast cancer clinical trial from the European Organisation for Research and Treatment of Cancer (EORTC), a randomised phase III trial comparing perioperative (periop) chemotherapy versus no perioperative chemotherapy for early breast cancer: 2795 patients are entered by 14 institutions (Legrand et al., 2005). The endpoint used is disease-free survival, which corresponds to the time from randomisation to time to death or recurrence, whatever comes first. Patients that are still at risk at the end of the study are censored at that time. Apart from the treatment effect, also the effect of prognostic factors at the level of the patient is studied. As an example, we consider nodal status: cancer cells are found already in the lymph nodes (nodal status=1) or not (nodal status=0). Additionally, the effect of factors at the institute level can be considered. Here we study the effect of country. The data for a few patients from the first centre and the last centre are given in Table 1.5. ∎

Table 1.4. Mastitis data set. The first column contains the cow identification number, the second, third, and fourth columns contain the time (in days) to infection (the lowerbound, upperbound, and midpoint of the interval, resp.), the fifth column gives the censoring status taking value one (status=1) if infection is observed and zero (status=0) otherwise. The last two columns give the parity (multiparous cow (heifer=0) or primiparous cow (heifer=1)) and the udder quarter (LF=Left-Front, LR=Left-Rear, RF=Right-Front, RR=Right-Rear).

	Time to infection					
Cowid	Lower	Upper	Midpoint	Status	Heifer	Quarter
1	261	297	279	0	1	LF
1	261	297	279	1	1	LR
1	48	78	63	1	1	RF
1	141	165	153	1	1	RR
2	303	330	316.5	0	0	LF
2	303	330	316.5	0	0	LR
2	303	330	316.5	0	0	RF
2	303	330	316.5	0	0	RR
...						
99	39	72	55.5	1	1	LF
99	189	228	208.5	1	1	LR
99	129	156	142.5	1	1	RF
99	72	129	100.5	1	1	RR
100	60	93	76.5	1	1	LF
100	60	93	76.5	1	1	LR
100	60	93	76.5	1	1	RF
100	60	93	76.5	1	1	RR

Table 1.5. Early breast cancer data set. The first column contains the patient identification number, the second column gives the time (in days) to death or recurrence,
the third column gives the censoring status taking value one (status=1) if death or
recurrence is observed and zero (status=0) otherwise. The fourth and fifth columns
give the institute where the patient was treated and the country in which the institute is located (country=F for France, ..., country=N for the Netherlands. The last
two columns give the treatment received (perioperative treatment (periop=1) or not
(periop=0)) and the nodal status (cancer cells in the lymph nodes (nodal status=1)
or not (nodal status=0)) of the patient.

Patid	Time to death/ recurrence	Status	Institute	Country	Periop	Nodal status
1	230	1	1	F	Y	1
2	3100	0	1	F	Y	0
3	560	1	1	F	N	1
...						
2793	1800	0	14	N	N	1
2794	130	1	14	N	N	0
2795	1900	0	14	N	Y	0

Example 1.6 DCIS data set: Breast conserving therapy with or without radiotherapy for ductal carcinoma in situ

Ductal carcinoma in situ (DCIS) is a not frequently occurring type of breast
cancer. The data set studied here is based on an EORTC randomised clinical
trial (Julien et al., 2000) in which all patients underwent breast conserving
therapy but half of them were randomly assigned to radiotherapy and the
other half to no further treatment. Due to the fact that this cancer type
is rather rare, a large number of institutes (equal to 46) recruit patients in
this study to obtain a sufficiently large number of patients. In total, 1010
patients are included in the study. We consider time to local recurrence as
main endpoint and investigate the effect of radiotherapy. As this cancer is a
benign form of breast cancer, only 155 events are observed after a median
follow-up time of 5.75 years. The data for a few patients are given in Table
1.6. ∎

Example 1.7 Culling data set: Culling of dairy heifer cows

The time to culling is studied in heifers as a function of the somatic cell count
(SCC) measured between 5 and 15 days (measurement day) after calving (De
Vliegher et al., 2005). High somatic cell count (we use the logarithm of somatic cell count as covariate) might be a surrogate marker for intramammary
infections. Heifers which have intramammary infections or which are expected
to develop intramammary infections in the future are quite expensive to keep

Table 1.6. Ductal carcinoma in situ (DCIS) data set. The first column contains the patient identification number, the second column gives the time (in days) to local recurrence, the third column gives the censoring status taking value one (status=1) if local recurrence is observed and zero (status=0) otherwise. The fourth column gives the institute where the patient is treated. The last column gives the treatment received (radiotherapy (radiotherapy=1) or not (radiotherapy=0)).

Patid	Time to local recurrence	Status	Institute	Radiotherapy
1	1996	1	1	0
2	1114	0	2	1
3	2535	0	2	0
...				
1000	428	1	46	1
1001	755	0	46	0
1002	771	0	46	0
1003	948	1	46	0
1004	1078	0	46	0
1005	1343	0	46	1
1006	1475	0	46	0
1007	1566	0	46	1
1008	1621	0	46	1
1009	3056	0	46	0
1010	893	0	46	1

due to the high costs for drugs and the loss in milk production. Cows are followed up for an entire lactation period (roughly 300–350 days) and if they are still alive at the end of the lactation period they are censored at that time. Cows are further clustered within herds (140 herds in total) and this clustering needs to be taken into account as culling policy and also SCC in early lactation might differ substantially between the herds. The data for a few heifer cows from the first and the last herd are given in Table 1.7. ∎

Example 1.8 Insemination data set: Time to first insemination in dairy heifer cows

In a dairy farm, the calving interval (the time between two calvings) should be optimally between 12 and 13 months. One of the main factors determining the length of the calving interval is the time from parturition to the time of first insemination. The objective of this study is to look for cow factors that might predict the time to first insemination, so that actions can be taken based on these predictors. As no inseminations take place in the first 29 days after calving, we subtract 29 days (and not 30 days as the first event would then have first insemination time zero) from the time to first insemination since at risk

Table 1.7. Culling data set. The first column contains the cow identification number, the second column gives the time (in days) to culling, the third column gives the censoring status taking value one (status=1) if the cow is culled and zero (status=0) otherwise. The fourth column gives the herd to which the cow belongs. The last two columns give the day on which the somatic cell count is assessed (between 5 and 15 days after parturition) and the logarithm of the observed somatic cell count on that day.

Cowid	Time to death	Status	Herd	Measurement day	log(SCC)
1	230	1	1	5	6.2
2	300	0	1	7	5.3
3	300	0	1	13	4.1
...					
14244	158	0	140	9	4.4
14245	65	1	140	6	5.9
14246	88	1	140	12	8.0

time starts only then. Cows which are culled without being inseminated are censored at their culling time. Furthermore, cows that are not yet inseminated 300 days after calving are censored at that time. The time to first insemination is studied in dairy cows as a function of two types of covariates. The first type of covariates is fixed over time. An example is the parity of the cow, corresponding to the number of calvings the cow has had already. As we observe only one lactation period for each cow in the study, it is indeed a constant cow characteristic within the time framework of the study. We dichotomise parity into primiparous cows or heifers (only one calving (heifer=1)) and multiparous cows (more than one calving (heifer=0)). Other covariates that are used in the analysis are the different milk constituents such as protein and ureum concentration at parturition (Duchateau and Janssen, 2004; Duchateau et al., 2005). For a few dairy cows from the first and the last herd the data with fixed covariates are given in Table 1.8.

The second type of covariates that is relevant in this study does change over time. The protein and ureum concentrations are measured, during the experiment, at a number of points in time. It might be more adequate to model the hazard at a particular time using the concentration at that particular point in time. In order to accommodate for time-varying covariates, the risk time for each cow is split into time intervals with a start and an end time and in each such interval a constant value for the concentration. We therefore have for each cow as many data lines as there are risk intervals. Using time-varying covariates the complete data information available for the first cow (cowid=1) in Table 1.8 is given in Table 1.9. ∎

Table 1.8. Insemination data set with fixed covariates. The first column contains the cow identification number, the second column gives the time (in days) to first insemination, the third column gives the censoring status taking value one (status=1) if the cow is inseminated and zero (status=0) otherwise. The fourth column gives the herd to which the cow belongs. The fifth and sixth columns give the milk ureum and protein concentration (%) at the start of the lactation period. The seventh and eighth columns contain the parity (number of calvings) and heifer information (multiparous cow (heifer=0) or primiparous cow (heifer=1)).

Cowid	Time	Status	Herd	Ureum (%)	Protein (%)	Parity	Heifer
1	69	1	1	3.12	3.22	6	0
2	201	0	1	6.60	3.02	5	0
3	22	1	1	3.97	2.74	5	0
4	24	0	1	4.04	3.00	4	0
...							
51	71	1	1	3.61	3.42	1	1
52	34	1	2	2.33	2.87	6	0
53	40	1	2	2.43	3.61	6	0
...							
10503	37	0	181	2.43	3.40	1	1
10504	27	1	181	2.44	3.11	1	1
10505	39	1	181	3.09	3.01	4	0
10506	61	1	181	2.64	2.91	1	1
10507	48	1	181	2.47	2.81	1	1
10508	45	1	181	2.56	3.02	1	1
10509	30	1	181	2.85	3.41	1	1
10510	55	1	181	2.95	3.13	1	1
10511	48	1	181	2.19	3.55	1	1
10512	78	1	181	3.53	3.52	1	1
10513	156	1	181	1.67	3.09	1	1

Example 1.9 Asthma data set: Recurrent asthma attacks in children

Asthma is occurring more and more frequently in very young children (between 6 and 24 months). Therefore, a new application of an existing anti-allergic drug is administered to children who are at higher risk to develop asthma in order to prevent it. A prevention trial is set up with such children randomised to placebo or drug, and the asthma events that developed over time are recorded in a diary. Typically, a patient has more than one asthma event. The different events are thus clustered within a patient and are ordered in time. This ordering can be taken into account in the model. Such data can be presented in different formats, but in Table 1.10, we choose to use the calendar time representation (see Duchateau et al. (2003) for a discussion on other data formats and a comparison of the different formats). In the calendar time representation, the time at risk for a particular event is the time from the end of the previous event (asthma attack) to the start of the next event

Table 1.9. Insemination data set with time-varying covariates. The first column contains the cow identification number, the second and third columns give the start and the end (in days) of the interval, the fourth column gives the censoring status taking value one (status=1) if the cow is inseminated at the end time of the interval and zero (status=0) otherwise. The fifth column gives the herd to which the cow belongs. The sixth and seventh columns give the milk ureum and protein concentration (%) at the begin time of the interval. The eighth column contains the heifer information (multiparous cow (heifer=0) or primiparous cow (heifer=1)).

Cowid	Start	End	Status	Herd	Ureum (%)	Protein (%)	Parity
1	0	9	0	1	3.12	3.22	6
1	10	18	0	1	3.23	3.13	6
1	19	27	0	1	3.34	3.05	6
1	28	33	0	1	3.44	2.97	6
1	34	42	0	1	3.51	2.92	6
1	43	50	0	1	3.57	3.01	6
1	51	58	0	1	3.62	3.09	6
1	59	63	0	1	3.68	3.17	6
1	64	69	1	1	3.71	3.22	6
2	0	7	0	1	6.60	3.02	5
2	8	14	0	1	6.01	3.03	5
...							

(start of the next asthma attack). In describing recurrent event data, we need a somewhat more complex data structure to keep track of the sequence of events within a patient. A particular patient has different periods at risk during the total observation period which are separated either by an asthmatic event that lasts one or more days or by a period in which the patient was not under observation. The start and end of each such risk period is required, together with the status indicator to denote whether the end of the risk period corresponds to an asthma attack or not. The data for a few patients are given in Table 1.10. ■

Example 1.10 Bladder cancer data set: Prognostic index evaluation for bladder cancer

Bladder cancer is a common urological malignancy and about 70–80% of all bladder cancers are superficial (stage Ta–T1). We consider a pooled database of seven trials conducted in this patient population by the EORTC Genito-Urinary Group. These trials are designed to investigate the use of prophylactic treatment following transurethral resection (TUR). A total of 2649 eligible patients are included in these trials. However, our analysis is restricted to the 2501 patients without missing information for the prognostic index we consider. These patients are recruited from 63 centres. Prognostic factors in superficial bladder cancer have been the subject of numerous publications

Table 1.10. Asthma data set. The first column contains the patient identification number, the second and third columns give the start and the end (in days) of the risk period, the fourth column gives the censoring status taking value one (status=1) if the patient experiences an asthma attack at the end time of the risk period and zero (status=0) otherwise. The fifth column contains the drug information (placebo (drug=P) or drug (drug=D)).

Patid	Start	End	Status	Drug
1	0	168	1	P
1	172	420	0	P
2	0	56	1	D
2	57	134	1	D
2	148	325	0	D
...				
111	0	465	0	D

over the past years (Sylvester et al., 2006) with the objective of adapting the treatment to the risk group in which a patient is classified. Allard et al. (1998) develop a prognostic index using the disease-free interval (DFI) as outcome variable. The disease-free interval corresponds to the time from randomisation until the time of disease or death, whatever comes first. They consider the following adverse tumour characteristics (ATC) present at initial resection: tumour multiplicity, tumour diameter > 3 cm, stage T1, and histological grade 2 or 3. The prognostic model is developed based on a cohort of 382 patients with primary Ta and T1 bladder cancer. They propose grouping the patients into four risk groups, each category being simply defined by the number of ATC: no ATC, 1 ATC, 2 ATC, 3–4 ATC. Along the same lines, we regroup patients to define only two risk groups, considering patients without any ATC at initial resection as good prognosis patients and patients with at least one ATC as poor prognosis patients. This leads to about a 15%–85% distribution of patients over prognostic groups and could therefore be used to save one sixth of the patients from more aggressive, more toxic, or more expensive treatment. Our interest is mainly focused on the heterogeneity of this prognostic index from centre to centre. The data for a few patients are given in Table 1.11. ∎

Example 1.11 Infant mortality data set: Infant mortality in Ethiopia

A large birth cohort study is conducted in southwest Ethiopia including 46 urban and 64 rural "kebeles" or villages, which further cluster into "woredas" or districts, with an estimated size of 300,200 persons (Asefa et al., 1996). The main focus is on studying possible causes of infant mortality in order to develop strategies for intervention (Asefa et al., 2000). The cohort study comprises in total 8162 newborns. From these 8162 newborns 856 infants died in their first year.

A whole set of sociodemographic, fertility history, and general hygiene factors are investigated in this study. We restrict attention to the impact of the gender of the infant on time to death using models that take the hierarchical structure of the data into account in a proper way. The data for a few infants are given in Table 1.12. ■

Table 1.11. Bladder cancer data set. The first column contains the patient identification number, the second column gives the time (in days) from randomisation to the time of disease/death, the third column gives the censoring status taking value one (status=1) if the patient experiences the disease or dies and zero (status=0) otherwise. The fourth column gives the centre where the patient is treated. The fifth and sixth columns give the prognostic group (good (PI=0) or bad (PI=1) prognosis) and the treatment received (prophylactic treatment (treatment=1) or not (treatment=0)).

Patid	Time	Status	Centre	PI	Treatment
1	310	1	1	1	0
2	1954	0	1	0	0
3	1758	1	1	1	1
...					
15	119	1	1	1	1
16	84	0	2	1	1
...					
2501	392	1	63	0	0

Table 1.12. Infant mortality data set. The first column contains the child identification number, the second column gives the time (in days) to death, the third column gives the censoring status taking value one (status=1) if the child dies and zero (status=0) otherwise. The fourth and fifth column give the district and village where the child is born. The sixth column gives the gender (male (gender=1) or female (gender=2)).

Childid	Time	Status	District	Village	Gender
1	363	0	1	1	2
2	361	0	1	1	1
...					
19	233	1	1	1	2
20	361	0	1	2	1
...					
841	361	0	1	4	1
842	360	0	1	4	1
...					
8162	240	1	4	1	1

1.4 Survival analysis

This section gives some important and typical characteristics of survival data and models in the absence of clustering.

The specific feature that makes survival analysis different from classical statistical analysis is data censoring. Typically, the survival time is unknown for some of the subjects; the only information available being that the subject has survived up to a certain time. Thereafter, the subject is no longer followed up. This type of censoring is called right censoring. It is the most common type of censoring. Different types of right censoring exist. In Type I censoring, the event is observed only if it occurs before a prespecified censoring time. For instance, in Example 1.3, the censoring time for each udder quarter is set equal to 6.5 days and is fixed by the investigator. These censoring times may differ from subject to subject. In the majority of our examples, however, the censoring times are not fixed but random. As will be shown in Section 1.4.1, these different right censoring mechanisms lead to the same survival likelihood functions, and can therefore be handled by the same survival analysis techniques. In our examples we mainly focus on right-censored data, although some examples are given of interval-censored data, where the survival time is known to be in a certain time interval. Many other censoring schemes are possible and are further discussed in Section 7.1; see Klein and Moeschberger (1997) for a detailed discussion and examples.

Throughout the book, we assume that the censoring time and the survival time are statistically independent random variables. This assumption is sufficient for the distribution of the event time to be identifiable in inference from the censored data (Fleming and Harrington, 1991).

For right-censored data, the actual information for subject i, $i = 1, \ldots, n$, is contained in the pair (y_i, δ_i), where y_i is the minimum of the event time t_i and the censoring time c_i, $y_i = \min(t_i, c_i)$ and δ_i is the censoring indicator, taking the value one if the event has been observed, otherwise δ_i takes value zero.

$$\delta_i = \begin{cases} 1 \text{ if } t_i \leq c_i \\ 0 \text{ if } t_i > c_i \end{cases}$$

Although the techniques discussed here are generally presented as survival analysis, they are not only useful to model time to death, but any outcome variable that describes the time to a particular event, especially if the event time is not observed for all subjects. In general, we use time to event and event time to denote the outcome variable, but depending on the example we may speak about time to death, time to recurrence, time to first insemination, etc. The observational unit for which the event time is observed is generally called the subject, and the observational units are grouped together in clusters. But, depending on the example, we often use more specific words such as patients clustered in centres or cows clustered in herds. Obviously in some examples a patient can be a subject whereas in other examples a patient is a cluster. In multicentre clinical trials patients are subjects clustered in centres (e.g., Example 1.5), whereas in recurrent event data, the recurrent event times are clustered within the patient (e.g., Example 1.9).

1.4.1 Survival likelihood

Due to censoring, the survival likelihood is quite different from the classical likelihood for independent data without censoring. We first introduce some notation that will enable us to write down the survival likelihood.

Let f be the probability density function of the event time T with corresponding cumulative distribution function

$$F(t) = P(T \le t) = \int_0^t f(u)du$$

and survival function

$$S(t) = 1 - F(t) = P(T > t)$$

Another important function in survival analysis is the hazard rate or instantaneous death rate $h(t)$. The hazard rate $h(t)$ is obtained from the conditional probability that an event occurs in the interval $[t, t + \Delta t[$ given that the event did not occur yet before time t. A rate is obtained by dividing this conditional probability by the time interval Δt (resulting in a conditional probability per time unit). The hazard rate is the limit of this ratio for Δt tending to zero:

$$h(t) = \lim_{\Delta t \to 0} \frac{P(t \le T < t + \Delta t \mid T \ge t)}{\Delta t} = \frac{f(t)}{S(t)} \qquad (1.1)$$

A related function is the cumulative or integrated hazard rate

$$H(t) = \int_0^t h(u)du$$

The survival function can be rewritten in terms of the integrated hazard rate. First we have, using (1.1),

$$h(t) = -\frac{d}{dt}\log(S(t))$$

and after integrating and exponentiating we obtain

$$S(t) = \exp\left(-\int_0^t h(u)du\right) = \exp\left(-H(t)\right)$$

Finally, in the case of random right censoring, we introduce g and G as notation for the density function and the cumulative distribution function of the censoring time.

The form of likelihood expression is determined by the type of data that is available. In this book, we consider complete data (all event times are observed), right-censored data (event times are subject to right censoring), and interval-censored data (event times are known to be contained in an observed interval). For right-censored data with random censoring, the likelihood contribution of an event time ($y_i = t_i$, $\delta_i = 1$) is given by

$$\lim_{\epsilon \to 0 \atop >} \frac{1}{2\epsilon} P\left(y_i - \epsilon < Y_i < y_i + \epsilon, \delta_i = 1\right)$$

$$= \lim_{\epsilon \to 0 \atop >} \frac{1}{2\epsilon} P\left(y_i - \epsilon < T_i < y_i + \epsilon, T_i \leq C_i\right)$$

$$= \lim_{\epsilon \to 0 \atop >} \frac{1}{2\epsilon} \int_{y_i-\epsilon}^{y_i+\epsilon} \int_t^\infty dG(c)dF(t) \quad \text{(due to independence)}$$

$$= \lim_{\epsilon \to 0 \atop >} \frac{1}{2\epsilon} \int_{y_i-\epsilon}^{y_i+\epsilon} (1 - G(t))dF(t)$$

$$= (1 - G(y_i))f(y_i)$$

On the other hand, for a right-censored observation ($y_i = c_i$, $\delta_i = 0$) with random censoring the contribution to the likelihood is given by

$$\lim_{\epsilon \to 0 \atop >} \frac{1}{2\epsilon} P\left(y_i - \epsilon < Y_i < y_i + \epsilon, \delta_i = 0\right)$$

$$= \lim_{\epsilon \to 0 \atop >} \frac{1}{2\epsilon} P\left(y_i - \epsilon < C_i < y_i + \epsilon, T_i > C_i\right)$$

$$= (1 - F(y_i))g(y_i)$$

Under random right censoring, survival data consist of a combination of event times and right-censored observations. The likelihood for a sample of size n is therefore given by

$$L = \prod_{i=1}^{n} [(1 - G(y_i))f(y_i)]^{\delta_i} [(1 - F(y_i))g(y_i)]^{1-\delta_i}$$

If we further assume that the distribution of the censoring times does not depend on the parameters of interest related to the survival function, called uninformative censoring (Liang et al., 1995; Fleming and Harrington, 1991), the factors $(1 - G(y_i))^{\delta_i}$ and $(g(y_i))^{1-\delta_i}$ are not informative for inference on the survival function and, therefore, they can be deleted from the likelihood resulting in

$$L = \prod_{i=1}^{n} (f(y_i))^{\delta_i} (S(y_i))^{1-\delta_i}$$

$$= \prod_{i=1}^{n} (h(y_i))^{\delta_i} S(y_i) \tag{1.2}$$

It is straightforward to see that the same survival likelihood (1.2) is also valid in the case of fixed censoring times.

Under interval censoring, a subject that is interval-censored, with an event time between times l_i and r_i, contributes the difference of the value of the survival functions at l_i and r_i, $S(l_i) - S(r_i)$.

1.4.2 Proportional hazards models

The proportional hazards model is the most popular model for survival data. For the simplest case of a treated and a control group with hazard functions $h_T(t)$ and $h_C(t)$, the proportional hazards model is given by

$$h_T(t) = \Psi h_C(t)$$

with Ψ the hazard ratio, i.e.,

$$\Psi = \frac{h_T(t)}{h_C(t)}$$

stating that the hazard of a treated subject over the hazard of a control subject does not change over time (proportional hazards assumption).

As the hazard ratio can never be negative, it is convenient to model Ψ as $\exp(\beta)$. In general in the presence of covariates the proportional hazards model can be written as

$$h_i(t) = h_0(t) \exp\left(\mathbf{x}_i^t \boldsymbol{\beta}\right) \tag{1.3}$$

with $h_0(t)$ the baseline hazard function corresponding to the hazard function of a subject with covariate information $\mathbf{x}_i$ equal to $\mathbf{0}$ and $\mathbf{x}_i^t$ the transpose of the vector $\mathbf{x}_i$. The introductory example above is a special case with $h_0(t) = h_C(t)$, $\mathbf{x}_i = 0$ if subject i is in the control group and $\mathbf{x}_i = 1$ if subject i is in the treatment group (then $h_i(t) = h_0(t) \exp(\beta) = h_T(t)$).

The baseline hazard function $h_0(t)$ either can be assumed to have a particular parametric form or can be left unspecified. The parametric case is described in the next section, followed by a section on the semiparametric model (a model that leaves the baseline hazard function unspecified).

Parametric proportional hazards models

In parametric proportional hazards models we assume a particular parametric function for the baseline hazard $h_0(t)$. A popular assumption for the baseline hazard corresponds to

$$h_0(t) = \lambda \rho t^{\rho - 1} \tag{1.4}$$

with $\lambda > 0$, $\rho > 0$. In the remainder of the text, λ is called the scale parameter and ρ the shape parameter. A scale parameter is a parameter that provides information on the way the hazard (or density) is stretched out; the shape parameter is a parameter that allows the density to take a variety of shapes, depending on the value of the shape parameter.

With ρ smaller than 1, the hazard decreases monotonically with time, with ρ larger than 1, the hazard increases monotonically with time. For $\rho = 1$, the hazard is constant over time (the exponential hazard).

Baseline hazard functions of form (1.4) are shown in Figure 1.1a-b for $\lambda = 1$ and $\lambda = 2$ and ρ taking values 0.5, 1, 2, and 3. For a fixed value of ρ, λ determines the overall height of the hazard function. For a fixed value of λ, ρ determines how fast the hazard function increases ($\rho > 1$) or decreases ($\rho < 1$). When making this parametric assumption (1.4) for the baseline hazard, it follows that the event times are Weibull distributed.

Indeed, with

$$h_i(t) = \lambda \rho t^{\rho - 1} \exp\left(\mathbf{x}_i^t \boldsymbol{\beta}\right)$$

it follows that

$$S_i(t) = \exp\left(-\int_0^t \lambda \rho s^{\rho - 1} \exp\left(\mathbf{x}_i^t \boldsymbol{\beta}\right) ds\right) = \exp\left(-\lambda t^\rho \exp\left(\mathbf{x}_i^t \boldsymbol{\beta}\right)\right) \tag{1.5}$$

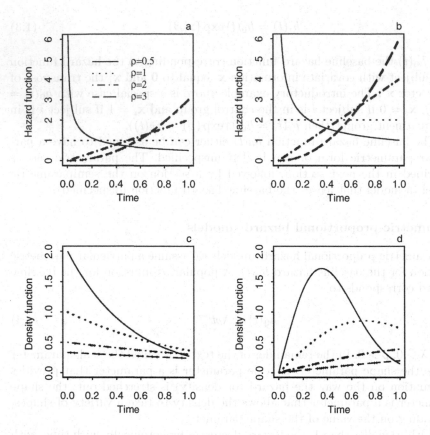

Fig. 1.1. Hazard and density functions for Weibull distributed event times. Hazard functions with different values for ρ are depicted with (a) $\lambda = 1$ and (b) $\lambda = 2$. The corresponding density functions are depicted in (c) for $\lambda = 1$ and in (d) for $\lambda = 2$.

and

$$f_i(t) = h_i(t)S_i(t) = \lambda \rho t^{\rho-1} \exp\left(\mathbf{x}_i^t \boldsymbol{\beta}\right) \exp\left(-\lambda t^\rho \exp\left(\mathbf{x}_i^t \boldsymbol{\beta}\right)\right) \qquad (1.6)$$

and therefore T_i is Weibull distributed, denoted as $T_i \sim W\left(\lambda \exp\left(\mathbf{x}_i^t \boldsymbol{\beta}\right), \rho\right)$.

Thus, all subjects are Weibull distributed with the same shape parameter ρ but differ with respect to the scale parameter. An important aspect of the Weibull distribution is therefore its proportional hazards property: Weibull distributed event times with the same parameter ρ lead to the proportional hazards model.

The Weibull density functions corresponding to the baseline hazard functions shown in Figure 1.1a-b are given in Figure 1.1c-d.

Weibull distributed event times are often used in practice because they seem to be able to describe the actual evolution of the hazard function in an appropriate way in many circumstances. We will often use this parametric assumption in the examples in this book.

Another parametric choice for $h_0(t)$ leads to event times with a Gompertz density function. The baseline hazard corresponds to

$$h_0(t) = \lambda \exp(\gamma t) \tag{1.7}$$

with $\lambda > 0$, $\gamma \in \mathbb{R}$. For $\gamma = 0$ the baseline hazard (1.7) reduces to the exponential hazard. The corresponding survival function is

$$S_0(t) = \exp\left[-\lambda\gamma^{-1}\left(\exp(\gamma t) - 1\right)\right]$$

We note that for $\gamma > 0$, $S_0(t)$ goes to zero for $t \to \infty$. With $\gamma < 0$, $S_0(t)$ goes to $0 < \exp\left(\lambda\gamma^{-1}\right) < 1$ for $t \to \infty$. Therefore, the event never occurs for a proportion $\exp\left(\lambda\gamma^{-1}\right)$ of the population. We therefore consider the case $\gamma > 0$. The resulting regression model

$$h_i(t) = \lambda \exp(\gamma t) \exp\left(\mathbf{x}_i^t \boldsymbol{\beta}\right)$$

is indeed a proportional hazards model with

$$S_i(t) = \exp\left(-\int_0^t \lambda\exp(\gamma s)\exp\left(\mathbf{x}_i^t\boldsymbol{\beta}\right) ds\right)$$

$$= \exp\left[-\lambda\gamma^{-1}\exp\left(\mathbf{x}_i^t\boldsymbol{\beta}\right)\left(\exp(\gamma t) - 1\right)\right]$$

and

$$f_i(t) = \lambda\exp(\gamma t)\exp\left(\mathbf{x}_i^t\boldsymbol{\beta}\right)\exp\left[-\lambda\gamma^{-1}\exp\left(\mathbf{x}_i^t\boldsymbol{\beta}\right)\left(\exp(\gamma t) - 1\right)\right]$$

Other parametric choices for $h_0(t)$ are of course possible, but in the sequel we mainly use the Weibull assumption for the event times in the parametric proportional hazards models.

Semiparametric proportional hazards models

Alternatively, we can leave the form of the baseline hazard $h_0(t)$ in (1.3) unspecified. Since, under this assumption, the model contains one parametric factor, $\exp(\mathbf{x}_i^t \boldsymbol{\beta})$, and one factor that is not specified in a parametric way, $h_0(t)$, we call the model semiparametric. Using the ideas that led to the survival likelihood (1.2), it is easy to see that for right-censored data with covariates the survival likelihood is

$$\prod_{i=1}^{n} (h_i(y_i))^{\delta_i} S_i(y_i) \tag{1.8}$$

where $(y_i, \delta_i, \mathbf{x}_i)$ with $y_i = \min(t_i, c_i)$ is the data information for subject i. Since $h_i(t)$ and $S_i(t)$ are defined in terms of $h_0(t)$ the use of the survival likelihood (1.8) becomes problematic. We therefore need an adapted version of the survival likelihood that does not contain the unspecified baseline hazard and that collects sufficient information to estimate the parameters of interest, the $\boldsymbol{\beta}$ vector, in a consistent way. This adaptation will result in the partial likelihood originally given by Cox (1972).

The partial likelihood can be derived as a profile likelihood, i.e., first $\boldsymbol{\beta}$ is fixed and the survival likelihood is maximised as a function of $h_0(t)$ only to find estimators for the baseline hazard in terms of $\boldsymbol{\beta}$.

We introduce new notation to be able to keep track of the ordering of the event times. Let, with r the number of observed event times (assuming no ties and thus $r = d$, the number of events), $y_{(1)} < y_{(2)} < \ldots < y_{(r)}$ denote the ordered event times with corresponding covariates $\mathbf{x}_{(1)}, \ldots, \mathbf{x}_{(r)}$. The survival likelihood can then be written as

$$\prod_{i=1}^{r} h_{0(i)} \exp\left(\mathbf{x}_{(i)}^t \boldsymbol{\beta}\right) \prod_{j=1}^{n} \exp\left(-H_0\left(y_j\right) \exp\left(\mathbf{x}_j^t \boldsymbol{\beta}\right)\right) \tag{1.9}$$

with $h_{0(i)} = h_0(y_{(i)})$. Based on nonparametric maximum likelihood estimation ideas for right-censored data it is natural to work with the following discrete version of the cumulative baseline hazard:

$$H_0^{Dis}\left(y_j\right) = \sum_{y_{(i)} \leq y_j} h_0\left(y_{(i)}\right) \tag{1.10}$$

This implies that we take $h_0(t)$ zero except for times at which an event occurs, as this choice leads to the largest contribution to the likelihood if a discrete hazard function is assumed. Using (1.10) with $\boldsymbol{\beta}$ fixed we obtain, after rearranging terms, that the survival likelihood (1.9) can be rewritten as

$$L\left(h_{0(1)}, \ldots, h_{0(r)} \mid \beta\right) =$$

$$\prod_{i=1}^{r} h_{0(i)} \prod_{i=1}^{r} \exp\left(\mathbf{x}_{(i)}^{t}\beta\right) \prod_{i=1}^{r} \exp\left(-h_{0(i)} \sum_{j \in R(y_{(i)})} \exp\left(\mathbf{x}_{j}^{t}\beta\right)\right) \quad (1.11)$$

where $R\left(y_{(i)}\right)$ is the risk set at time $y_{(i)}$ containing all the subjects that are still at risk to experience the event at that time. We can now maximise this survival likelihood with respect to $h_{0(i)}$ by setting the partial derivatives with respect to $h_{0(i)}$ equal to zero.

Taking, e.g., the partial derivative with respect to $h_{0(1)}$ we obtain

$$\frac{\partial L\left(h_{0(1)}, \ldots, h_{0(r)} \mid \beta\right)}{\partial h_{0(1)}} = \prod_{i=1}^{r} \exp\left(\mathbf{x}_{j}^{t}\beta\right) \prod_{i=1}^{r} \exp\left(-h_{0(i)}b_{i}\right)$$

$$\times \exp\left(h_{0(2)} \ldots h_{0(r)} - h_{0(1)}h_{0(2)} \ldots h_{0(r)}b_{1}\right)$$

with $b_{i} = \sum_{j \in R(y_{(i)})} \exp\left(\mathbf{x}_{j}^{t}\beta\right)$. It easily follows that equating this partial derivative to zero is equivalent to

$$1 - h_{0(1)}b_{1} = 0$$

This holds in general: equating the partial derivatives of the likelihood $L\left(h_{0(1)}, \ldots, h_{0(r)} \mid \beta\right)$ with respect to $h_{0(i)}$, $i = 1, \ldots, r$, to zero results in the set of equations

$$1 - h_{0(i)}b_{i} = 0$$

Solving for $h_{0(i)}$ gives

$$h_{0(i)} = \frac{1}{b_{i}} = \frac{1}{\sum_{j \in R(y_{(i)})} \exp\left(\mathbf{x}_{j}^{t}\beta\right)}$$

Plugging in this solution into the survival likelihood expression (1.11), we obtain, upon a factor $\exp(-d)$ which does not contain any of the parameters,

$$L(\beta) = \prod_{i=1}^{r} \frac{\exp\left(\mathbf{x}_{(i)}^{t}\beta\right)}{\sum_{j \in R(y_{(i)})} \exp\left(\mathbf{x}_{j}^{t}\beta\right)}$$

$L(\beta)$ is called the partial likelihood. This expression is used to estimate β through maximisation. The partial likelihood can also be interpreted in terms of conditional probabilities (Klein and Moeschberger, 1997). The properties (consistency, asymptotic normality) of the partial likelihood estimator for β are well established (Gill, 1984; Fleming and Harrington, 1991).

1.4.3 Accelerated failure time models

The accelerated failure time model is an alternative if the proportional hazards assumption does not hold. Different diagnostic tests have been developed to evaluate the proportional hazards assumption (Klein and Moeschberger, 1997). In contrast to the proportional hazards model, the accelerated failure time model is best characterised in terms of the survival function. We first discuss the simple case of a treated and a control group. With $S_T(t)$ and $S_C(t)$ the survival functions in the treated and the control population, the accelerated failure time model specifies that, with $\Phi > 0$,

$$S_T(t) = S_C(\Phi t)$$

The interpretation is as follows: the percentage of subjects in the treatment group that lives longer than t equals the percentage of subjects in the control group that lives longer than Φt. The parameter Φ is called the acceleration factor, values below one are in favour of the treatment, as the survival time is then prolonged under the treatment.

An alternative interpretation is in terms of the median survival times. With M_T and M_C the median survival times in the treated and control group, we have that

$$S_T(M_T) = S_C(M_C) = 0.5$$

From the accelerated failure time assumption it follows that

$$S_T(M_T) = S_C(\Phi M_T) = 0.5$$

and therefore $\Phi M_T = M_C$. For $\Phi < 1$ the median survival time in the treatment group is larger than the median survival time in the control group. This is demonstrated in Figure 1.2. The survival function of the control group is based on Weibull distributed event times with $\lambda = 2$ and $\rho = 2$. With $\Phi = 0.5$, the hazard rate (see (1.12)) is lower in the treated group compared to the control group, and the median event time in the treated group is twice the median event time in the control group.

From the expression of the accelerated failure time model in terms of the survival, it follows that

$$f_T(t) = \Phi f_C(\Phi t) \text{ and } h_T(t) = \Phi h_C(\Phi t)$$

Since $\Phi > 0$, it is convenient to set $\Phi = \exp(\beta)$, $\beta \in I\!R$, leading to

$$h_T(t) = \exp(\beta) h_C(\exp(\beta)t)$$

For general covariates (so far we only considered the binary covariate 0–1) the accelerated failure time model can be written as

$$h_i(t) = \exp\left(\mathbf{x}_i^t \boldsymbol{\beta}\right) h_0\left(\exp\left(\mathbf{x}_i^t \boldsymbol{\beta}\right) t\right) \tag{1.12}$$

Again we will assume a particular parametric form for the baseline hazard function $h_0(t)$. A first proposal is to use the same parametric form as in the parametric proportional hazards model, $h_0(t) = \lambda \rho t^{\rho-1}$. Note, however, that the argument of the baseline hazard in (1.12) differs from the proportional hazards model as it also contains the covariate information $\exp\left(\mathbf{x}_i^t \boldsymbol{\beta}\right)$. When making this parametric assumption for the baseline hazard, it again follows that the event times are Weibull distributed.

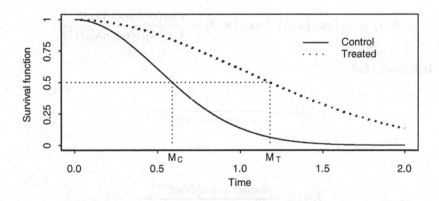

Fig. 1.2. Survival functions of the control group with Weibull distributed event times ($\lambda = 2$ and $\rho = 2$) and of the treated group with the acceleration factor in the accelerated failure time model equal to 0.5. M_C and M_T are the median event times for the control and treated group.

As the hazard for this parametric model can be written as

$$h_i(t) = \left(\exp\left(\mathbf{x}_i^t\boldsymbol{\beta}\right)\right)^\rho \lambda\rho t^{\rho-1} \tag{1.13}$$

it follows that

$$S_i(t) = \exp\left(-\lambda t^\rho \exp\left(\rho\mathbf{x}_i^t\boldsymbol{\beta}\right)\right) \tag{1.14}$$

and

$$f_i(t) = \lambda\rho t^{\rho-1} \exp\left(\rho\mathbf{x}_i^t\boldsymbol{\beta}\right) \exp\left(-\lambda t^\rho \exp\left(\rho\mathbf{x}_i^t\boldsymbol{\beta}\right)\right)$$

and therefore $T_i \sim W\left(\lambda\exp\left(\rho\mathbf{x}_i^t\boldsymbol{\beta}\right),\rho\right)$. Thus, all subjects have Weibull distributed event times with the same shape parameter ρ but differ with respect to the scale parameter. Note that the scale parameter differs from the scale parameter in the parametric proportional hazards model (1.6).

Another useful parametric form for the baseline hazard is the following:

$$h_0(t) = \frac{\exp(\alpha)\kappa t^{\kappa-1}}{1+\exp(\alpha)t^\kappa}$$

with $\kappa > 0$ and $\alpha \in I\!R$. The hazard function of subject i with covariate information $\mathbf{x}_i$ is then given by

$$h_i(t) = h_0\left(\exp\left(\mathbf{x}_i^t\boldsymbol{\beta}\right)t\right)\exp\left(\mathbf{x}_i^t\boldsymbol{\beta}\right) = \frac{\exp\left(\alpha + \kappa\mathbf{x}_i^t\boldsymbol{\beta}\right)\kappa t^{\kappa-1}}{1+\exp\left(\alpha+\kappa\mathbf{x}_i^t\boldsymbol{\beta}\right)t^\kappa}$$

It follows that

$$S_i(t) = \frac{1}{1+\exp\left(\alpha + \kappa\mathbf{x}_i^t\boldsymbol{\beta}\right)t^\kappa}$$

and

$$f_i(t) = \frac{\exp(\alpha + \kappa\mathbf{x}_i^t\boldsymbol{\beta})\kappa t^{\kappa-1}}{\left(1+\exp\left(\alpha + \kappa\mathbf{x}_i^t\boldsymbol{\beta}\right)t^\kappa\right)^2}$$

This corresponds to the loglogistic distribution with parameters κ and $\alpha + \kappa\mathbf{x}_i^t\boldsymbol{\beta}$.

Another density function corresponds to the lognormal density function, which is summarised in Table 1.13.

Table 1.13. Hazard function $h_0(t)$, density function $f_0(t)$, and survival function $S_0(t)$ of some distributions used for modelling survival time. In the presence of covariates $\mathbf{x}_i$ the corresponding hazard function $h_i(t)$ for the proportional hazards model is obtained by multiplying the hazard function by $\exp\left(\mathbf{x}_i^t\beta\right)$. From the hazard function, the survival function can be obtained as $\exp(-H_i(t))$ with the cumulative hazard $H_i(t) = \int_0^t h_i(s)ds$. The density function is given by $h_i(t)S_i(t)$.

Distribution	Parameter range	Function	Expression
Exponential	$\lambda > 0$	$h_0(t)$	λ
		$f_0(t)$	$\lambda \exp(-\lambda t)$
		$S_0(t)$	$\exp(-\lambda t)$
Weibull	$\rho, \lambda > 0$	$h_0(t)$	$\lambda \rho t^{\rho-1}$
		$f_0(t)$	$\rho \lambda t^{\rho-1} \exp\left(-\lambda t^\rho\right)$
		$S_0(t)$	$\exp\left(-\lambda t^\rho\right)$
Gompertz	$\gamma, \lambda > 0$	$h_0(t)$	$\lambda \exp(\gamma t)$
		$f_0(t)$	$\lambda \exp(\gamma t) \exp\left[-\lambda\gamma^{-1}\left(\exp(\gamma t) - 1\right)\right]$
		$S_0(t)$	$\exp\left[-\lambda\gamma^{-1}\left(\exp(\gamma t) - 1\right)\right]$
Loglogistic	$\alpha \in \mathbb{R}, \kappa > 0$	$h_0(t)$	$\dfrac{\exp(\alpha)\kappa t^{\kappa-1}}{1 + \exp(\alpha)t^\kappa}$
		$f_0(t)$	$\dfrac{\exp(\alpha)\kappa t^{\kappa-1}}{\left(1 + \exp(\alpha)t^\kappa\right)^2}$
		$S_0(t)$	$\dfrac{1}{1 + \exp(\alpha)t^\kappa}$
Lognormal	$\mu \in \mathbb{R}, \gamma > 0$	$h_0(t)$	$f(t)/S(t)$
		$f_0(t)$	$\dfrac{1}{t\sqrt{2\pi\gamma}} \exp\left[-\dfrac{1}{2\gamma}\left(\log(t) - \mu\right)^2\right]$
		$S_0(t)$	$1 - F_N\left(\dfrac{\log(t) - \mu}{\sqrt{\gamma}}\right)$

1.4.4 The loglinear model representation

Instead of modelling the hazard function or the survival function, we can also model the survival time directly. The loglinear model is an example of such direct modelling. It is given by

$$\log T_i = \mu + \mathbf{x}_i^t \boldsymbol{\alpha} + \sigma E_i \tag{1.15}$$

with T_i the event time for subject i, μ the intercept, $\mathbf{x}_i$ the vector of covariates for subject i, $\boldsymbol{\alpha}$ the vector containing the covariate effects, σ the scale parameter, and finally E_i the random error term for subject i. The random error term is assumed to have a fully specified distribution. For instance, assuming a normal, logistic, and Gumbel (see (1.16)) distribution for E_i, we obtain respectively the lognormal, loglogistic, and Weibull distributions for the event times.

As Weibull is the most popular choice for the distribution of the event times, we now demonstrate the link between the loglinear model and both the Weibull proportional hazards model and the accelerated failure time model, together with the relationships between the parameter estimates of the loglinear model and the two other models. These relationships are important because most software packages, e.g., R and SAS, only supply the parameter estimates for the loglinear model.

In model (1.15), we assume that the random error term E_i has a Gumbel distribution

$$E_i \sim f_E(e) = \exp\left(e - \exp(e)\right) \quad \text{for } -\infty < e < \infty \tag{1.16}$$

In the remainder, the density of $\exp(E_i)$ is required. By simple transformation, it can be shown that it has an exponential density with mean one, $\exp(E_i) \sim \text{Exp}(1)$. The model representation (1.15) can be rewritten in terms of the survival function

$$
\begin{aligned}
S_i(t) = \mathrm{P}\left(T_i > t\right) &= \mathrm{P}\left(\log T_i > \log t\right) \\
&= \mathrm{P}\left(\mu + \mathbf{x}_i^t \boldsymbol{\alpha} + \sigma E_i > \log t\right) \\
&= \mathrm{P}\left(E_i > \left(\log t - \mu - \mathbf{x}_i^t \boldsymbol{\alpha}\right)/\sigma\right) \\
&= \mathrm{P}\left[\exp(E_i) > \exp\left(\left(\log t - \mu - \mathbf{x}_i^t \boldsymbol{\alpha}\right)/\sigma\right)\right] \\
&= \exp\left[-\exp\left(\left(\log t - \mu - \mathbf{x}_i^t \boldsymbol{\alpha}\right)/\sigma\right)\right]
\end{aligned}
$$

This last expression can be rewritten as

$$S_i(t) = \exp\left[-\exp\left(-\mu/\sigma\right) t^{1/\sigma} \exp\left(\mathbf{x}_i^t \left(-\boldsymbol{\alpha}/\sigma\right)\right)\right] \qquad (1.17)$$

The Weibull accelerated failure time model can be written in terms of the survival function (see (1.14))

$$S_i(t) = \exp\left(-\lambda t^\rho \exp\left(\rho \mathbf{x}_i^t \boldsymbol{\beta}\right)\right) \qquad (1.18)$$

Comparing (1.17) and (1.18) it is easy to see that the two models correspond with

$$\lambda = \exp(-\mu/\sigma) \quad \rho = \sigma^{-1} \quad \boldsymbol{\beta} = -\boldsymbol{\alpha}$$

On the other hand, the survival function for the Weibull proportional hazards model is given by (see (1.5))

$$S_i(t) = \exp\left(-\lambda t^\rho \exp\left(\mathbf{x}_i^t \boldsymbol{\beta}\right)\right) \qquad (1.19)$$

Comparing (1.17) and (1.19) it is easy to see that the two models correspond with

$$\lambda = \exp(-\mu/\sigma) \quad \rho = \sigma^{-1} \quad \boldsymbol{\beta} = -\boldsymbol{\alpha}/\sigma$$

Therefore, the parameter estimates from the loglinear model can easily be transformed into parameter estimates for either the Weibull accelerated failure time model or the Weibull proportional hazards model.

Obtaining, for the Weibull accelerated failure time model and the Weibull proportional hazards model, variance estimates based on the variance estimates of the parameters of the loglinear model is not straightforward. We demonstrate how this can be done for one of the components of the parameter vector of interest $\boldsymbol{\beta}$. Obviously for the accelerated failure time model $\text{Var}(\hat{\beta}_j) = \text{Var}(\hat{\alpha}_j)$. For the proportional hazards model, however, we need to derive the variance of a ratio of two parameter estimates

$$\text{Var}(\hat{\beta}_j) = \text{Var}\left(\frac{\hat{\alpha}_j}{\hat{\sigma}}\right)$$

This can be approximated by using the delta method. We first discuss the delta method generally.

The original parameters are contained in the vector $\boldsymbol{\zeta}^t = (\zeta_1, \ldots, \zeta_k)$ and interest is in a univariate continuous function $g(\boldsymbol{\zeta})$. The delta method starts from the one-term Taylor expansion of $g(\hat{\boldsymbol{\zeta}})$, with $\hat{\boldsymbol{\zeta}}$ the maximum likelihood estimator of ζ,

$$g(\hat{\zeta}) \approx g(\zeta) + \gamma^t(\hat{\zeta} - \zeta) \tag{1.20}$$

with

$$\gamma^t = \left(\frac{\partial g\,(\zeta)}{\partial \zeta_1}, \ldots, \frac{\partial g\,(\zeta)}{\partial \zeta_k} \right)$$

the vector of the first partial derivatives evaluated at ζ. From (1.20) we obtain

$$\mathrm{Var}(g(\hat{\zeta})) \approx \gamma^t \mathrm{Var}(\hat{\zeta} - \zeta)\gamma \approx \gamma^t \mathrm{Var}(\hat{\zeta})\gamma$$

where in the last approximation we ignore the bias contribution. $\mathrm{Var}(\hat{\zeta})$ is the variance–covariance matrix of $\hat{\zeta}$. For the specific case of the Weibull proportional hazards model we have $\zeta^t = (\mu, \alpha, \sigma)$ and $\hat{\beta}_j = -\hat{\alpha}_j/\hat{\sigma}$. We therefore have

$$\gamma^t = \left(0, 0, \ldots, \frac{-1}{\sigma}, \ldots, 0, \frac{\alpha_j}{\sigma^2} \right)$$

Given the many zeros it is easily observed that

$$\mathrm{Var}(\hat{\beta}_j) \approx \gamma^t \mathrm{Var}(\hat{\zeta})\gamma$$

$$= \left(-\frac{1}{\sigma} \quad \frac{\alpha_j}{\sigma^2} \right) \left(\begin{array}{cc} \mathrm{Var}\,(\hat{\alpha}_j) & \mathrm{Cov}\,(\hat{\alpha}_j, \hat{\sigma}) \\ \mathrm{Cov}\,(\hat{\alpha}_j, \hat{\sigma}) & \mathrm{Var}\,(\hat{\sigma}) \end{array} \right) \left(-\frac{1}{\sigma} \quad \frac{\alpha_j}{\sigma^2} \right)^t$$

$$= \frac{1}{\sigma^2} \mathrm{Var}\,(\hat{\alpha}_j) - 2\frac{\alpha_j}{\sigma^3} \mathrm{Cov}\,(\hat{\alpha}_j, \hat{\sigma}) + \frac{\alpha_j^2}{\sigma^4} \mathrm{Var}\,(\hat{\sigma}) \tag{1.21}$$

An estimate for $\mathrm{Var}(\hat{\beta}_j)$ is obtained by using in (1.21) as estimates for $\mathrm{Var}\,(\hat{\alpha}_j)$, $\mathrm{Var}\,(\hat{\sigma}_j)$, and $\mathrm{Cov}\,(\hat{\alpha}_j, \hat{\sigma})$ the corresponding entries of the inverse of the observed information matrix and by replacing in (1.21) α_j and σ by their corresponding estimates $\hat{\alpha}_j$ and $\hat{\sigma}$ obtained by fitting the loglinear model.

1.5 Semantics and history of the term frailty

In the medical field frailty is a term that is used more frequently than it is defined (Rockwood, 2005). The term originates from gerontology where it is used to indicate that frail people have an increased risk for morbidity and mortality (Gillick, 2001).

There is a lack of consensus on how to determine the frailty status of an individual. A variety of tests have been developed to measure this status. As an example we mention a timed version of the "Get-Up and Go" (TAG) test; the test measures functional mobility for frail elderly people as the time that a patient needs to rise from an armchair, walk three meters, turn, walk back, and sit down again (Podsiadlo and Richardson, 1991). Other tests have been developed; see Lundin-Olsson et al. (1998) and Morley et al. (2002).

The previous examples consider frailty at the individual level. Frailty, however, can also be considered at a higher aggregation level. If in a multicentre trial some hospitals perform better than other hospitals (e.g., the median survival time varies over hospitals) one can try to quantify the "frailty" of a hospital.

This quantification idea brings us to frailty models where frailty is defined as a random effect. For the TAG example each patient has his or her own frailty (univariate frailty model). The interpretation is similar to what is aimed at in the medical field: patients with a high frailty value have an increased risk for morbidity or mortality. For the multicentre trial example hospitals that perform poorly have a high frailty value.

At the same time it is good to realise that quantifying a frailty as a random effect does not completely cover the way frailty is used in the gerontology examples. There are important differences. First, the frailty in a frailty model is considered to be constant for a particular individual, whereas in the medical context, one expects frailty to increase with age. Second, the frailty term is included in the univariate frailty model mainly to describe heterogeneity. Determining which subjects are frail is less important in frailty models. On the contrary, in the medical literature, the main objective is to find a surrogate marker for frailty to select the frail patients.

Additionally, with clusters containing different subjects, the situation is quite different. In the shared frailty model, we assume that persons in the same cluster share the same frailty term. Although we do not know the frailty term, due to the fact that persons in the same cluster share the same frailty term, we can predict the value of the frailty term for that cluster.

The introduction of a random effect to model survival data (in a univariate way, i.e., each person has a particular frailty) is due to Beard (1959). The purpose of introducing the random effect was to improve the modelling of mortality in a population. Beard (1959) used the term longevity factor rather than frailty. The proposed model is based on Makeham's law (Makeham, 1867)

$$h(t) = \alpha + \beta \exp(\lambda t)$$

with α ($\alpha > 0$) the basic hazard which is constant over age. Additionally the hazard function evolves over time through the function $\exp(\lambda t)$ with coefficient β. For appropriate choices of β and λ (i.e., $\beta > 0$, $\lambda > 0$), the hazard function will continue to increase with age.

In the approach of Beard (1959) a longevity factor is added to this model for each subject, resulting in

$$h_i(t) = \alpha + u_i \beta \exp(\lambda t) \tag{1.22}$$

with u_i the actual value of a random variable with density f_U with support $[0, \infty)$. For subjects with a small value for the longevity factor, the hazard function will increase slower compared to subjects with a large value for the longevity factor as

$$\frac{dh_i(t)}{dt} = u_i \beta \lambda \exp(\lambda t)$$

The population survival function can be obtained from (1.22) by integrating out the longevity factor using its distribution

$$S_f(t) = \int_0^\infty \exp(-\alpha t) \exp\left(-u\beta \int_0^t \exp(\lambda v) dv\right) f_U(u) du \tag{1.23}$$

The subindex f is added to the population survival function in (1.23) to denote that it originates from a conditional model including a frailty term or longevity factor. The subindex f will be used in that sense throughout the book.

Starting from (1.23) the population hazard function is

$$h_f(t) = \frac{-d \log S_f(t)}{dt}$$

$$= \frac{\int_0^\infty (\alpha + u\beta \exp(\lambda t)) \exp(-\alpha t) \exp\left(-u\beta \int_0^t \exp(\lambda v) dv\right) f_U(u) du}{\int_0^\infty \exp(-\alpha t) \exp\left(-u\beta \int_0^t \exp(\lambda v) dv\right) f_U(u) du}$$

$$\tag{1.24}$$

It can easily be deduced from (1.24) that the population hazard function is a weighted mean of all the possible hazard values $\alpha + u\beta \exp(\lambda t)$ in the population. The weight for a particular hazard with actual frailty u changes over time through the function $\exp(-\alpha t) \exp\left(-u\beta \int_0^t \exp(\lambda v) dv\right)$ which corresponds to the survival at time t for that particular frailty u. The relative weight therefore becomes smaller and smaller over time for high frailty values u, corresponding to low survival. Therefore, the population hazard function

$h_f(t)$ diverges more and more from (and becomes substantially smaller than) $h(t)$.

Beard (1959) proposes a two-parameter gamma distribution to model longevity. We restrict our attention to a one-parameter gamma distribution with mean one and variance θ, which is the classical choice for the parameters when using gamma frailties (see Section 2.1). The gamma density function with mean one is given by

$$f_U(u) = \frac{u^{1/\theta-1} \exp(-u/\theta)}{\theta^{\frac{1}{\theta}} \Gamma(1/\theta)} \tag{1.25}$$

with Γ the gamma function. The support of f_U is $[0, \infty)$. For this particular choice of longevity factor distribution, the population survival function is given by

$$S_f(t) = \exp(-\alpha t) \left[1 + \frac{\beta\theta}{\lambda} (\exp(\lambda t) - 1)\right]^{-1/\theta}$$

and the population hazard function is given by

$$h_f(t) = -\frac{d \log S_f(t)}{dt} = \alpha + \frac{B \exp(\lambda t)}{1 + C \exp(\lambda t)}$$

with

$$B = \frac{\beta\lambda\theta^{-1}}{\lambda\theta^{-1} - \beta} \text{ and } C = \frac{\beta}{\lambda\theta^{-1} - \beta}$$

This expression corresponds to a Perks logistic curve (Perks, 1932). With $B > 0$ and $C > 0$ the hazard function starts at α and increases over time towards the horizontal asymptotic line with value

$$\alpha + \frac{B}{C} = \alpha + \frac{\lambda}{\theta} \tag{1.26}$$

The Perks logistic curve often describes mortality curves well. An example of such a curve with values proposed by Beard (1959), i.e., $\alpha = 0.003$, $\lambda = 0.1$, $\theta = 0.167$, $\beta = 0.01$ with asymptotic horizontal line at $\alpha + \lambda\theta^{-1} = 0.602$, is given in Figure 1.3.

The term frailty was introduced by Vaupel et al. (1979) in order to interpret mortality data more appropriately. The proposed model is again a univariate frailty model with each individual having its own frailty term thus allowing for individual differences in mortality hazard rate. They discuss the

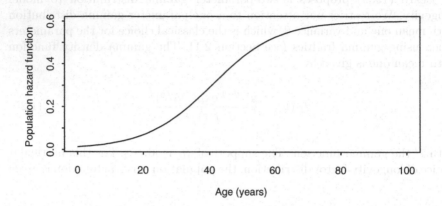

Fig. 1.3. The population hazard function for a Makeham model with $\alpha = 0.003$, $\lambda = 0.1$, and $\beta = 0.01$ and a gamma distributed longevity factor with mean one and variance $\theta = 0.167$.

case with no covariates and define the frailty as follows:

$$\frac{h_i(t)}{h_j(t)} = \frac{u_i}{u_j}$$

with the u_i's the actual values of a sample from a density f_U. Thus, the ratio of the hazard rates of two different individuals at any time corresponds to the ratio of their time-constant frailties. An alternative model representation is

$$h_i(t) = u_i h_0(t)$$

with $h_0(t)$ the hazard rate for an individual with frailty equal to one, which might be called a reference individual. An individual with a frailty term equal to two is, at an arbitrary timepoint, twice as likely to die as the reference individual. For an individual with 0.5 as frailty value we have that, at any arbitrary point in time, the risk of death is only one half of the reference risk.

The main objective of Vaupel et al. (1979) was to demonstrate that population mortality hazard rates do not reflect the mortality hazard rates of individuals from that population. Mortality rates for individuals typically increase faster with age than the observed mortality rate of the whole population. Therefore, Vaupel et al. (1979) explain how mortality hazard rates for individuals at any specified level of frailty can be estimated based on the population hazard rates obtained from life tables. For the model

$$h_i(t) = u_i h_0(t)$$

they consider the u_i's as the actual values of a sample from a gamma distribution with mean one and variance θ and show (as will be explained in (3.40) in Chapter 3) that

$$h_0(t) = h_f(t) S_f^{-\theta}(t)$$

and therefore

$$h_i(t) = u_i h_f(t) S_f^{-\theta}(t) \tag{1.27}$$

with $h_f(t)$ and $S_f(t)$ the population hazard and survival function. We can rewrite (1.27) (see (3.41) for details) as

$$h_i(t) = \frac{u_i h_f(t)}{\mathrm{E}\,(U \mid T > t)} \tag{1.28}$$

with $\mathrm{E}\,(U \mid T > t)$ the mean of the frailty at time t. It is clear from (1.28) that the hazard rate for a reference individual becomes larger in time relative to the population hazard rate due to the fact that the conditional mean of the frailty is decreasing over time as, on average, more frail individuals die sooner. Therefore, the percentage of less frail individuals increases over time.

Instead of considering the hazard it is also possible to look at the probability of dying in a particular interval Δt (taken to be one day), conditional on having survived up to the start of the interval for a subject i with frailty u_i

$$P_i(t) - \mathrm{P}\,(t \le T_i < t + \Delta t \mid T_i \ge t) = \frac{S_i(t) - S_i(t + \Delta t)}{S_i(t)} \tag{1.29}$$

Using (1.27) we have

$$S_i(t) = \exp\left(-\int_0^t u_i h_f(v) S_f^{-\theta}(v) dv\right)$$

$$= \exp\left[u_i \int_0^t \left(\frac{d}{dv} \log S_f(v)\right) S_f^{-\theta}(v) dv\right]$$

$$= \exp\left[-\frac{1}{\theta} u_i \left(S_f^{-\theta}(t) - 1\right)\right] \tag{1.30}$$

Using (1.30) in (1.29) we obtain

$$P_i(t) = 1 - \exp\left[-\frac{u_i}{\theta}\left(S_f^{-\theta}(t + \Delta t) - S_f^{-\theta}(t)\right)\right] \qquad (1.31)$$

As an example, we use the mortality data of the population of Swedish females and males over two centuries described by Vaupel et al. (1979). The probability (1.31) is depicted in Figure 1.4 for different values of θ for a reference individual, i.e., $u_i = 1$, using the probabilities observed for the population as a whole.

As the variability decreases, the probability of dying for a reference individual becomes more similar to the probability of dying in the population as a whole. However, even for rather small values of θ, the differences are still substantial.

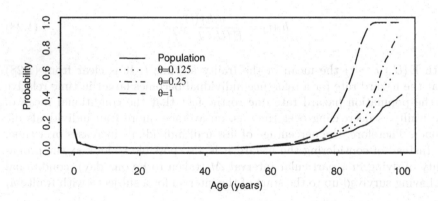

Fig. 1.4. The probability of dying in an interval $[t, t + \Delta t[$ for a reference individual ($u_i = 1$) assuming different values for the variance θ of the frailty term based on the observed probability of dying for the population depicted as a solid line.

The probability of dying for individuals with different frailty values with $\theta = 1$ is shown in Figure 1.5. Even for an individual with a low frailty value equal to 0.25, the probability of dying increases faster with time than the probability of dying in the population.

So it is clear from these examples that population hazard functions have to be interpreted with care.

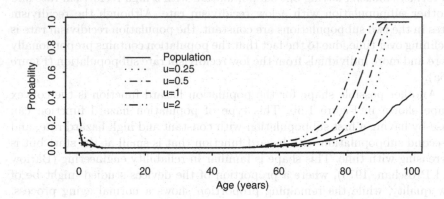

Fig. 1.5. The probability of dying in an interval $[t, t + \Delta t[$ for individuals with different actual frailty values assuming $\theta = 1$ based on the observed probability of dying for the population depicted as a solid line.

Vaupel and Yashin (1985) show that caution is also needed in populations where heterogeneity is present through the existence of two subpopulations (where each subpopulation is assumed to be homogeneous). This is different from using a frailty distribution to describe the heterogeneity present in the population. They assume that each subpopulation has its own hazard function, and demonstrate that the mixture of these two subpopulations can lead to quite unexpected results at the population level. We discuss a few examples after having defined the population hazard function.

Assume that the two subpopulations are characterised by the hazard functions $h_{1,p}(t)$ and $h_{2,p}(t)$ with corresponding survival functions $S_{1,p}(t)$ and $S_{2,p}(t)$, and let $\pi(t)$ be the proportion of individuals that are still alive at time t in the first subpopulation, i.e.,

$$\pi(t) = \frac{\pi(0)S_{1,p}(t)}{\pi(0)S_{1,p}(t) + (1 - \pi(0))S_{2,p}(t)}$$

with $\pi(0)$ the proportion of individuals in the first subpopulation at time zero. Then it easily follows that the population hazard function is

$$h_p(t) = \pi(t)h_{1,p}(t) + (1 - \pi(t))h_{2,p}(t)$$

In the first example we consider two subpopulations having a constant but different hazard rate. This might happen when considering the recidivism rate for former smokers, having one subpopulation with a high recidivism rate and another subpopulation with a low recidivism rate. Although the recidivism rates in the two subpopulations are constant, the population recidivism rate is declining over time, due to the fact that the population contains proportionally more and more individuals from the low recidivism rate subpopulation (Figure 1.6a).

Another possible shape for the population hazard function is the convex shape shown in Figure 1.6b. This type of population hazard function can arise by having a first subpopulation with constant and high hazard rate, and a second subpopulation with hazard function that is small at the start but is increasing with time. This shape is familiar in reliability engineering (Barlow and Proschan, 1975), where a proportion of the devices studied might be of low quality, while the remaining proportion shows a normal aging process. Due to the fact that the first subpopulation is disappearing quickly from the population, the hazard decreases for small values of age. After some time, however, the hazard starts to increase since at higher age the population mainly consists of devices from the second subpopulation that has a hazard function that increases with age.

Mixing two subpopulations having increasing hazard functions with a different slope results in the population hazard function shown in Figure 1.6c. The population hazard function is first increasing, but due to the fact that the proportion of the first subpopulation with a more steeply increasing hazard function is decreasing, with the population hazard function mainly determined by the second subpopulation, the population hazard function decreases at a certain point in time, to increase again after some time because the hazard rate is also increasing with time in the second subpopulation.

The fourth example is presented in Figure 1.6d. The hazard rate of the two subpopulations increases at the same rate but the first subpopulation starts from a higher value. The hazard rate is increasing at a faster rate in the two subpopulations than the population hazard rate.

For the above examples, Vaupel and Yashin (1985) propose to maximise the likelihood

$$\prod_{i=1}^{n} (h_p(t_i))^{\delta_i} S_p(t_i)$$

for $\pi(0)$, the proportion of individuals in the first subpopulation, and possibly also for other parameters related to the hazard functions of the two subpopulations if they are unknown.

The important message that follows from all these examples is that heterogeneity in the hazard function of different individuals should not be neglected. Starting from these findings, a whole series of techniques has been developed for frailty models, also for clustered survival data, which is the topic of this book.

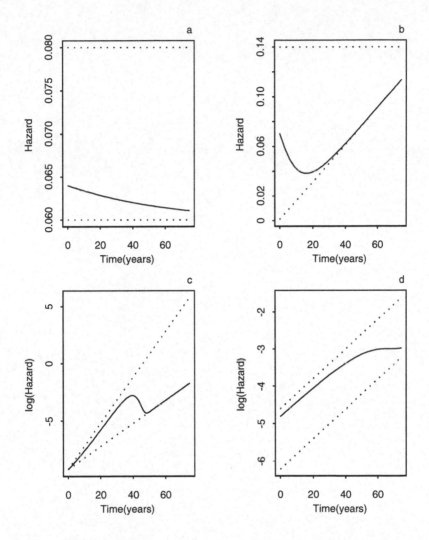

Fig. 1.6. The population hazard function (solid line) and the hazard functions of the two subpopulations (dotted lines) for four different situations:
(a) $h_{1,p}(t) = 0.06$, $h_{2,p}(t) = 0.08$, and $\pi(0) = 0.8$,
(b) $h_{1,p}(t) = 0.14$, $h_{2,p}(t) = 0.001 + 0.0015t$, and $\pi(0) = 0.5$,
(c) $h_{1,p}(t) = 0.0001 \exp(0.2t)$, $h_{2,p}(t) = 0.0001 \exp(0.1t)$, and $\pi(0) = 0.5$, and
(d) $h_{1,p}(t) = 0.01 \exp(0.04t)$, $h_{2,p}(t) = 0.02 \exp(0.04t)$, and $\pi(0) = 0.8$.
Note that the hazard functions in (c) and (d) are depicted on the logarithmic scale.

2

Parametric proportional hazards models with gamma frailty

This chapter discusses the parametric shared frailty model, with a one-parameter gamma frailty factor. The simplicity of this model is twofold: (i) the choice of a gamma frailty makes it possible to formally integrate out the frailties in the conditional survival likelihood resulting in an explicit and simple expression for the marginal likelihood. Although the integration is also feasible for some other frailty distributions, it leads to much more complex expressions (see Chapter 4); (ii) the choice of a parametric baseline hazard means that the marginal likelihood is fully parametric so that we can rely on classical maximum likelihood techniques to estimate the parameters. For most of the examples in this chapter we assume a baseline hazard corresponding to Weibull distributed event times; in a number of practical situations this is an appropriate assumption. The methodology presented in this chapter can easily be extended to other parametric models.

In Section 2.1, the proportional hazards model with frailty is introduced. In Section 2.2, the model is fitted based on the frequentist approach. First, it is shown how the gamma frailties can be integrated out from the conditional survival likelihood, leading to a marginal likelihood that contains only the parameters of interest, and no longer the frailties. This marginal likelihood is then maximised for the parameters of interest; standard errors can be obtained from the inverse of the Hessian of the marginal likelihood. In Section 2.3, it is shown that also in the case of interval-censored data, the frailties can still be integrated out analytically, although it leads to a more complex expression for the marginal likelihood. In Section 2.4, the frailty model for right-censored data with gamma distributed frailties is fitted but now using a Bayesian approach. By integrating out the frailties in a similar way as before, we can obtain the joint posterior density of the parameters of interest. In a genuine Bayesian analysis, however, inference is based on the posterior density of each specific parameter. Therefore, the other parameters need to be integrated out from the joint posterior density. Since closed form integration is not possible, approximation techniques are needed. A first technique consists of approximating this integral by Laplacian integration. A second technique is based on sampling using the Markov Chain Monte Carlo algorithm. In this chapter, the Metropolis algorithm is used to perform this task.

2.1 The parametric proportional hazards model with frailty term

The proportional hazards model is most commonly used to fit survival data. We introduce this model for the time to first insemination data (Example 1.8). The time to first insemination in dairy cows is studied as a function of different parameters. In this section, the effect of parity on the time to first insemination is studied. The parity is the number of calvings a cow has already had. We dichotomise the parity covariate to obtain a binary covariate: a heifer has had one calving and a multiparous cow more than one calving.

For subject (cow) j, $j = 1, \ldots, n_i$, from cluster (herd) i, $i = 1, \ldots, s$, we observe y_{ij}, the minimum of the censoring time c_{ij} and the event (insemination) time t_{ij}, and δ_{ij}, the censoring indicator ($\delta_{ij} = I(t_{ij} \leq c_{ij})$). The t_{ij}'s and the c_{ij}'s are assumed to be independent. The number of observed events in the ith cluster is $d_i = \sum_{j=1}^{n_i} \delta_{ij}$. The shared frailty model is defined as

$$h_{ij}(t) = h_0(t) \exp(\mathbf{x}_{ij}^t \boldsymbol{\beta} + w_i) \tag{2.1}$$

where $h_{ij}(t)$ is the conditional hazard function for the jth subject from the ith cluster (conditional on w_i); $h_0(t)$ is the baseline hazard, $\boldsymbol{\beta}$ is the fixed effects vector of dimension p, $\mathbf{x}_{ij}$ is the vector of covariates, and w_i is the random effect for the ith cluster. The w_i's, $i = 1, \ldots, s$, are the actual values of a sample from a density f_W. This model can be rewritten as

$$h_{ij}(t) = h_0(t) u_i \exp(\mathbf{x}_{ij}^t \boldsymbol{\beta}) \tag{2.2}$$

where $u_i = \exp(w_i)$ is called the frailty for the ith cluster. The u_i's, $i = 1, \ldots, s$, are the actual values of a sample from a density f_U.

Model (2.2) is called the shared frailty model because subjects in the same cluster all share the same frailty factor. Both models (2.1) and (2.2) are conditional hazard models (given the w_i's, respectively the u_i's). A mathematically convenient choice for the distribution of the u_i's, and the one that is considered throughout this chapter, is the one-parameter gamma distribution already defined in (1.25)

$$f_U(u) = \frac{u^{1/\theta - 1} \exp(-u/\theta)}{\theta^{\frac{1}{\theta}} \Gamma(1/\theta)} \tag{2.3}$$

with Γ the gamma function. Note that $\mathrm{E}(U) = 1$ and $\mathrm{Var}(U) = \theta$. This gives the following interpretation: individuals in a group i with $u_i > 1$ ($u_i < 1$) are frail (strong) (higher risk, respectively lower risk). The parameter θ provides information on the variability (the heterogeneity) in the population of clusters.

Different parametric forms can be assumed for the baseline hazard (see Table 1.13). In most examples a Weibull baseline hazard is assumed, but the theory is developed in general, so that other parametric baseline hazards can be used in the examples.

2.2 Maximising the marginal likelihood: the frequentist approach

In a frequentist approach, estimates of the parameters of interest are obtained by maximising the marginal loglikelihood. Estimated standard errors of the parameters are on the diagonal of the inverse of the Hessian matrix.

To obtain the marginal loglikelihood we proceed as follows. Within the context of clustered survival data we typically have observed information $\mathbf{z}$ containing the observed (event or censoring) times $\mathbf{y} = (y_{11}, \ldots, y_{sn_s})^t$ and the censoring indicators $(\delta_{11}, \ldots, \delta_{sn_s})^t$, the covariate information $\mathbf{x} = (\mathbf{x}_{11}, \ldots, \mathbf{x}_{sn_s})^t$, and finally the unobserved information $\mathbf{u} = (u_1, \ldots, u_s)^t$, also called the latent information.

From (2.2) and following ideas from Section 1.4.1, it is easy to see that the conditional likelihood for the ith cluster, with $H_0(t)$ the cumulative baseline hazard, is

$$L_i(\boldsymbol{\xi}, \boldsymbol{\beta} \mid u_i) = \prod_{j=1}^{n_i} (h_0(y_{ij})u_i \exp(\mathbf{x}_{ij}^t\boldsymbol{\beta}))^{\delta_{ij}} \exp(-H_0(y_{ij})u_i \exp(\mathbf{x}_{ij}^t\boldsymbol{\beta})) \quad (2.4)$$

with $\boldsymbol{\xi}$ containing the parameters of the baseline hazard. For instance, in case of a Weibull baseline hazard we have $\boldsymbol{\xi} = (\lambda, \rho)$. With $\boldsymbol{\zeta} = (\boldsymbol{\xi}, \theta, \boldsymbol{\beta})$ it follows that the marginal likelihood $L_{marg,i}(\boldsymbol{\zeta})$ for the ith cluster is

$$L_{marg,i}(\boldsymbol{\zeta}) = \int_0^\infty \prod_{j=1}^{n_i} (h_0(y_{ij})u \exp(\mathbf{x}_{ij}^t\boldsymbol{\beta}))^{\delta_{ij}} \exp(-H_0(y_{ij})u \exp(\mathbf{x}_{ij}^t\boldsymbol{\beta}))$$

$$\times \frac{u^{1/\theta-1}}{\theta^{1/\theta}\Gamma(1/\theta)} \exp\left(-u/\theta\right) du \quad (2.5)$$

There exists a closed form expression for this integral. With $z = 1/\theta + \sum_{j=1}^{n_i} H_0(y_{ij}) \exp(\mathbf{x}_{ij}^t\boldsymbol{\beta})$, we can write the previous expression of the marginal likelihood as

$$L_{marg,i}(\zeta) = \frac{\prod_{j=1}^{n_i}(h_0(y_{ij})\exp(\mathbf{x}_{ij}^t\boldsymbol{\beta}))^{\delta_{ij}}}{z^{1/\theta+d_i}\theta^{1/\theta}\Gamma(1/\theta)} \int_0^\infty (zu)^{1/\theta+d_i-1}\exp(-zu)d(zu)$$

and working out the integral gives

$$L_{marg,i}(\zeta) = \frac{\Gamma(d_i+1/\theta)\prod_{j=1}^{n_i}(h_0(y_{ij})\exp(\mathbf{x}_{ij}^t\boldsymbol{\beta}))^{\delta_{ij}}}{\left(1/\theta+\sum_{j=1}^{n_i}H_0(y_{ij})\exp\left(\mathbf{x}_{ij}^t\boldsymbol{\beta}\right)\right)^{1/\theta+d_i}\theta^{1/\theta}\Gamma(1/\theta)} \quad (2.6)$$

By taking the logarithm of this expression and summing over the s clusters, we obtain the marginal loglikelihood $l_{marg}(\zeta)$ (Klein, 1992):

$$l_{marg}(\zeta) = \sum_{i=1}^s \left[d_i\log\theta - \log\Gamma(1/\theta) + \log\Gamma(1/\theta+d_i) \right.$$

$$\left. -(1/\theta+d_i)\log\left(1+\theta\sum_{j=1}^{n_i}H_{ij,c}(y_{ij})\right) + \sum_{j=1}^{n_i}\delta_{ij}\left(\mathbf{x}_{ij}^t\boldsymbol{\beta}+\log h_0(y_{ij})\right) \right] \quad (2.7)$$

where $H_{ij,c}(y_{ij}) = H_0(y_{ij})\exp\left(\mathbf{x}_{ij}^t\boldsymbol{\beta}\right)$. We note that, since $H_{ij}(y_{ij}) = u_i H_{ij,c}(y_{ij})$, $H_{ij,c}(y_{ij})$ denotes the unconditional part of $H_{ij}(y_{ij})$.

Maximum likelihood estimators for $\boldsymbol{\xi}$, θ, and $\boldsymbol{\beta}$ can be found by maximising this loglikelihood. The asymptotic variance–covariance matrix can also be derived from the loglikelihood expression. We first define $\mathbf{H}(\zeta)$, the Hessian matrix of the mixed partial second derivatives of $l_{marg}(\zeta)$.

With $\zeta = (\zeta_1, \ldots, \zeta_q)$, the $(i,j)^{\text{th}}$ element of the $(q \times q)$ Hessian matrix is given by

$$\frac{\partial^2}{\partial\zeta_i\partial\zeta_j}l_{marg}(\zeta) \quad (2.8)$$

The Fisher information matrix, on the other hand, is the negative of the expected value of the Hessian matrix

$$\mathcal{I}(\zeta) = -\mathrm{E}(\mathbf{H}(\zeta))$$

and the observed information matrix, or in short the information matrix, is the negative of the Hessian matrix

$$\mathbf{I}(\zeta) = -\mathbf{H}(\zeta) \tag{2.9}$$

The asymptotic variance–covariance matrix of the vector of parameter estimates is the inverse of the Fisher information matrix; the estimated variance–covariance matrix is obtained as the inverse of the observed information matrix (evaluated at $\hat{\zeta}$, the vector with the actual values of the maximum likelihood estimators).

As an example, we work out the Hessian matrix for the frailty model with Weibull baseline hazard and one covariate. We give the first- and second-order derivatives of the loglikelihood with respect to the parameters $\zeta = (\lambda, \rho, \theta, \beta)$ as they are required in later chapters. Below, we show the contribution to the first derivative of the marginal loglikelihood of a particular cluster i. These contributions can then be summed over all clusters to obtain the first derivative of the marginal loglikelihood.

$$\frac{\partial l_{marg,i}(\zeta)}{\partial \lambda} = \frac{-(d_i\theta + 1)\sum_{j=1}^{n_i} \lambda^{-1}H_{ij,c}(y_{ij})}{1 + \theta\sum_{j=1}^{n_i} H_{ij,c}(y_{ij})} + d_i\lambda^{-1} \tag{2.10}$$

$$\frac{\partial l_{marg,i}(\zeta)}{\partial \rho} = \frac{-(d_i\theta + 1)\sum_{j=1}^{n_i} H_{ij,c}(y_{ij})\log y_{ij}}{1 + \theta\sum_{j=1}^{n_i} H_{ij,c}(y_{ij})}$$
$$+ \sum_{j=1}^{n_i} \delta_{ij}\left(\rho^{-1} + \log y_{ij}\right) \tag{2.11}$$

$$\frac{\partial l_{marg,i}(\zeta)}{\partial \theta} = \frac{-(d_i + \theta^{-1})\sum_{j=1}^{n_i} H_{ij,c}(y_{ij})}{1 + \theta\sum_{j=1}^{n_i} H_{ij,c}(y_{ij})} + \theta^{-2}\log\left(1 + \theta\sum_{j=1}^{n_i} H_{ij,c}(y_{ij})\right)$$
$$-I(d_i > 0)\sum_{l=0}^{d_i-1}\left(\theta + l\theta^2\right)^{-1} + d_i\theta^{-1} \tag{2.12}$$

$$\frac{\partial l_{marg,i}(\zeta)}{\partial \beta} = \frac{-(d_i\theta + 1)\sum_{j=1}^{n_i} H_{ij,c}(y_{ij})x_{ij}}{1 + \theta\sum_{j=1}^{n_i} H_{ij,c}(y_{ij})} + \sum_{j=1}^{n_i} \delta_{ij}x_{ij} \tag{2.13}$$

The second derivatives with respect to the four parameters are given by

$$\frac{\partial^2 l_{marg,i}(\zeta)}{\partial \lambda^2} = \frac{\left(d_i + \theta^{-1}\right)}{\left(\theta^{-1} + \sum_{j=1}^{n_i} H_{ij,c}(y_{ij})\right)^2} \left(\sum_{j=1}^{n_i} y_{ij}^{\rho} \exp\left(\mathbf{x}_{ij}^t \beta\right)\right)^2 - d_i \lambda^{-2}$$

(2.14)

$$\frac{\partial^2 l_{marg,i}(\zeta)}{\partial \rho^2} = \frac{\left(d_i + \theta^{-1}\right)}{\left(\theta^{-1} + \sum_{j=1}^{n_i} H_{ij,c}(y_{ij})\right)^2} \left[\left(\sum_{j=1}^{n_i} H_{ij,c}(y_{ij}) \log y_{ij}\right)^2\right.$$
$$\left. - \left(\theta^{-1} + \sum_{j=1}^{n_i} H_{ij,c}(y_{ij})\right) \sum_{j=1}^{n_i} H_{ij,c}(y_{ij}) (\log y_{ij})^2\right] - d_i \rho^{-2} \qquad (2.15)$$

$$\frac{\partial^2 l_{marg,i}(\zeta)}{\partial \theta^2} = I\left(d_i > 0\right) \sum_{l=0}^{d_i - 1} \frac{1 + 2l\theta}{\left(l\theta^2 + \theta\right)^2} - \frac{2 \log \theta - 3}{\theta^3}$$
$$- \frac{2}{\theta^3} \log\left(\sum_{j=1}^{n_i} H_{ij,c}(y_{ij}) + 1/\theta\right)$$
$$- \frac{3/\theta + d_i + (4 + 2\theta d_i) \sum_{j=1}^{n_i} H_{ij,c}(y_{ij})}{\left(\theta + \theta^2 \sum_{j=1}^{n_i} H_{ij,c}(y_{ij})\right)^2} \qquad (2.16)$$

$$\frac{\partial^2 l_{marg,i}(\zeta)}{\partial \beta^2} = \frac{\left(d_i + \theta^{-1}\right)}{\left(\theta^{-1} + \sum_{j=1}^{n_i} H_{ij,c}(y_{ij})\right)^2} \left[\left(\sum_{j=1}^{n_i} H_{ij,c}(y_{ij}) x_{ij}\right)^2\right.$$
$$\left. - \sum_{j=1}^{n_i} H_{ij,c}(y_{ij}) x_{ij}^2 \left(\theta^{-1} + \sum_{j=1}^{n_i} H_{ij,c}(y_{ij})\right)\right] \qquad (2.17)$$

and finally the remaining second derivatives are given by

$$\frac{\partial^2 l_{marg,i}(\boldsymbol{\zeta})}{\partial\lambda\partial\rho} = \frac{(d_i\theta+1)}{\left(1+\theta\sum_{j=1}^{n_i}H_{ij,c}\left(y_{ij}\right)\right)^2}\left(-\sum_{j=1}^{n_i}\lambda^{-1}H_{ij,c}\left(y_{ij}\right)\log y_{ij}\right)$$

(2.18)

$$\frac{\partial^2 l_{marg,i}(\boldsymbol{\zeta})}{\partial\lambda\partial\theta} = \frac{\left(-d_i+\sum_{j=1}^{n_i}H_{ij,c}\left(y_{ij}\right)\right)}{\left(1+\theta\sum_{j=1}^{n_i}H_{ij,c}\left(y_{ij}\right)\right)^2}\left(\sum_{j=1}^{n_i}\lambda^{-1}H_{ij,c}\left(y_{ij}\right)\right) \qquad (2.19)$$

$$\frac{\partial^2 l_{marg,i}(\boldsymbol{\zeta})}{\partial\lambda\partial\beta} = \frac{(d_i\theta+1)}{\left(1+\theta\sum_{j=1}^{n_i}H_{ij,c}\left(y_{ij}\right)\right)^2}\left(-\sum_{j=1}^{n_i}\lambda^{-1}x_{ij}H_{ij,c}\left(y_{ij}\right)\right) \quad (2.20)$$

$$\frac{\partial^2 l_{marg,i}(\boldsymbol{\zeta})}{\partial\rho\partial\theta} = \frac{\left(-d_i+\sum_{j=1}^{n_i}H_{ij,c}\left(y_{ij}\right)\right)}{\left(1+\theta\sum_{j=1}^{n_i}H_{ij,c}\left(y_{ij}\right)\right)^2}\left(\sum_{j=1}^{n_i}H_{ij,c}\left(y_{ij}\right)\log y_{ij}\right) \qquad (2.21)$$

$$\frac{\partial^2 l_{marg,i}(\boldsymbol{\zeta})}{\partial\rho\partial\beta} = \frac{(d_i\theta+1)}{\left(1+\theta\sum_{j=1}^{n_i}H_{ij,c}\left(y_{ij}\right)\right)^2}$$
$$\left[-\left(1+\theta\sum_{j=1}^{n_i}H_{ij,c}\left(y_{ij}\right)\right)\sum_{j=1}^{n_i}x_{ij}H_{ij,c}\left(y_{ij}\right)\log y_{ij}\right.$$
$$\left.+\theta\sum_{j=1}^{n_i}H_{ij,c}\left(y_{ij}\right)\log y_{ij}\sum_{j=1}^{n_i}H_{ij,c}\left(y_{ij}\right)x_{ij}\right] \qquad (2.22)$$

$$\frac{\partial^2 l_{marg,i}(\boldsymbol{\zeta})}{\partial\theta\partial\beta} = \frac{-d_i\sum_{j=1}^{n_i}H_{ij,c}\left(y_{ij}\right)x_{ij}+\sum_{j=1}^{n_i}H_{ij,c}\left(y_{ij}\right)x_{ij}\sum_{j=1}^{n_i}H_{ij,c}\left(y_{ij}\right)}{\left(1+\theta\sum_{j=1}^{n_i}H_{ij,c}\left(y_{ij}\right)\right)^2}$$

(2.23)

Example 2.1 The parametric proportional hazards frailty model for time to first insemination based on marginal likelihood maximisation

For the time to first insemination data presented in Example 1.8, the following simple model is fitted:

$$h_{ij}(t) = h_0(t)u_i \exp(x_{ij}\beta) \tag{2.24}$$

where $h_{ij}(t)$ is the hazard function for the jth cow from the ith herd with x_{ij} the heifer covariate (0=multiparous cow, 1=heifer), β the heifer effect, and u_i the frailty term for herd i. Given the frailty u_i we assume that the event times follow a Weibull distribution $W(\lambda u_i \exp(x_{ij}\beta), \rho)$, i.e., given u_i the conditional density of T_{ij} is

$$f_{ij}(t) = \rho\lambda u_i \exp(x_{ij}\beta) t^{\rho-1} \exp(-\lambda u_i \exp(x_{ij}\beta) t^\rho) \tag{2.25}$$

and the survival function is

$$S_{ij}(t) = \exp(-\lambda u_i \exp(x_{ij}\beta) t^\rho) \tag{2.26}$$

We can then maximise the marginal loglikelihood (2.7) with respect to $\zeta = (\lambda, \rho, \theta, \beta)$. We transform the time from days to months as too small values for the estimate of the parameter λ typically lead to convergence problems. Therefore, the estimate $\hat{\lambda}$ refers to months rather than days, but the parameter estimate can be easily back-transformed to days, as is shown later. This transformation does not have an effect on any of the other parameters (see (2.27)).

This leads to the estimates $\hat{\lambda} = 0.174$ (s.e. $= 0.009$), $\hat{\rho} = 1.769$ (s.e. $= 0.014$), $\hat{\theta} = 0.394$ (s.e. $= 0.041$), and $\hat{\beta} = -0.153$ (s.e. $= 0.023$). The standard errors are given by the square root of the diagonal elements of the inverse of the information matrix of the marginal likelihood evaluated at $(\hat{\lambda}, \hat{\rho}, \hat{\theta}, \hat{\beta})$, i.e., at the arguments that maximise the marginal likelihood.

In a herd with $u_i = 1$, the hazard ratio for heifers compared to multiparous cows is therefore given by $\exp(-0.153) = 0.858$ with 95% confidence interval given by $[\exp(-0.153 - 1.96 \times 0.023); \exp(-0.153 + 1.96 \times 0.023)] = [0.820; 0.897]$: the hazard of first insemination is significantly lower for heifers. In order to express the results above in terms of median first insemination time, we can back-transform the parameter estimate $\hat{\lambda}$ referring to monthly hazard rates to the parameter corresponding to the daily hazard rate $\hat{\lambda}_d$ as follows. The cumulative hazard at any time is required to be the same, and thus

$$\lambda u_i \exp(x_{ij}\beta) t^\rho = \lambda_d u_i \exp(x_{ij}\beta) (t \times 365.25/12)^\rho \tag{2.27}$$

and thus it follows that $\lambda_d = \lambda \times (365.25/12)^{-\rho}$, and therefore $\hat{\lambda}_d = 0.000413$.

From (2.26) it is immediate that, in a herd with $u_i = 1$, the median time to first insemination is $[\log 2/ (\lambda_d \exp{(x_{ij}\beta)})]^{1/\rho}$. Using the estimates for the parameters we have for multiparous cows ($x_{ij} = 0$) an estimated median time to first insemination of 66.5 days, for heifers ($x_{ij} = 1$) we obtain 72.5 days. As risk time starts only 29 days after calving (no inseminations take place before that day), the actual median times to first insemination equal 95.5 and 101.5 days for multiparous cows and heifers, respectively.

The hazard functions for multiparous cows and heifers are depicted in Figure 2.1. Although this figure gives us an idea about variability between herds, it is difficult to understand heterogeneity at the level of the hazard function. We can, however, translate heterogeneity in terms of the hazard function to heterogeneity in terms of the median time to first insemination or in terms of the proportion of the cows with time to first insemination before a particular point in time (Duchateau and Janssen, 2005).

Since, with M_{i1} (M_{i0}) the median time to first insemination for herd i in heifers (multiparous cows), (2.24) and (2.25) imply that $M_{i1} = g(U_i) = [\log 2/ (U_i \lambda_d \exp(\beta))]^{1/\rho}$, we obtain the density function for M_{i1}

$$f_{M_{i1}}(m) = \rho \left(\frac{\log 2}{\theta \lambda_d \exp(\beta)} \right)^{1/\theta} \frac{1}{\Gamma(1/\theta)} \left(\frac{1}{m} \right)^{1+\rho/\theta} \exp \left(\frac{-\log 2}{\theta m^\rho \lambda_d \exp(\beta)} \right)$$

with a similar expression for M_{i0} where β is set to zero. In Figure 2.2, the density function for the median time to first insemination over the different herds is depicted for multiparous cows and heifers. As values for λ_d, ρ, β, and θ the estimates are used. The density functions for the median time to first insemination for the two groups do not only differ with respect to the mode but also with respect to the shape. Although both density functions are based on the same variance component estimate $\hat{\theta}$, it is clear from Figure 2.2 that the density function is more flat for heifers than for multiparous cows. The variance of the median time to first insemination, therefore, shows a different behaviour compared to the variance at the loghazard level

$$\log h_{ij}(t) = \log h_0(t) + \log u_i + x_{ij}\beta$$

Indeed, the variance is the same for multiparous cows and heifers at the loghazard level, and therefore independent of β; this is no longer true for the variance of the median time to first insemination. The spread of the median event time generally depends on the covariates.

Heterogeneity in hazard rates can also be translated in $P_{t,i1}$ ($P_{t,i0}$), the proportion of heifers (multiparous cows) with first insemination before a particular timepoint t: $P_{t,i1} = 1 - \exp{(-t^\rho \lambda_d \exp(\beta)U_i)}$. The density function of $P_{t,i1}$ is given by

$$f_{P_{t,i1}}(p_t) = \frac{1}{t^\rho \lambda_d \exp(\beta)\theta^{1/\theta}\Gamma(1/\theta)}(1-p_t)^{(t^\rho\lambda_d\exp(\beta)\theta)^{-1}-1}$$
$$\times\left(\frac{-\log(1-p_t)}{t^\rho\lambda_d\exp(\beta)}\right)^{1/\theta-1}$$

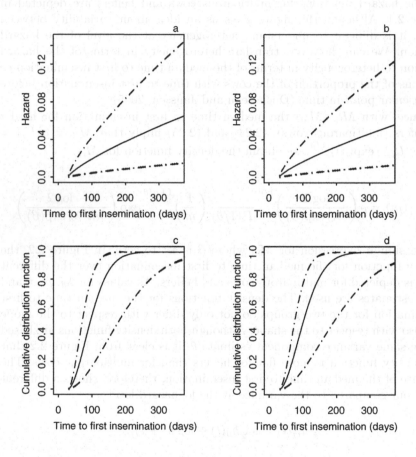

Fig. 2.1. Hazard functions for time to first insemination for (a) multiparous cows and for (b) heifers, with corresponding cumulative distribution functions for (c) multiparous cows and for (d) heifers. The full line corresponds to the hazard function in herds with frailty equal to one, the lower and upper lines correspond to the hazard functions of herds with frailty equal to the 5th and the 95th percentiles of the gamma distribution with mean one and variance $\theta = 0.394$.

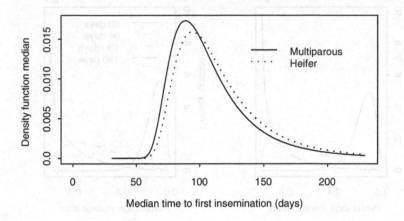

Fig. 2.2. Density functions for the median time to first insemination in multiparous cows and heifers.

Obviously, the density function of the percentage of animals with first insemination before a particular timepoint over the different herds shows most spread for that timepoint where the mode of the density function is close to 50%, corresponding to the percentage considered at 95.5 days for the multiparous cows (Figure 2.3). The density function of the percentage of first insemination before either an earlier (e.g., 60 days) or a later timepoint (e.g., 180 days) is more concentrated as at those timepoints most herds have respectively low and high proportions of first insemination. ∎

Example 2.2 The accelerated failure time model for time to first insemination based on marginal likelihood maximisation

The marginal likelihood maximisation approach can also be used for the accelerated failure time model in case of the Weibull baseline hazard. The parameter estimates for the accelerated failure time model can be obtained by simple transformation from the parameter estimates for the proportional hazards model given in Example 2.1. Rewriting the proportional hazards model (2.24) in terms of the accelerated failure time model (1.13), with the random effect introduced in the model in the same way as the fixed effects covariates

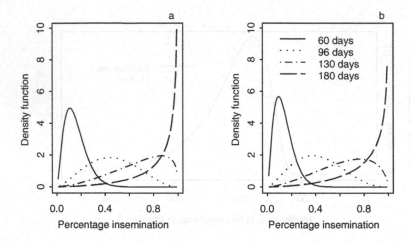

Fig. 2.3. Density functions for the percentage insemination at different timepoints (see legend: timepoints 60, 96, 130, and 180 days) for (a) multiparous cows (with median event time 95.5 days) and (b) heifers (with median event time 101.5 days).

we have

$$h_{ij}(t) = \lambda \rho t^{\rho-1} \left(\exp \left(x_{ij} \beta \rho^{-1} + w_i \rho^{-1} \right) \right)^\rho$$

$$= \lambda \rho t^{\rho-1} u_i \left(\exp \left(x_{ij} \beta \rho^{-1} \right) \right)^\rho \qquad (2.28)$$

From (2.28) it follows that λ, ρ, and the u_i's with corresponding θ remain the same in the accelerated failure time model, and therefore we have, as in Example 2.1, $\hat{\lambda} = 0.174$, $\hat{\rho} = 1.769$, and $\hat{\theta} = 0.394$. The estimated accelerator becomes $\exp(\hat{\beta}/\hat{\rho}) = 0.916$.

The software package STATA contains functions to fit parametric frailty models. The possible choices for the baseline hazard form are exponential, Weibull, Gompertz, lognormal, loglogistic, and gamma; for the frailty distribution the possible choices are the gamma or the inverse Gaussian distribution (see Sections 4.2 and 4.3 for detailed discussions). STATA allows the choice between the proportional hazards and the accelerated failure time representation with the Weibull baseline hazard assumption. ∎

As shown in the example above, parametric models are easy to fit (compared to semiparametric model fitting, a topic discussed in Chapter 5).

The disadvantage of parametric models is that they are not flexible in describing for example changes in the shape of the hazard function, e.g., Weibull hazards are monotone by definition. Parametric models can be made more flexible: divide the time axis in intervals and allow the parameters of the model to be different on each interval. Such models can still be fitted by maximising the marginal likelihood. We discuss two such examples below. The two examples differ in the way the intervals are specified.

In the first example the at risk period is split into different intervals and each interval has its own baseline hazard function. Such models are called piecewise models. In Example 2.3 we assume constant baseline hazards within each interval. The second example deals with recurrent events. An interval corresponds to the time since the last event (or since the entry of the subject in the study for the first event) to the next event. The length of the intervals therefore differs from subject to subject. So the intervals arise here in a more natural and data-driven way. Each interval in the sequence of events has now its own conditional hazard function described by a different Weibull distribution. In Example 2.4 these risk functions are defined, for different timescales, starting from a Weibull baseline hazard.

Example 2.3 The piecewise constant baseline hazard frailty model for the time to culling data based on marginal likelihood maximisation

For the time to culling data presented in Example 1.7, the following simple model is fitted:

$$h_{ij}(t) = h_0(t)u_i \exp\left(\beta \log(SCC_{ij})\right)$$

with $h_0(t)$ the baseline hazard function, assumed to be constant $h_0(t) = \lambda$, u_i the frailty term for herd i, and β the risk coefficient explaining the linear effect of the logarithm of the somatic cell count on the loghazard of culling. Again, we use as time unit month rather than day to avoid convergence problems.

The constant baseline hazard is estimated by $\hat{\lambda} = 0.016$ (s.e. $= 0.001$), $\hat{\theta} = 0.062$ (s.e. $= 0.024$), and $\hat{\beta} = 0.088$ (s.e. $= 0.015$). Thus, as expected, the culling hazard is increasing with increasing values for the logarithm of the somatic cell count. The loglikelihood at the maximum likelihood estimators is equal to -15125.74.

The model above is probably too simple to be realistic, as it is well known that the baseline hazard function is not constant over time in this type of data. The economic value of a dairy cow is highest at the start of the lactation at calving time, as she produces milk in the next 300 days. Peak milk production occurs around 70 days after calving. A farmer is reluctant to cull a dairy cow at the start of the lactation period, even when she is sick and needs expensive medical care. We can, however, expect that after 70 days farmers might decide to cull cows that produce much less milk compared to what could be expected at that time of high milk production. However, the highest culling rate is expected when the lactation period finishes (around 300 days after calving) and the dairy cow does not produce milk anymore for a few months. Farmers then cull cows that produced little milk or had a lot of health problems. In order to accommodate for this expected pattern in the culling rate, time is split into three periods: 0 to 70 days after calving, 70 to 300 days after calving, and more than 300 days after calving. This gives the following model:

$$h_{ij}(t) = (\lambda_1 I(t \leq 70) + \lambda_2 I(70 < t \leq 300) + \lambda_3 I(t > 300))$$

$$\times u_i \exp\left(\beta \log(SCC_{ij})\right)$$

with λ_1, λ_2, and λ_3 the baseline hazards in the first, second, and third period, respectively. The parameter estimates for this extended model are given by $\hat{\lambda}_1 = 0.007$ (s.e. $= 0.001$), $\hat{\lambda}_2 = 0.011$ (s.e. $= 0.001$), $\hat{\lambda}_3 = 0.097$ (s.e. $= 0.008$) with the baseline hazard, as expected, increasing with number of days in lactation. The effect of the logarithm of the somatic cell count on the loghazard is the same as in the other model, $\hat{\beta} = 0.088$ (s.e. $= 0.016$), but the estimate of the between herds variance increases to $\hat{\theta} = 0.144$ (s.e. $= 0.029$). Note that, despite the extension of the model with two additional parameters, the variance increases. The parameter θ refers to the variability between herds, whereas the additional parameters of the extended model relate to the hazard functions of individual animals. The more adequate modelling of the risk at the individual cow level has apparently led to a greater separation between the herds (cluster effect).

Finally, the loglikelihood at these maximum likelihood estimates equals -13608.52. We can compare the extended model with the original model by the likelihood ratio (LR) test, which corresponds to minus two times the difference in loglikelihood between the original and extended model:

$$\text{LR} = 2\,(-15125.74 + 13608.52) = 3034$$

The corresponding p-value (using a chi-square distribution with 2 degrees of freedom) is less than 0.00001. Therefore, the extended model fits the data far better than the original model. ∎

Example 2.4 The frailty model with Weibull baseline hazard for the recurrent asthma data based on marginal likelihood maximisation

We now analyse the recurrent asthma data presented in Example 1.9. We need some additional notation in order to keep track of the ordering. Assume we have in total s patients. A patient is at risk in different periods, which are separated from each other by either an asthmatic event or a timespan, during which the patient is not under observation. The number of such risk periods for patient i is denoted by n_i. The complete information for patient i can then be presented by the n_i triplets

$$(y_{i11}, y_{i12}, \delta_{i1}), \ldots, (y_{in_i1}, y_{in_i2}, \delta_{in_i})$$

where, for triplet j, y_{ij1} is the start of at risk period j, y_{ij2} is the end of at risk period j, δ_{ij} is the censoring indicator, and $y_{i11} = 0$. The main objective is to compare the placebo group ($x_i = 0$) with the drug group ($x_i = 1$). Compared to the previous example, the covariate information in this example is cluster specific, i.e., x_{ij} does not change with j: $x_{ij} \equiv x_i = 0$ or 1.

Different timescales can be used to model recurrent event data. In the gap time representation, the time at risk starts at 0, but the length of the time at risk now corresponds to the time since the end of the previous event (or entry to the study in the case of the first event) until the time of the particular event. In the calendar time representation, the length of the at risk period is the same, but the start of the at risk period is not reset to 0 but to the actual time since entry to the study (see Figure 2.4).

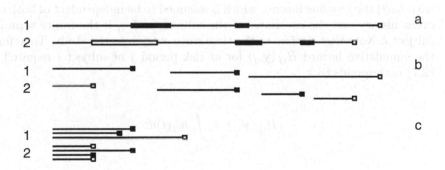

Fig. 2.4. (a) Event history for two subjects where a line denotes time at risk, a filled box corresponds to asthma attack time, and an empty box is censored time with (b) the calendar time representation and (c) the gap time representation.

We first analyse the recurrent event data using each of these two timescales separately, but eventually combine the two timescales in one and the same model. For convenience, the same notation $(\lambda, \rho, \theta, \beta)$ will be used in each of the models, although the parameters have different meaning in the different models. The marginal likelihood that needs to be maximised is given by (see (2.7))

$$
l_{marg}(\zeta) = \sum_{i=1}^{s} \left[d_i \log \theta - \log \Gamma(1/\theta) + \log \Gamma(1/\theta + d_i) \right.
$$
$$
\left. -(1/\theta + d_i) \log \left(1 + \theta \sum_{j=1}^{n_i} H_{ij,c}(y_{ij}) \right) + \sum_{j=1}^{n_i} \delta_{ij} \log h_{ij,c}(y_{ij}) \right] \quad (2.29)
$$

with now s standing for the number of patients. The different models below are specified in terms of the conditional hazard function and conditional cumulative hazard function. The unconditional parts of these functions, $h_{ij,c}(y_{ij})$ and $H_{ij,c}(y_{ij})$, present in (2.29), can easily be obtained by setting u_i equal to one in the conditional expressions.

The frailty model based on calendar time (model 1: calendar) is given by

$$
h_{ij}(t) = \begin{cases} h_0(t)u_i \exp\left(\beta x_i\right) & \text{for } y_{ij1} \leq t \leq y_{ij2}, j = 1, \ldots, n_i \\ 0 & \text{otherwise} \end{cases}
$$

with $h_0(t)$ the baseline hazard, which is assumed to be independent of both the event history and the covariates of the subject, and u_i is the frailty term for subject i. Note that t refers to the time since entry into the study. Therefore, the cumulative hazard $H_{ij}(\mathbf{y}_{ij})$ for at risk period j of subject i required in (2.7) corresponds to

$$
H_{ij}(\mathbf{y}_{ij}) = \int_{y_{ij1}}^{y_{ij2}} h_{ij}(t)dt
$$

with $\mathbf{y}_{ij} = (y_{ij1}, y_{ij2})^t$ referring to the start and the end of the interval j. We further assume a Weibull baseline hazard $h_0(t) = \lambda \rho t^{\rho-1}$.

Maximising the marginal likelihood with respect to the parameters λ, ρ, θ, and β gives the estimates shown in Table 2.1. The estimate of ρ is close to one resulting in a hazard function that is almost constant (Figure 2.5a).

Alternatively, recurrent event data can be modelled as gap time data. In the case of gap time, part of the information in the triplets is abundant and we can summarise the information in the triplets as

$$
(y_{i12} - y_{i11}, \delta_{i1}), \ldots, (y_{in_i2} - y_{in_i1}, \delta_{in_i})
$$

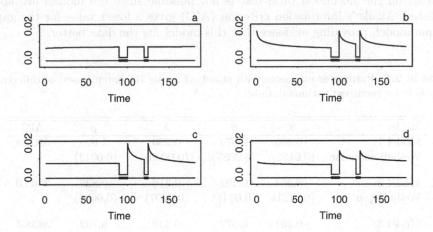

Fig. 2.5. The hazard as a function of time for a subject with event history depicted at the bottom of the picture according to (a) Model 1: calendar, (b) Model 2: gap, (c) Model 3: gap but first event exp, and (d) Model 4: gap calendar.

In other words, only the length of the time at risk is needed, and not the particular time (relative to the time of entry in the study) when the patient is at risk.

The frailty model for the gap time data (model 2: gap) is given by

$$
h_{ij}(t) = \begin{cases} h_0(t - y_{ij1})u_i \exp{(\beta x_i)} & \text{for } y_{ij1} \leq t \leq y_{ij2}, j = 1, \ldots, n_i \\ 0 & \text{otherwise} \end{cases}
$$

The cumulative hazard $H_{ij}(\mathbf{y}_{ij})$ for at risk period j of subject i required in (2.7) now corresponds to

$$
H_{ij}(\mathbf{y}_{ij}) = \int_0^{y_{ij2}-y_{ij1}} h_{ij}(t)dt
$$

We again assume a Weibull baseline hazard $h_0(t) = \lambda \rho t^{\rho-1}$.

Maximising the marginal likelihood with respect to the parameters λ, ρ, θ, and β gives the estimates shown in Table 2.1. The estimate of ρ is equal to 0.829 and thus substantially smaller than one. The hazard function decreases with time. This means that the asthma event rate is larger immediately after an event and decreases with time since the last event (Figure 2.5b). A goodness of fit comparison between the calendar time and gap time models based on the likelihood ratio test is not possible since the models are not nested. Akaike's information criterion (AIC) gives a lower value for the gap time model, providing evidence that this model fits the data better.

Table 2.1. Parameter estimates with standard errors (in parentheses) of different models for recurrent asthma data set.

Model	β	θ	λ	ρ	AIC
Model 1:	−0.300	0.574	0.230	1.029	3906.8
Weibull-calendar	(0.0152)	(0.0055)	(0.0009)	(0.0013)	
Model 2:	−0.254	0.402	0.316	0.829	3863.0
Weibull-gap	(0.0121)	(0.0041)	(0.0007)	(0.0006)	
Model 3:	−0.251	0.372	0.346	0.762	3838.4
Weibull-gap but	(0.0117)	(0.0040)	(0.0008)	(0.0007)	
first event exp			$\hat{\lambda}_f = 0.217$		
			(0.0005)		
Model 4:	−0.245	0.421	0.134	0.687	3885.4
Weibull-gap	(0.0126)	(0.0045)	(0.0007)	(0.0020)	
calendar			$\hat{\lambda}_f = 0.210$	$\hat{\rho}_f = 0.946$	
			(0.0020)	(0.0008)	

In the gap time model, we assume the same hazard function regardless of the ordering of the event in the sequence. The first event, however, is different from the other events. It is assumed that the subject at the time of study entry did not experience an asthmatic event yet. Therefore, it is inappropriate to model the rate for the first event in the same way as the common rate for the other events, namely, as a function of the time since the last event. A more appropriate assumption is a constant hazard rate λ_f for the first event leading to the following model (model 3: gap but first event exp)

$$
h_{ij}(t) = \begin{cases} \lambda_f u_i \exp(\beta x_i) & \text{for } 0 \leq t \leq y_{i12} \\ \lambda \rho(t - y_{ij1})^{\rho-1} u_i \exp(\beta x_i) & \text{for } y_{ij1} \leq t \leq y_{ij2}, j = 2, \ldots, n_i \\ 0 & \text{otherwise} \end{cases}
$$

As Akaike's information criterion decreases further from 3863.0 to 3838.4, the model with a separate (constant) hazard rate for the first event is preferable. The parameter estimates for this model are similar, but the decrease in the recurrent event rate with time since the last event is more pronounced

($\hat{\rho} = 0.762$) and the constant hazard rate for the first event is substantially smaller ($\hat{\lambda}_f = 0.217$) than for the subsequent events ($\hat{\lambda} = 0.346$).

Since we focus both on what happens over calendar time with children aged between 6 and 24 months, and on the asthma event rate after an asthma event has taken place, it seems appropriate to combine both timescales in one and the same model (model 4: gap calendar) as follows:

$$
h_{ij}(t) = \begin{cases} \lambda_f \rho_f t^{\rho_f - 1} u_i \exp\left(\beta x_i\right) & \text{for } 0 \leq t \leq y_{i12} \\ \left(\lambda_f \rho_f t^{\rho_f - 1} + \lambda \rho (t - y_{ij1})^{\rho - 1}\right) u_i \exp\left(\beta x_i\right) & \text{for } y_{ij1} \leq t \leq y_{ij2}, \\ & \qquad\qquad j = 2, \ldots, n_i \\ 0 & \text{otherwise} \end{cases}
$$

The cumulative hazard $H_{ij}\left(\mathbf{y}_{ij}\right)$ for at risk period j of subject i corresponds now to

$$
H_{ij}\left(\mathbf{y}_{ij}\right) = \begin{cases} \lambda_f y_{i12}^{\rho_f} u_i \exp\left(\beta x_i\right) & \text{for } j = 1 \\ \left(\lambda_f \left(y_{ij2}^{\rho_f} - y_{ij1}^{\rho_f}\right) + \lambda \left(y_{ij2} - y_{ij1}\right)^{\rho}\right) u_i \exp\left(\beta x_i\right) \\ & \text{for } j = 2, \ldots, n_i \end{cases}
$$

An example of this model for a particular subject in the placebo group is given in Figure 2.5d. The part of the baseline hazard rate that is due to calendar time ($\lambda_f \rho_f t^{\rho_f - 1}$) decreases over time (even before the first event). We superimpose on the calendar time hazard rate the part of the baseline hazard rate that is due to gap time ($\lambda \rho (t - y_{ij1})^{\rho - 1}$), i.e., a hazard that changes as a function of the time at risk since the last event. The gap time hazard rate decreases with time at risk since the last event. The parameter estimates of the last model show a further decrease in treatment effect. The hazard rate now decreases as a function of time since study entry as well ($\hat{\rho}_f = 0.946$) and the decrease of the recurrent event rate with time since the last event is more pronounced ($\hat{\rho} = 0.687$). This model, however, has a much higher Akaike's information criterion, so it is not the preferred model for the actual data set.

■

2.3 Extension of the marginal likelihood approach to interval-censored data

In the previous section, we looked at right-censored data and we demonstrated how we arrived at a closed form expression for $L_{marg,i}(\zeta)$, the marginal likelihood, by integrating out the one-parameter gamma frailty density in the conditional likelihood $L_i\left(\xi, \beta \mid u_i\right)$. In this section we show that a parallel discussion can be given for interval-censored data (Goethals et al., 2007). We use the following notation. Within cluster i there are r_i right-censored subjects and g_i interval-censored subjects collected respectively in subsets R_i and

G_i. For subject j in R_i the right-censored times are denoted by y_{ij}. The event time of a subject j in G_i is contained in an interval with start time l_{ij} and end time r_{ij}.

The conditional likelihood of cluster i is then given by

$$L_i\left(\boldsymbol{\xi}, \boldsymbol{\beta} \mid u_i\right) = \prod_{j \in R_i} S_{ij}\left(y_{ij}\right) \prod_{j \in G_i} \left(S_{ij}\left(l_{ij}\right) - S_{ij}\left(r_{ij}\right)\right)$$

with $\boldsymbol{\xi}$ containing the parameters of the baseline hazard. For a Weibull baseline hazard we have

$$L_i\left(\boldsymbol{\xi}, \boldsymbol{\beta} \mid u_i\right) = \exp\left(-\sum_{j \in R_i} \lambda y_{ij}^\rho u_i \exp\left(\mathbf{x}_{ij}^t \boldsymbol{\beta}\right)\right)$$

$$\times \prod_{j \in G_i} \left[\exp\left(-\lambda l_{ij}^\rho u_i \exp\left(\mathbf{x}_{ij}^t \boldsymbol{\beta}\right)\right) - \exp\left(-\lambda r_{ij}^\rho u_i \exp\left(\mathbf{x}_{ij}^t \boldsymbol{\beta}\right)\right)\right]$$

$$= \exp\left(-u_i q_i\right) \times \prod_{j \in G_i} \left(\exp\left(-u_i l_{ij}^*\right) - \exp\left(-u_i r_{ij}^*\right)\right) \qquad (2.30)$$

with $q_i = \sum_{j \in R_i} \lambda y_{ij}^\rho \exp\left(\mathbf{x}_{ij}^t \boldsymbol{\beta}\right)$, $l_{ij}^* = \lambda l_{ij}^\rho \exp\left(\mathbf{x}_{ij}^t \boldsymbol{\beta}\right)$, and $r_{ij}^* = \lambda r_{ij}^\rho \exp\left(\mathbf{x}_{ij}^t \boldsymbol{\beta}\right)$.

To obtain the marginal likelihood we integrate out the unobserved frailties in (2.30) assuming a one-parameter gamma frailty distribution. Before we do this analytic (closed form) integration it is convenient to rewrite the conditional likelihood in matrix notation. We first define the following column vector $\mathbf{a}_i$ of length 2^{g_i}:

$$\mathbf{a}_i = \left({}_c a_{ik}\right)_{k=1}^{2^{g_i}} = \bigotimes_{j \in G_i} \left(\begin{array}{c} \exp(-u_i l_{ij}^*) \\ -\exp(-u_i r_{ij}^*) \end{array}\right)$$

where $\mathbf{A} \bigotimes \mathbf{B}$ is the Kronecker or direct product of the matrices $\mathbf{A}$ and $\mathbf{B}$. For $\mathbf{A}$ an $(r \times c)$ matrix and $\mathbf{B}$ a $(p \times q)$ matrix we have that $\mathbf{A} \bigotimes \mathbf{B} = (a_{ij}\mathbf{B})$ an $(rp \times cq)$ matrix. The first element of this column vector, for example, is $\exp\left(-u_i \sum_{j \in G_i} l_{ij}^*\right)$. The last element is $\pm \exp\left(-u_i \sum_{j \in G_i} r_{ij}^*\right)$ with a positive sign if the number of r_{ij}^*'s in the sum of the exponent is even and a negative sign if the number is odd. The number of r_{ij}^*'s in a_{ik} will be denoted as n_{ik}. Expression (2.30) can then be rewritten as

$$L_i\left(\boldsymbol{\xi}, \boldsymbol{\beta} \mid u_i\right) = \exp\left(-u_i q_i\right) \left(\sum_{k=1}^{2^{g_i}} a_{ik}\right)$$

Starting from this form of the conditional likelihood we integrate out the gamma distributed frailties to obtain the following expression for the marginal likelihood:

$$L_{marg,i}(\zeta) = \int_0^\infty \frac{u^{1/\theta-1}\exp(-u/\theta)}{\theta^{1/\theta}\Gamma(1/\theta)} \exp(-uq_i) \left(\sum_{k=1}^{2^{g_i}} a_{ik}\right) du$$

$$= \frac{1}{\theta^{1/\theta}\Gamma(1/\theta)} \sum_{k=1}^{2^{g_i}} \int_0^\infty u^{1/\theta-1} \exp\left(-u\left(q_i + \frac{1}{\theta}\right)\right) a_{ik} du$$

$$= \sum_{k=1}^{2^{g_i}} \frac{(-1)^{n_{ik}}}{(q_i + \log p_{ik} + 1/\theta)^{1/\theta}\,\theta^{1/\theta}} \tag{2.31}$$

with $\mathbf{p}_i$ the column vector

$$\mathbf{p}_i = (_c p_{ik})_{k=1}^{2^{g_i}} = \bigotimes_{j\in G_i} \left(\begin{array}{c} \exp(l_{ij}^*) \\ \exp(r_{ij}^*) \end{array}\right)$$

To obtain the full marginal likelihood we take the product of the s cluster-specific marginal likelihoods $\prod_{i=1}^s L_{marg,i}(\zeta)$. Since the second partial derivatives can be obtained for all parameters, an explicit expression for the Hessian matrix is available (see the Appendix in Goethals et al. (2007)), from which an estimate of the asymptotic variance–covariance matrix can be obtained.

Example 2.5 The parametric proportional hazards frailty model for the interval-censored udder quarter infection data based on marginal likelihood maximisation

We consider the interval-censored udder quarter infection times described in Example 1.4, and investigate the effect of the location of the udder quarter (front or rear) and parity. The estimated hazard ratio of front versus rear udder quarters equals 1.197 with the 95% confidence interval [0.943; 1.520]. The baseline hazard parameter estimates are $\hat{\lambda} = 0.896$ (s.e. $= 0.165$) and $\hat{\rho} = 1.929$ (s.e. $= 0.110$), and the hazard is increasing with time both for the front (Figure 2.6a) and the rear (Figure 2.6b) udder quarters.

The variance component estimate is $\hat{\theta} = 1.784$ (s.e. $= 0.303$). Thus, infection times within the cow are highly correlated with Kendall's τ estimated as $\hat{\theta}/(\hat{\theta}+2)=0.471$ (see (4.28) for the definition of Kendall's τ for the gamma frailty distribution). An estimate of the standard error of τ can be obtained by applying the delta method

$$\mathrm{Var}(\hat{\tau}) = \mathrm{Var}\left(\frac{\hat{\theta}}{\hat{\theta}+2}\right) \approx \frac{4}{\left(\hat{\theta}+2\right)^4}\mathrm{Var}(\hat{\theta})$$

leading to the standard error estimate 0.042.

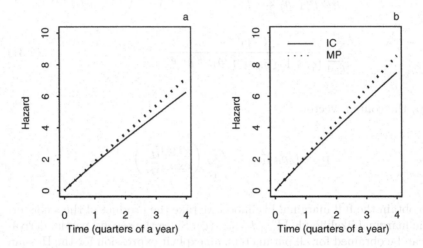

Fig. 2.6. Hazard functions for time to infection based on the interval-censored data (IC) and on the midpoint (MP) imputation for (a) the front udder quarters and (b) the rear udder quarters.

Alternatively, the midpoint of the interval can be imputed and can be considered to be the exact infection time; then the more simple techniques of the previous section can be used. For the imputed data, the estimated hazard ratio of front versus rear udder quarters equals 1.194 with the 95% confidence interval [0.945; 1.509], the variance component estimate is $\hat{\theta} = 1.798$ (s.e. = 0.304), and the baseline hazard parameter estimates are $\hat{\lambda} = 0.926$ (s.e. = 0.171) and $\hat{\rho} = 1.981$ (s.e. = 0.106). The hazard function is increasing with time for both the front (Figure 2.6a) and the rear (Figure 2.6b) udder quarters.

In this particular case, using the interval-censored data or the midpoint imputation leads to only small differences. Especially with the hazard function decreasing over time ($\rho < 1$), parameter estimates can, however, differ substantially (Goethals et al., 2007).

The estimated hazard ratio of multiparous versus primiparous cows equals 1.369 with the 95% confidence interval $[0.717; 2.613]$. The variance component estimate is $\hat{\theta} = 1.772$ (s.e. $= 0.303$). Thus, infection times within the cow are highly correlated with Kendall's τ estimated as $\hat{\theta}/(\hat{\theta}+2)=0.470$ (s.e. $= 0.043$). The baseline hazard parameter estimates are $\hat{\lambda} = 0.811$ (s.e. $= 0.209$) and $\hat{\rho} = 1.924$ (s.e. $= 0.110$), and the hazard is increasing with time for both the primiparous and the multiparous cows. ∎

2.4 Posterior densities: the Bayesian approach

In this section, we introduce some basic Bayesian terminology and apply it to the frailty model. For a detailed account of Bayesian methodology, we refer to Gelman et al. (2004). In Section 2.4.1 we explain in a practical way for the parametric gamma frailty model how the Metropolis algorithm can be used as a resampling technique to obtain a sample from the posterior densities of the parameters of interest. The Bayesian analysis is then based on this sample. The theoretical foundations of the Metropolis algorithm are given in Section 2.4.2.

In the approach presented here, the gamma distributed frailties are first integrated out so that the frailty terms do not appear in the Bayesian analysis. In the classical Bayesian approach, discussed in Section 6.2.2, the frailties will be considered as parameters. Integrating out the frailties, however, reduces the parameter space. In a low-dimensional parameter space, it is convenient to apply the Metropolis algorithm. The proposed approach also enables us to compare, in a simple setting, the frequentist approach discussed in Section 2.1 and the Bayesian analysis presented in this section.

2.4.1 The Metropolis algorithm in practice for the parametric gamma frailty model

Bayesian statistical inference on a parameter of interest is made in terms of probability statements. The probability statements are conditional on the observed information $\mathbf{y}$. The density function of the parameter of interest, conditional on the observations $\mathbf{y}$, is called the posterior density function of the parameter. Statistical analysis can be based on the posterior density. For instance, the mode of this density is taken as an estimate of the parameter. Also credible sets or Bayesian confidence intervals, the Bayesian analogues of frequentist confidence intervals, are derived from the posterior density function.

A $100(1 - \alpha)\%$ credible set C for parameter ν with parameter space N is formally defined as

$$1 - \alpha \leq \mathrm{P}(C \mid \mathbf{y}) = \int_C f(\nu \mid \mathbf{y})d\nu$$

so that the probability that ν lies in C given the observed data $\mathbf{y}$ is at least $1 - \alpha$ (Carlin and Louis, 1996).

In our case, the parameters of interest are $\boldsymbol{\xi}$, θ, and $\boldsymbol{\beta}$ with $\boldsymbol{\xi}$ an $(a \times 1)$ vector containing the parameters related to the baseline hazard, e.g., for the Weibull $\boldsymbol{\xi} = (\lambda, \rho)$, and therefore interest will be in the posterior density functions of each of these parameters (using f as generic notation):

$$f\left(\xi_1 \mid \mathbf{y}\right), \ldots, f\left(\xi_a \mid \mathbf{y}\right), f\left(\theta \mid \mathbf{y}\right), f\left(\beta_1 \mid \mathbf{y}\right), \ldots, f\left(\beta_p \mid \mathbf{y}\right)$$

To obtain these posterior densities, we start from the joint density function of the observed information $\mathbf{y}$ and latent information $\mathbf{u}$

$$f\left(\mathbf{y}, \mathbf{u} \mid \boldsymbol{\zeta}\right)$$

with $\boldsymbol{\zeta} = (\boldsymbol{\xi}, \theta, \boldsymbol{\beta})$. This expression can be rewritten as

$$f\left(\mathbf{y} \mid \mathbf{u}, \lambda, \rho, \boldsymbol{\beta}\right) f\left(\mathbf{u} \mid \theta\right)$$

We have demonstrated in the previous section how the gamma frailties $\mathbf{u}$ can be integrated out from this expression to obtain $f\left(\mathbf{y} \mid \boldsymbol{\zeta}\right)$. According to the Bayes theorem, we have

$$f\left(\boldsymbol{\zeta} \mid \mathbf{y}\right) = \frac{f\left(\mathbf{y} \mid \boldsymbol{\zeta}\right) f\left(\boldsymbol{\zeta}\right)}{f\left(\mathbf{y}\right)} \tag{2.32}$$

where $f\left(\mathbf{y} \mid \boldsymbol{\zeta}\right)$ is called the sampling density and $f\left(\boldsymbol{\zeta}\right)$ is the prior density function of the parameters. The sampling density $f\left(\mathbf{y} \mid \boldsymbol{\zeta}\right)$ actually corresponds to the marginal likelihood $L_{marg}\left(\boldsymbol{\zeta}\right)$ obtained in the frequentist approach. The prior density models the prior belief on the parameters, i.e., the information already available before sampling has taken place. Furthermore, $f\left(\mathbf{y}\right) = \int_{\Xi} f\left(\mathbf{y} \mid \boldsymbol{\zeta}\right) f\left(\boldsymbol{\zeta}\right) d\boldsymbol{\zeta}$ with Ξ the parameter space of $\boldsymbol{\zeta}$.

In Bayesian terminology, $f\left(\mathbf{y}\right)$ is called the normalising constant. It is often hard to obtain $f\left(\mathbf{y}\right)$ in an explicit way. However, since $f\left(\mathbf{y}\right)$ does not depend on $\boldsymbol{\zeta}$, it can be dropped from the expression for the posterior density, i.e., we can work with the unnormalised posterior density

$$f\left(\boldsymbol{\zeta} \mid \mathbf{y}\right) \propto f\left(\mathbf{y} \mid \boldsymbol{\zeta}\right) f\left(\boldsymbol{\zeta}\right) \tag{2.33}$$

Using this expression and assuming independence between the prior density functions of the parameters, we have that

$$f\left(\boldsymbol{\xi}, \theta, \boldsymbol{\beta} \mid \mathbf{y}\right) \propto L_{marg}\left(\boldsymbol{\zeta}\right) \times \prod_{i=1}^{a} f\left(\xi_i\right) \times f\left(\theta\right) \times \prod_{j=1}^{p} f\left(\beta_j\right) \tag{2.34}$$

We still need to make assumptions with respect to the prior density functions in (2.34). The option we take here is to assume a noninformative prior for each of these density functions: we assume that the density functions have a constant value over the whole parameter space. This also means that the prior density functions are proportional to one and thus we can write

$$f\left(\boldsymbol{\beta}\right) = \prod_{j=1}^{p} f(\beta_j) \propto 1, f\left(\boldsymbol{\xi}\right) = \prod_{i=1}^{a} f(\xi_i) \propto 1, f\left(\theta\right) \propto 1 \qquad (2.35)$$

Noninformative priors have the advantage that they give the same weight to each possible value, and therefore the posterior distribution will be more influenced by the data and less by the prior distribution function. Note that θ takes values in $[0, +\infty)$ and β_j, $j = 1 \ldots, p$, in $(-\infty, +\infty)$. Therefore, the prior distributions in (2.35) are called improper, as they do not integrate to one over the parameter space but have an infinite integral. We can make use of improper prior density functions as long as they lead to proper posterior density functions (Jeffreys, 1961). Plugging in these prior density functions, (2.34) simplifies to

$$f\left(\boldsymbol{\xi}, \theta, \boldsymbol{\beta} \mid \mathbf{y}\right) \propto L_{marg}\left(\boldsymbol{\xi}, \theta, \boldsymbol{\beta}\right)$$

Obviously, taking the mode of this joint posterior density leads to the same solution as the maximisation of the marginal likelihood discussed in Section 2.2. Now we further have to derive the univariate posterior density for each of the parameters individually, starting from the joint posterior density. This can be achieved either through numerical integration or by approximating the integral using Laplacian integration whenever exact integration is impossible. Alternatively, different sampling techniques can be used to draw samples from the joint posterior density, from which then parameters of interest of the univariate posterior densities can be estimated. We will demonstrate here how characteristics of the univariate posterior densities can be obtained through the Metropolis algorithm. We will first describe the different steps of the algorithm.

The basic idea behind the Metropolis algorithm is to draw a multivariate sample from the joint posterior density. A univariate sample of the univariate posterior density corresponding to a particular parameter is then obtained by taking the relevant component of the multivariate sample. Bayesian inference of each individual parameter is then based on the univariate sample for that parameter. It will be demonstrated in the next section that the Metropolis algorithm will generate univariate sequences of random points whose distributions converge to the univariate posterior densities.

The Metropolis algorithm is useful for a low-dimensional parameter space such as the particular case presented in this chapter, and when the joint posterior density function is known up to a proportionality constant. In the particular setting studied here, the parameter estimates and the Hessian obtained from the frequentist approach are used in the algorithm (initialisation step and observed information matrix). In other settings, alternative techniques exist to initialise the Metropolis algorithm (Gelman et al., 2004). Note that the parameter estimates correspond to the mode of the joint posterior density. In Bayesian analysis, we work with the posterior distribution of the parameters. This is in contrast with the frequentist approach. There we assume the parameters to be fixed and we use point estimates and their corresponding standard errors.

We use below the Metropolis algorithm to generate a sample from the joint posterior distribution. This sample will provide information on specific characteristics of the univariate posterior distributions.

The algorithm for our particular setting goes as follows:

1. Select an initial value $\zeta^{(0)}$. We can take for instance the mode of the joint posterior density $\hat{\zeta}$. Any other value with $f\left(\zeta^{(0)} \mid \mathbf{y}\right) > 0$ will do.

   To obtain a sample from the joint posterior density we generate the sequence of points $\zeta^{(1)}$, $\zeta^{(2)}$, ... by applying Step 2 and Step 3 for $j = 1, 2, \ldots$

2. For a fixed j generate ζ^* at random from the density that is derived from an appropriate symmetric transition kernel $J_j\left(\zeta^* \mid \zeta^{(j-1)}\right)$ (see Section 2.4.2), e.g., ζ^* can be generated from a multivariate normal density with mean $\zeta^{(j-1)}$ and variance–covariance matrix $\mathbf{V} = \mathbf{T}\mathbf{I}^{-1}(\hat{\zeta})\mathbf{T}$ with $\mathbf{I}(\hat{\zeta})$ the observed information matrix (see (2.9)) evaluated at the mode of the joint posterior density $\hat{\zeta}$ and $\mathbf{T}$ a diagonal tuning matrix (see the discussion following the description of the algorithm). The transition kernel has to be symmetric, i.e., $J_j\left(\zeta^a \mid \zeta^b\right) = J_j\left(\zeta^b \mid \zeta^a\right)$.

3. Obtain the following ratio (r_j is called the acceptance rate):

$$r_j = \frac{f\left(\zeta^* \mid \mathbf{y}\right)}{f\left(\zeta^{(j-1)} \mid \mathbf{y}\right)} \qquad (2.36)$$

   Accept ζ^* as new value, i.e., put $\zeta^{(j)} = \zeta^*$, with probability $\min(r_j, 1)$ and let $\zeta^{(j)} = \zeta^{(j-1)}$ with probability $1 - \min(r_j, 1)$.

In Section 2.4.2 it will be explained that for n_B large enough $\left\{\zeta^{(j)} : j \geq n_B\right\}$ can be considered as a sample from the posterior density. The period from $j = 1$ to $j = n_B$ is called the burn-in period. As explained in Gelman et al. (1995) a tuning matrix is useful to make sure that n_B is not too large, i.e., to make the burn-in period not too long. The tuning matrix has especially an effect on the acceptance rate (in Step 3). The matrix is a diagonal matrix. There is a tuning parameter for each of the parameters of interest. As a rule of thumb, the diagonal elements are 2.4 divided by the square root of the number of parameters, e.g., for our example we take $2.4/\sqrt{a+p+1}$ (see Gelman et al. (1995) for more details).

The transition kernel $J_j\left(\zeta^* \mid \zeta^{(j-1)}\right)$ has the subindex j to denote that it possibly depends on the iteration number j. This is not the case in the example given below where the multivariate normal distribution with the variance–covariance matrix based on the observed information matrix is used throughout the iterations.

Example 2.6 The parametric proportional hazards frailty model for time to first insemination based on the Metropolis algorithm

We reconsider the time to first insemination data set (Example 1.8). The general scheme of the Metropolis algorithm presented above is now adapted in a number of ways. First, a different parameterisation is used. Since $\lambda, \rho,$ and θ have range $[0, +\infty)$, it is better to work with the logarithm for data simulation so that no problems arise regarding range preservation. Whatever value in $(-\infty, +\infty)$ is generated for the logarithm of these three parameters, it always corresponds with a value for the actual parameters in the interval $[0, +\infty)$.

Therefore, we also need to rewrite the joint posterior density in terms of this new parameterisation $(\log \lambda, \log \rho, \log \theta, \beta) \equiv (l\lambda, l\rho, l\theta, \beta)$. In general, if $f_{\mathbf{Z}}(\zeta)$ is a density function for the parameter vector $\mathbf{Z}$, and $\mathbf{N} = \mathbf{g}(\mathbf{Z})$ is a one to one transformation, then the density function of $\mathbf{N}$ is

$$f_{\mathbf{N}}(\boldsymbol{\nu}) = \mid \mathbf{J} \mid f_{\mathbf{Z}}\left(\mathbf{g}^{-1}(\boldsymbol{\nu})\right)$$

where $\mid \mathbf{J} \mid$ is the absolute value of the determinant of the Jacobian of the transformation $\boldsymbol{\nu} = \mathbf{g}(\zeta)$, i.e., $\mathbf{J}$ is the square matrix of partial derivatives with $(i, j)^{\text{th}}$ entry the value for $\partial \zeta_i / \partial \nu_j$. In our particular case, we have $\zeta = (\lambda, \rho, \theta, \beta)$ and $\boldsymbol{\nu} = (l\lambda, l\rho, l\theta, \beta)$ and thus

$$\zeta = \mathbf{g}^{-1}(\boldsymbol{\nu}) = (\exp(l\lambda), \exp(l\rho), \exp(l\theta), \beta)$$

Furthermore, the determinant of the Jacobian is given by

$$\mid \mathbf{J} \mid = \det \begin{pmatrix} \exp(l\lambda) & 0 & 0 & 0 \\ 0 & \exp(l\rho) & 0 & 0 \\ 0 & 0 & \exp(l\theta) & 0 \\ 0 & 0 & 0 & 1 \end{pmatrix} = \exp(l\lambda)\exp(l\rho)\exp(l\theta)$$

and therefore the posterior density function in terms of the new parameterisation is the same as in (2.34) but now with $\lambda, \rho,$ and θ replaced by $\exp(l\lambda), \exp(l\rho),$ and $\exp(l\theta),$ respectively, and we furthermore have to multiply with the term $\exp(l\lambda)\exp(l\rho)\exp(l\theta).$

Second, we work with unnormalised posterior densities, for which we have a closed form expression. The posterior densities are only needed in the ratio presented in Step 3, so that there is no difference between taking the normalised or unnormalised posterior densities.

Third, we rather work with the logarithm of the ratio of the posterior densities. This corresponds to the difference in the logarithm of the posterior densities

$$\log\left(f\left(\zeta^* \mid \mathbf{y}\right)\right) - \log\left(f\left(\zeta^{(j-1)} \mid \mathbf{y}\right)\right)$$

Working with the posterior densities themselves leads to very small values, so that it is better to work with the logarithm. For the actual generation of the sequence, it turns out that, in order to evaluate convergence of the sequence, it is better to generate a series of independent sequences rather than one long sequence. We will discuss this issue at the end of the example. We generate four such independent sequences.

In order to have good starting values for the sequences we can use the mode of the joint posterior density function which is given by (see Example 2.1) $\left(\log(\hat{\lambda}), \log(\hat{\rho}), \log(\hat{\theta}), \hat{\beta}\right) = (\log(0.174), \log(1.769), \log(0.394), -0.153).$

In the algorithm, we also need the Hessian matrix at this mode, which can also be obtained from the frequentist approach, and which is given by

$$\begin{bmatrix} 419.15264 & -5.18558 & 152.15192 & 820.28050 \\ -5.18558 & 74.46179 & 0.54133 & -102.17770 \\ 152.15192 & 0.54133 & 1900.14616 & 622.05440 \\ 820.28055 & -102.17773 & 622.05436 & 18004.74200 \end{bmatrix}$$

Minus the inverse of the Hessian matrix is

$$\begin{bmatrix} 0.00268 & 0.00003 & -0.00018 & -0.00012 \\ 0.00003 & 0.01354 & -0.00003 & 0.00008 \\ -0.00018 & -0.00003 & 0.00054 & -0.00001 \\ 0.00012 & 0.00008 & -0.00001 & 0.00006 \end{bmatrix}$$

Finally, we use as tuning parameter $2.4/2=1.2$ ($\sqrt{a+p+1} = \sqrt{4} = 2$) for each of the parameters, according to the recommendation by Gelman et al.

(1995), leading to the following tuning matrix:

$$\begin{bmatrix} 1.2 & 0 & 0 & 0 \\ 0 & 1.2 & 0 & 0 \\ 0 & 0 & 1.2 & 0 \\ 0 & 0 & 0 & 1.2 \end{bmatrix}$$

Each of the four sequences is started by drawing an initial value from the multivariate normal distribution with mean equal to the mode of the joint posterior density and variance equal to $\mathbf{V} = \mathbf{TI}^{-1}\left(\hat{\zeta}\right)\mathbf{T}$. Each sequence consists of 5000 draws. In order to assess whether convergence has been obtained we can depict the sequence of values, called the trace. According to Figure 2.7, the stable behaviour of the sequences suggests that convergence has been obtained.

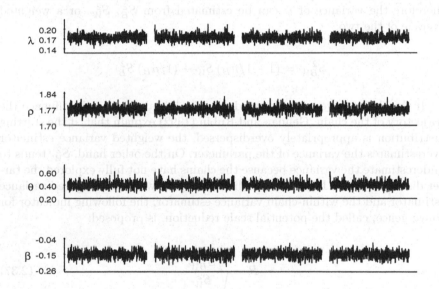

Fig. 2.7. The traces of the four sequences for each of the four parameters of the time to first insemination data set.

Alternatively, the convergence diagnostic proposed by Gelman and Rubin (1992) can be used. Assume there are m sequences or chains, all of length $2n_B$ and starting from different points that are overdispersed relative to the target distribution. Only the second half of the $2n_B$ chain iterations are used in the convergence diagnostic.

Denote the jth iteration for chain i by ψ_{ij}, the mean of the last n_B chain iterations of chain i by $\bar{\psi}_{i.}$ and let $\bar{\psi}_{..}$ be the overall mean over the m different chain means $\bar{\psi}_{i.}, i = 1, \ldots, m$. The within-chain variance is

$$S_W^2 = \frac{1}{m(n_B - 1)} \sum_{i=1}^{m} \sum_{j=n_B+1}^{2n_B} \left(\psi_{ij} - \bar{\psi}_{i.}\right)^2$$

and the between-chain variance is

$$S_B^2 = \frac{n_B}{m - 1} \sum_{i=1}^{m} \left(\bar{\psi}_{i.} - \bar{\psi}_{..}\right)^2$$

If the chains have converged (say after the first n_B chain iterations), all values that are subsequently drawn, come from the posterior density, and therefore the variance of ψ can be estimated from S_B^2, S_W^2, or a weighted average of the two:

$$S_{BW}^2 = (1 - 1/n_B) S_W^2 + (1/n_B) S_B^2$$

If the chains have not converged yet, the initial values still influence the trajectory of the chain. Gelman and Rubin (1992) explain that, if the starting distribution is appropriately overdispersed, the weighted variance estimator overestimates the variance of the parameter. On the other hand, S_W^2 tends to underestimate the variance because the chains have not fully explored the target distribution yet. Based on this discrepancy between the weighted variance estimator and the within-chain variance estimator, the following indicator for convergence, called the potential scale reduction, is proposed:

$$\hat{R} = \sqrt{\frac{S_{BW}^2}{S_W^2}} \tag{2.37}$$

Upon convergence, we expect this value to be close to one. In our example, $\hat{R}$ is between 1.00 and 1.01 for any of the four parameters considered, which is an additional and more formal indication of convergence. The posterior densities of the four parameters are depicted in Figure 2.8 and are based on the last 2500 values of each of the four sequences, using the first 2500 runs as burn-in period. In Table 2.2 we also present the different quantiles that are obtained from the posterior densities and from which credible sets can be obtained. The results are very similar to the results obtained by the frequentist approach (see Example 2.1). ■

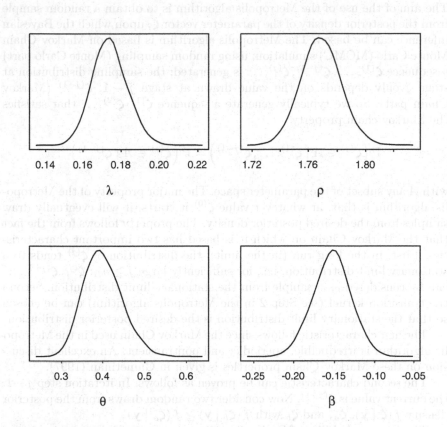

Fig. 2.8. The estimated posterior densities of the four parameters of the time to first insemination data set.

Table 2.2. Summary statistics of posterior density functions for time to first insemination data set.

Parameter	Mean	s.e.	Quantiles				
			2.5%	25%	50%	75%	97.5%
λ	0.174	0.009	0.157	0.168	0.174	0.180	0.192
ρ	1.769	0.014	1.742	1.759	1.768	1.778	1.797
θ	0.400	0.047	0.320	0.367	0.396	0.429	0.496
β	−0.153	0.023	−0.198	−0.168	−0.152	−0.138	−0.108

2.4.2* Theoretical foundations of the Metropolis algorithm

The aim of the use of the Metropolis algorithm is to obtain a random sample from the posterior density of the parameter vector ζ, upon which the Bayesian inference can be based. The Metropolis algorithm is based on Markov Chain Monte Carlo (MCMC) simulation: using random sampling (Monte Carlo part) a sequence $\zeta^{(1)}, \ldots, \zeta^{(j-1)}, \zeta^{(j)}, \ldots$ is generated; the sampling distribution at stage j only depends on the value drawn at stage $j-1$, $\zeta^{(j-1)}$ (Markov Chain part). So we typically generate a sequence $\zeta^{(1)}, \zeta^{(2)}, \ldots$ that satisfies the Markov chain property

$$P\left(\zeta^{(j)} \in A \mid \zeta^{(1)}, \ldots, \zeta^{(j-1)}\right) = P\left(\zeta^{(j)} \in A \mid \zeta^{(j-1)}\right)$$

with A any subset of the parameter space. The major property of the Metropolis algorithm is that, at whatever value $\zeta^{(0)}$ it starts, it will eventually draw samples from the desired posterior density. The property follows from the fact that the Markov Chain on which it is based has two important characteristics. First, in the long run (in the limit), the distribution of $\zeta^{(j)}$ tends to a stationary limit distribution, i.e., for sufficiently large $j \geq n_B$: $\zeta^{(j)}, \zeta^{(j+1)}, \ldots$ can be considered as a sample from the stationary limit distribution. Second the transition kernel (see Step 2 in the Metropolis algorithm) can be chosen so that the stationary limit distribution is the desired posterior distribution.

The first characteristic follows since the Markov Chain used in the Metropolis algorithm is irreducible, aperiodic, and nontransient. An excellent discussion on these Markov Chain properties is given in Gamerman (1997).

The second characteristic can be proven as follows. In iteration step $j-1$, the current value is $\zeta^{(j-1)}$. Now consider two random draws from the posterior density $f(\zeta \mid \mathbf{y})$, ζ_a, and ζ_b with $f(\zeta_b \mid \mathbf{y}) \geq f(\zeta_a \mid \mathbf{y})$.

The joint probability of having first ζ_a and next ζ_b is given by

$$f\left(\zeta^{(j-1)} = \zeta_a, \zeta^{(j)} = \zeta_b\right) = f(\zeta_a \mid \mathbf{y}) J_j(\zeta_b \mid \zeta_a)$$

as the acceptance probability is one since

$$\min(r_j, 1) = \min\left(\frac{f(\zeta_b \mid \mathbf{y})}{f(\zeta_a \mid \mathbf{y})}, 1\right) = 1$$

On the other hand, the joint probability of having first ζ_b and next ζ_a is given by

$$f\left(\zeta^{(j-1)} = \zeta_b, \zeta^{(j)} = \zeta_a\right) = f(\zeta_b \mid \mathbf{y}) J_j(\zeta_a \mid \zeta_b) \frac{f(\zeta_a \mid \mathbf{y})}{f(\zeta_b \mid \mathbf{y})}$$

$$= f(\zeta_a \mid \mathbf{y}) J_j(\zeta_a \mid \zeta_b)$$

but this is exactly the same as the previous expression due to the symmetry of the kernel. Since the joint distribution is symmetric, $\zeta^{(j-1)}$ and $\zeta^{(j)}$ have the same marginal distribution, and therefore $f(\zeta \mid \mathbf{y})$ is the stationary distribution of the Markov Chain.

An important generalisation of the Metropolis algorithm is the Metropolis–Hastings algorithm. It differs from the Metropolis algorithm in that the transition kernel is no longer required to be symmetric. To correct for the asymmetry in the kernel, the ratio r_j in (2.36) is replaced by

$$r_j = \frac{f\left(\zeta^* \mid \mathbf{y}\right)/J_j\left(\zeta^* \mid \zeta^{(j-1)}\right)}{f\left(\zeta^{(j-1)} \mid \mathbf{y}\right)/J_j\left(\zeta^{(j-1)} \mid \zeta^*\right)}$$

It can also be proven, in a similar way as before, that the Metropolis–Hastings algorithm generates, after a burn-in period, a sample from a stationary limit distribution that is the desired posterior distribution (see Gelman et al. (2004), Chapter 11 for a more detailed discussion).

2.5 Further extensions and references

The methods discussed in this chapter can be applied for any baseline hazard that is specified in a parametric way (in Chapter 5 we will discuss semiparametric models, where the baseline hazard remains unspecified). The Weibull baseline hazard is a common choice. An alternative and flexible parametric approach is to use a piecewise constant baseline hazard (see Example 2.3). Other approaches include Box–Cox transformed hazard functions (Yin and Ibrahim, 2005) and the use of splines to model the baseline hazard (He and Lawless, 2003). Jeong et al. (2003) propose an alternative family of functions for the baseline hazard.

3

Alternatives for the frailty model

There are several alternatives for the frailty model that somehow take into account the clustering of observations. These alternatives are in most cases computationally simpler, but have also major drawbacks compared to the frailty model.

In the first section, we will discuss the fixed effects model. The clusters are introduced in the model as fixed effects rather than as random effects. Another approach is to model the clusters by using stratification; this is demonstrated in Section 3.2. Throughout Section 3.2 we consider paired data (clusters of size two). For bivariate data it is easier to compare the different models in a clear way. We note, however, that our findings generalise to clusters with larger cluster size.

In Section 3.3, the copula model is introduced. The copula is a function that describes the relationship between the population survival functions of the different subjects in a cluster and their joint survival function. It is often claimed in the literature that there is equivalence between a copula model and a particular frailty model, but we demonstrate in Section 3.3.4 that this claim is incorrect using as an example the Clayton copula and the shared gamma frailty model.

In Section 3.4, we discuss marginal models. To obtain estimates for the fixed covariate effects the survival model is first fitted without taking into account the correlation between observations within a cluster. To estimate the variances of the fixed effect estimators the correlation between survival times within a cluster is taken into account by using sandwich estimators. Finally, in Section 3.5, we discuss model and parameter interpretation for marginal and conditional (frailty) models.

3.1 The fixed effects model

3.1.1 The model specification

Assume that the cluster effect is modelled by a fixed rather than by a random effect, as in the following model:

$$h_{ij}(t) = h_0(t) \exp(\mathbf{x}_{ij}^t \boldsymbol{\beta} + c_i) \qquad (3.1)$$

where c_i is the fixed effect for the ith cluster. This model is overparameterised; we therefore add the restriction $c_1 = 0$.

Below we demonstrate that introducing the cluster effect as a fixed effect has some serious drawbacks such as less efficient estimation of the parameters and a less natural model interpretation. In order to evaluate the efficiency of the parameter estimates from the fixed effects model and compare it to the frailty model, we give, in (3.4) and (3.5), the likelihood expression for these two models. Additionally we give the likelihood for the unadjusted model that does not take into account clustering in the data

$$h_{ij}(t) = h_0(t) \exp(\mathbf{x}_{ij}^t \boldsymbol{\beta}) \qquad (3.2)$$

This model is also useful in our discussion on the comparison between fixed effects models and frailty models. For simplicity, we assume constant baseline hazard $h_0(t) = \lambda$ and consider a single covariate x_{ij}. Then the likelihood for the model without cluster effects is given by

$$L_1(\lambda, \beta) = \prod_{i=1}^{s} \lambda^{d_i} \exp\left(\beta \sum_{j=1}^{n_i} \delta_{ij} x_{ij} - \lambda \sum_{j=1}^{n_i} y_{ij} \exp(x_{ij}\beta)\right) \qquad (3.3)$$

with d_i the number of events in cluster i. This likelihood ignores the dependence between observations in the same cluster. In Section 3.4 it is shown that parameter estimates from this model are consistent, but that the variance estimators of the parameter estimates need to be adjusted.

On the other hand, the likelihood for the fixed effects model is given by

$$L_2(\boldsymbol{\lambda}, \beta) = \prod_{i=1}^{s} \lambda_i^{d_i} \exp\left(\beta \sum_{j=1}^{n_i} \delta_{ij} x_{ij} - \lambda_i \sum_{j=1}^{n_i} y_{ij} \exp(x_{ij}\beta)\right) \qquad (3.4)$$

with $\boldsymbol{\lambda}^t = (\lambda_1, \ldots, \lambda_s)$ and $\lambda_i = \lambda \exp(c_i), i = 1, \ldots, s$.

Finally, the marginal likelihood for the frailty model with gamma frailty distribution can be obtained from the general expression (2.6) leading to

$$L_3(\lambda, \theta, \beta) = \prod_{i=1}^{s} \frac{\Gamma(d_i + 1/\theta)\lambda^{d_i} \exp\left(\beta \sum_{j=1}^{n_i} \delta_{ij} x_{ij}\right)}{\Gamma(1/\theta)\theta^{1/\theta}\left(1/\theta + \lambda \sum_{j=1}^{n_i} y_{ij} \exp\left(x_{ij}\beta\right)\right)^{d_i+1/\theta}} \quad (3.5)$$

Example 3.1 The fixed effects and frailty model for the time to blood–milk barrier reconstitution: the treatment effect

We investigate the treatment effect on the time to blood–milk barier reconstitution in Example 1.3, where the udder quarters are clustered within cow. We first fit the unadjusted model which does not take into account the clustering:

$$h_{ij}(t) = \lambda \exp\left(x_{ij}\beta\right)$$

with λ the constant baseline hazard, x_{ij} the covariate for udder quarter j from cow i, taking the value zero if the quarter is treated with placebo and the value one if the quarter is treated with the active compound. The parameter β is therefore the treatment effect at the loghazard level.

This model is then extended to the fixed effects model

$$h_{ij}(t) = \lambda \exp\left(x_{ij}\beta + c_i\right)$$

where c_i is the fixed effect for cow i. The frailty model is given by

$$h_{ij}(t) = \lambda u_i \exp(x_{ij}\beta)$$

where now the frailty term u_i for cow i is assumed to come from a one-parameter gamma distribution with mean one and variance θ. The parameter estimates and their standard errors are given in Table 3.1 for the unadjusted, the fixed effects, and the frailty model, together with the results of the stratified model to be discussed in Section 3.2.

When fitting these models in R, the parameter estimates refer to the loglinear model representation as given in Section 1.4.4. Therefore, we need to transform these parameters to the proportional hazards model representation. For the unadjusted model the loglinear model representation is

$$\log T_{ij} = \mu + x_{ij}\alpha + \sigma E_{ij}$$

with $\exp(E_{ij}) \sim \text{Exp}(1)$, $\sigma = 1$, and α the treatment effect (see Section 1.4.4). The parameter estimates for the unadjusted model in this representation are

Table 3.1. Parameter estimates with standard errors (in parentheses) for the time to blood–milk barrier reconstitution based on the unadjusted, fixed effects, frailty, and stratified model.

Model	$\hat{\beta}$ (s.e.)	$\hat{\lambda}$ (s.e.)	$\hat{\theta}$ (s.e.)
Unadjusted	0.176 (0.162)	0.216 (0.025)	
Fixed effects	0.185 (0.190)	7×10^{-10} (2×10^{-6})	
Frailty	0.171 (0.168)	0.256 (0.038)	0.286 (0.141)
Stratified	0.131 (0.209)		

given by $\hat{\mu} = 1.531$ (s.e. $= 0.118$) and $\hat{\alpha} = -0.176$ (s.e. $= 0.162$). The corresponding proportional hazards model representation is

$$h_{ij}(t) = \lambda \exp\left(x_{ij}\beta\right)$$

for which we have that $\hat{\beta} = -\hat{\alpha} = 0.176$ with obviously the same standard error 0.162 and $\hat{\lambda} = \exp(-\hat{\mu}) = 0.216$ with the approximate standard error given by

$$\text{s.e.}(\hat{\lambda}) = \exp\left(-\hat{\mu}\right)\text{s.e.}\left(\hat{\mu}\right) = 0.216 \times 0.118 = 0.025$$

The parameter estimate $\hat{\lambda} = 0.216$ results in an estimate of the median time to reconstitution in untreated udder quarters of 3.2 days. The median time to reconstitution in treated udder quarters reduces to 2.7 days, but this difference is not significant. The hazard ratio is equal to 1.19 with 95% confidence interval $[0.87; 1.64]$.

For the fixed effects model the loglinear model representation is

$$\log T_{ij} = \mu + x_{ij}\alpha + k_i + E_{ij}$$

with k_i the fixed effect of cow i. The parameter estimates for the fixed effects model in this representation with cow introduced as categorical fixed effect can be obtained by the survreg function in R and are shown in Table 3.2.

The corresponding proportional hazards model representation is

$$h_{ij}(t) = \lambda \exp\left(x_{ij}\beta + c_i\right)$$

for which we have that $\hat{c}_i = -\hat{k}_i$ with the same standard error. The treatment effect estimate corresponds to $\hat{\beta} = -\hat{\alpha} = 0.185$ with standard error equal to 0.190. The parameter λ is now estimated as $\exp\left(-\hat{\mu}\right) = 7 \times 10^{-10}$ with standard error equal to $\exp\left(-\hat{\mu}\right)\text{s.e.}\left(\hat{\mu}\right) = 2 \times 10^{-6}$. This parameter, however,

Table 3.2. Parameter estimates with standard errors for the time to blood–milk barrier reconstitution based on the fixed effects model in loglinear model representation with treatment and cow as categorical fixed effects.

Parameter	Estimate	Standard error
(Intercept)	21.0	3331.69
trt	−0.185	0.19
cowid2	−18.8	3331.69
...		
cowid65	2×10^{-6}	0.00
...		
cowid100	−18.6	3331.69

corresponds to the constant hazard rate for the untreated udder quarter of the first cow, as c_1 has been put equal to zero (or equivalently $k_1=0$). The first cow has two censored observations (see Table 1.3), which results in this very small estimated hazard rate. The hazard rate can actually not be determined for this cow as no event has been observed; it can only be concluded that the particular cow seems to have a low hazard rate as no events occur during the observation period. Therefore, the hazard for the untreated udder quarter of this cow is set to an arbitrary low value.

The cow effect estimates $\hat{c}_i = -\hat{k}_i$ of other cows with two censored observations are equal to zero (e.g., cowid=65). Therefore, these cows have the same small value for the hazard rate of the untreated udder quarter as the first cow as the hazard rate of the untreated udder quarter of a particular cow is obtained by adding the cow effect to the intercept μ and then taking the exponential of minus this value, i.e., $\exp\left(-\hat{\mu} - \hat{k}_i\right)$.

All other cow effect estimates have large negative values to counteract the fact that the untreated udder quarter of the first cow has a low hazard rate and that their hazard rate is given by $\exp\left(-\hat{\mu} - \hat{k}_i\right)$. For instance, the second cow has a time to reconstitution equal to 0.93 day for the placebo-treated udder quarter, whereas the time to reconstitution for the active compound udder quarter was censored at 6.5 days (see Table 1.3). For this cow, the hazard rate in the placebo-treated quarter corresponds to $\exp\left(-21 + 18.8\right) = 0.11$.

Finally, the standard errors are very large for any of these cow effects. This can be expected since only two observations are available to estimate them; moreover for some cows we only have censored observations. For such cows the hazard cannot really be estimated. The fact that the variance estimates are high due to the presence of the censoring can be demonstrated as follows: give all the observed times to reconstitution in Table 1.3 censoring status=1 (i.e., act as if there is no censoring) and refit the model. For this "modified" data set the estimated standard errors take more reasonable values.

For the frailty model, the treatment effect estimate corresponds to $\hat{\beta} = 0.171$ (s.e. = 0.168). We now have only two additional parameters, with estimates $\hat{\lambda} = 0.256$ (s.e. = 0.038) and $\hat{\theta} = 0.286$ (s.e. = 0.141). ∎

Example 3.2 The fixed effects and frailty model for the time to blood–milk barrier reconstitution: the heifer effect

It is further also of interest to look at the heifer effect in Example 1.3. There is an important difference between this covariate and the treatment covariate considered in Example 3.1, in that the heifer covariate is a cow characteristic and is therefore the same for each of the two udder quarters of a cow. The heifer effect estimate in the unadjusted model equals 0.118 (s.e. = 0.162), resulting in a hazard ratio of 1.125 with 95% confidence interval [0.82; 1.55]. The hazard of reconstitution is thus larger for heifers, although not in a significant way.

If the fixed effects model is fitted containing both the cow effects and the heifer effect, results for the loglinear model representation obtained from the survreg function in R differ depending on the order in which the two covariates are introduced in the model.

The results obtained when introducing the heifer covariate first in the model are shown in Table 3.3.

Table 3.3. Parameter estimates with standard errors for the time to blood–milk barrier reconstitution based on the fixed effects model in loglinear model representation with heifer (introduced first in the model) and cow as categorical fixed effects.

Parameter	Estimate	Standard error
Intercept	20.90	4723
heifer	−20.10	6680
cowid2	1.21	4723
...		
cowid100	−18.50	4723

The heifer effect is estimated as $\hat{\alpha} = -20.1$, resulting in an impossibly high hazard ratio given by $\exp(-\hat{\alpha})$. It is obvious that this result does not make sense; R is not able to handle the confounding in the covariates (cow effect and heifer effect) in a correct way.

On the contrary, the heifer covariate can be introduced in the model after the cow covariate, which results in the estimates given in Table 3.4. This results in an estimate of the heifer effect equal to zero.

None of these two results actually make sense. There is complete confounding between the cow covariate and the heifer covariate: the heifer covariate can be written as a linear combination of the cow covariate. Consider the

Table 3.4. Parameter estimates with standard errors for the time to blood–milk barrier reconstitution based on the fixed effects model in loglinear model representation with cow (introduced first in the model) and heifer as categorical fixed effects.

Parameter	Estimate	Standard error
Intercept	20.90	4723
cowid2	−18.90	4723
...		
cowid100	−18.50	4723
heifer	0.00	6680

covariate matrix for the first three cows

$$
\begin{array}{cccccc}
\text{Intercept} & \text{Cowid2} & \text{Cowid3} & \text{Heifer} & \text{Parity} & \text{Treatment} \\
\left[\begin{array}{cccccc}
1 & 0 & 0 & 1 & 1 & 1 \\
1 & 0 & 0 & 1 & 1 & 0 \\
1 & 1 & 0 & 0 & 3 & 1 \\
1 & 1 & 0 & 0 & 3 & 0 \\
1 & 0 & 1 & 1 & 1 & 1 \\
1 & 0 & 1 & 1 & 1 & 0
\end{array}\right]
\end{array} \tag{3.6}
$$

The first two rows correspond to the active compound-treated (row 1) and placebo-treated (row 2) udder quarter of the first cow. The first column is the intercept, the next two columns are the indicators for cow 2 and cow 3, the fourth column corresponds to the heifer covariate, the fifth column indicates the parity, and finally the last column contains the treatment information. It is clear that the heifer column can be obtained by subtracting the Cowid2 column from the Intercept column. Similarly, the parity column can be obtained by adding two times the Cowid2 column to the Intercept column. On the contrary, the treatment column cannot be obtained as a linear combination of the other columns.

In other words, we allow each cow to have its own hazard through the introduction of the fixed cow effect, so that no remaining variability at the cow level is left for the heifer covariate which is only changing from cow to cow. In the frailty model, however, the cow effect is introduced as a frailty with a particular variance describing the cow variability. By introducing the heifer covariate we might be able to explain part of the cow variability. The heifer effect estimate in the frailty model equals 0.122 (s.e. = 0.202), resulting in a hazard ratio of 1.130 with 95% confidence interval [0.76; 1.68]. ■

In the example above, we observe that the estimated β parameter is largest for the fixed effects model. Furthermore, the largest value for the standard error is found for the fixed effects model, the smallest for the unadjusted model with the frailty model taking a value in between the two models. These differences are not haphazard and we demonstrate in the next section for a simple setting that the asymptotic variance of $\hat{\beta}$ obtained from the frailty model is indeed between the asymptotic variances obtained from the unadjusted and fixed effects model.

3.1.2* Asymptotic efficiency of fixed effects model parameter estimates

In deriving the asymptotic efficiency of the parameter estimates of the different models, we consider clusters of size two without censoring. Furthermore, it is assumed that the covariate is centred so that $\sum_{i=1}^{s}\sum_{j=1}^{2} x_{ij} = 0$. We first simplify the likelihood expression of the fixed effects model as it contains a set of λ_i's that are actually nuisance parameters. We can replace the λ_i's by their maximum likelihood expression in terms of β, which can be obtained by taking the first partial derivatives of the log likelihood to λ and equating them to zero. For instance for λ_i, we have

$$\frac{\partial \log L_2(\boldsymbol{\lambda}, \beta)}{\partial \lambda_i} = \frac{d_i}{\lambda_i} - \sum_{j=1}^{2} y_{ij} \exp\left(x_{ij}\beta\right) = 0$$

and

$$\lambda_i = \frac{d_i}{\sum_{j=1}^{2} y_{ij} \exp\left(x_{ij}\beta\right)}$$

Plugging in these expressions in the likelihood expression we obtain

$$L_2(\beta) = \prod_{i=1}^{s} d_i^{d_i} \exp(-d_i) \frac{\exp\left(\beta \sum_{j=1}^{2} \delta_{ij} x_{ij}\right)}{\left(\sum_{j=1}^{2} y_{ij} \exp\left(x_{ij}\beta\right)\right)^{d_i}}$$

It can be shown that $L_2(\beta)$ corresponds to the likelihood of the ratios $y_{i2}/y_{i1}, i = 1, \ldots, s$, which, according to the definition of Barnard (1963), is marginally sufficient for β in the absence of knowledge of $\boldsymbol{\lambda}$.

Expressions for the expected information for β

$$\boldsymbol{\mathcal{I}}(\beta) = -\mathrm{E}\left(\frac{\partial^2 \log L}{\partial \beta^2}\right)$$

for the three models are given in Wild (1983). As for each model $\hat{\beta}$ is asymptotically independent from the other estimated parameters (Wild, 1983), we have that $(\boldsymbol{\mathcal{I}}(\beta))^{-1}$ is the asymptotic variance of $\hat{\beta}$.

The expected information for β in the first model corresponds to

$$\mathcal{I}_1(\beta) = \sum_{i=1}^{s} \left(x_{i1}^2 + x_{i2}^2 \right) \tag{3.7}$$

whereas for the fixed effects model we have that

$$\mathcal{I}_2(\beta) = 2 \sum_{i=1}^{s} \frac{(x_{i1} - \bar{x}_{i\cdot})^2 + (x_{i2} - \bar{x}_{i\cdot})^2}{3} \tag{3.8}$$

and finally for the frailty model

$$\mathcal{I}_3(\beta) = \sum_{i=1}^{s} \left[\frac{1/\theta \left(x_{i1}^2 + x_{i2}^2 \right)}{1/\theta + 3} + \frac{2 \left((x_{i1} - \bar{x}_{i\cdot})^2 + (x_{i2} - \bar{x}_{i\cdot})^2 \right)}{1/\theta + 3} \right]$$

Therefore, we have that

$$\mathcal{I}_3(\beta) = \frac{1/\theta}{1/\theta + 3} \mathcal{I}_1(\beta) + \frac{3}{1/\theta + 3} \mathcal{I}_2(\beta)$$

Thus, $\mathcal{I}_3(\beta)$ is a linear combination of $\mathcal{I}_1(\beta)$ and $\mathcal{I}_2(\beta)$ with equal weights if $\theta = 1/3$. For $\theta > 1/3$, $\mathcal{I}_2(\beta)$ has more weight than $\mathcal{I}_1(\beta)$ in determining $\mathcal{I}_3(\beta)$ and the other way around for $\theta < 1/3$.

These efficiency comparisons can be extended further in an approximate way to the Weibull model; see Wild (1983) for a further discussion. The findings above on efficiency of the estimates of β are based on expected information and are therefore asymptotic in nature. To investigate the efficiency of the estimated fixed effects of these three models in finite sample size situations, we run some simulations as described below.

Data are generated from the frailty model assuming exponentially distributed event times with $\lambda = 0.23, \beta = 0.18$, and $\theta = 0.3$ (the choice of parameter values is inspired by parameter estimates in Table 3.1). We generate 2000 data sets each consisting of 100 pairs of two subjects. In the first setting, each pair has a treated and an untreated subject and the actual event times are observed. In the second setting, 80% of the pairs have a treated and an untreated subject, but in 10% of the pairs the two subjects are treated and in another 10% the two subjects are untreated. In the third setting, subjects are censored if the event time is longer than 6.5 days after the treatment corresponding on average to 20% censoring. For this setting covariates within a pair are assumed to be different.

For each of the 2000 data sets in each of the settings, the three models are fitted and the estimate for β and its standard error are obtained. We determine the median, 5% and 95% quantiles of these estimates and determine also the coverage percentage as the percentage of data sets for which the true value for β, equal to 0.18, is contained in the asymptotic confidence interval given by $[\hat{\beta} - 1.96 \times \text{s.e.}(\hat{\beta}); \hat{\beta} + 1.96 \times \text{s.e.}(\hat{\beta})]$.

For the first setting, the median of the estimates is close to the true value of 0.18 (see Table 3.5). The standard error of the parameter estimates is largest for the fixed effects model, smallest for the unadjusted model whereas the frailty model is, as expected, in between the two models. The coverage for the 95% confidence interval is equal to 95% for the fixed effects model but not for the frailty model and unadjusted model. The coverage for the frailty model, however, is just below 95% which might be explained by the fact that we use the asymptotic confidence interval based on the normal distribution. The unadjusted model, on the other hand, is well below 95% which is due to the fact that the standard error of the estimate is too low.

In the second setting, only 80% of the pairs have different covariate information for the two subjects within a pair. This leads to an inefficient analysis for the fixed effects model since all pairs in which the two individuals share the same covariate information are not used. This has an impact on the standard error of the estimate in the fixed effects model, which is increasing more compared to the frailty model. The information in pairs where the two individuals share the same covariate can be recovered in a frailty model as it also makes use of differences between clusters, the so-called recovery of interblock information, first introduced by Patterson and Thompson (1971) in the context of mixed models and extended for survival data by Wild (1983).

In extreme situations, where covariate information only changes at the level of the cluster (i.e., each individual within a cluster has the same covariate information) the fixed effects model is completely useless, as these covariates are entirely confounded with the fixed cluster effect (McGilchrist and Aisbett, 1991), as is demonstrated in Example 3.2 for the analysis of the heifer effect.

In the presence of censoring, the main problem arises with the fixed effects model. The estimate for β is biased away from the true value. The slight increase in the standard error is insufficient so that the coverage is well below 95% and the treatment effect estimate is systematically larger than the true value. On the other hand, although we observe an increase of the standard error in the unadjusted model, we observe at the same time less extreme quantiles for β so that in the presence of censoring the coverage of the unadjusted model is above 95%.

It is clear from these simulation results that the frailty model performs better than the fixed effects model, even if there is no censoring and if the covariate information is differing between the two subjects within each pair. In the presence of censoring and in the case that for some of the pairs the two subjects share the same covariate information, differences are even more pronounced which makes the frailty model even more preferable.

In a study with many small clusters, a lot of parameters need to be estimated compared to the total number of available observations. Due to this fact, the asymptotics might break down. In the context of binary outcomes, this has long been known to result in estimates of the parameters which are strongly biased away from null (Glidden and Vittinghoff, 2004).

Lastly, there is also a difference in interpretation of the fixed effects and frailty model. In most cases, we are not really interested in the cluster effect by itself, but rather in its variance, or we merely want to adjust for the correlation in the data. In the fixed effects model, however, the particular clusters are considered to be important by themselves. Therefore, no estimate of the variability between clusters is available from the fixed effects model. Furthermore, it seems that the fixed effects model is not adequate to test for the presence of cluster effects as the size of the usual tests are typically above the nominal significance level even for quite large studies with a large number of reasonably large clusters (Andersen et al., 1999).

3.2 The stratified model

A second approach is to use a different and unspecified baseline hazard for each of the clusters. This gives the semiparametric stratified model

$$h_{ij}(t) = h_{i0}(t) \exp\left(\mathbf{x}_{ij}^t \boldsymbol{\beta}\right) \tag{3.9}$$

with $h_{i0}(t)$ the baseline risk for cluster i. In this model we assume that the baseline hazards are completely unrelated nuisance functions and that the regression coefficients are the same in each stratum. Thus, this model is even more flexible than the fixed effects model as the baseline hazard can evolve independently over time within each cluster, whereas in the fixed effects model it is restricted to be of form $h_0(t) \exp(c_i)$ where c_i is the constant specific effect for cluster i.

To estimate $\boldsymbol{\beta}$ we adapt the partial likelihood idea developed in Section 1.4.2. With

$$R_i(y_{ij}) = \{l : y_{il} \geq y_{ij}\}$$

the risk set for cluster i at time y_{ij} containing all the subjects in cluster i who are still at risk at time y_{ij}, the partial likelihood for this model is

$$\prod_{i=1}^{s} \prod_{j=1}^{n_i} \left(\frac{\exp\left(\mathbf{x}_{ij}^t \boldsymbol{\beta}\right)}{\sum_{l \in R_i(y_{ij})} \exp\left(\mathbf{x}_{il}^t \boldsymbol{\beta}\right)} \right)^{\delta_{ij}}$$

Example 3.3 The stratified model for the time to blood–milk barrier reconstitution data and its likelihood

For the specific example considered in Section 3.1 with only two subjects per cluster and assuming no ties within a cluster, the partial likelihood expression for the stratified model simplifies to

$$
L_4\left(\beta\right) = \prod_{i=1}^{s} \left[\left(\frac{\exp\left(x_{i1}\beta\right) I\left(y_{i1} < y_{i2}\right)}{\exp\left(x_{i1}\beta\right) + \exp\left(x_{i2}\beta\right)} \right)^{\delta_{i1}} + \left(\frac{\exp\left(x_{i2}\beta\right) I\left(y_{i2} < y_{i1}\right)}{\exp\left(x_{i1}\beta\right) + \exp\left(x_{i2}\beta\right)} \right)^{\delta_{i2}} \right]
$$

It is clear from this expression that a cluster only has a contribution if an event for a subject is observed while the other subject is still at risk. Additionally, pairs where the subjects share the same covariate information do not contribute to the likelihood. Therefore, in many practical situations, this model is inefficient. The parameter estimate (see Table 3.1) for β equals 0.131 with a standard error of 0.209, larger than in any of the other models considered previously.

The inefficiency is further demonstrated in Table 3.5. The stratified model is the least efficient having the largest value for the standard error in any of the three settings studied. ∎

Example 3.4 Stratified model for time to first insemination with time-varying covariates

One of the aims of the time to first insemination study (Example 1.8) is to find a constituent in milk that is predictive for the hazard of first insemination. One possible predictor is the ureum concentration in the milk. Obviously, the milk ureum concentration of a particular cow changes over time. This type of predictor is called a time-varying covariate. Such variables can easily be incorporated in the semiparametric model: for each event time the risk set must be considered and the contribution of a subject at risk depends on the value of the covariate at that event time.

The relevant information for an individual cow j $(j = 1, \ldots, n_i)$ from herd i $(i = 1, \ldots, s)$ is contained in the vector

$$
\left(y_{ij}, \delta_{ij}, x_{ij}\left(t_{ij1}\right), \ldots, x_{ij}\left(t_{ijk_{ij}}\right)\right)
$$

with y_{ij} the time to first insemination or censoring, δ_{ij} the censoring indicator, and $x_{ij}\left(t_{ij1}\right), \ldots, x_{ij}\left(t_{ijk_{ij}}\right)$ the values for the covariate recorded at different timepoints $t_{ij1}, \ldots, t_{ijk_{ij}}$.

As the covariate is only determined once a month, its value at a particular timepoint t, $x_{ij}(t)$, is determined by linear interpolation based on the measurements immediately before and after time t.

Table 3.5. Simulation results for the unadjusted, fixed effects, frailty, and stratified models based on 2000 data sets each consisting of 100 pairs assuming exponentially distributed event times with $\lambda = 0.23, \beta = 0.18$, and $\theta = 0.3$. First setting: no censoring and covariates within pair different. Second setting: no censoring and only for 80% of the pairs covariates within pair different. Third setting: 20% censoring and covariates within pair different. The third column $(\hat{\beta})$ contains the median for $\hat{\beta}$ and the 5%-95% quantiles in brackets, the fourth column (s.e.$(\hat{\beta})$) contains the median for the standard error of $\hat{\beta}$, and the last column the actual coverage of the 95% confidence interval.

	Model	$\hat{\beta}$ Median (5%-95% quantile)	s.e.$(\hat{\beta})$ Median	Coverage 95% CI
First setting	$\lambda \exp(\beta x_{ij})$	0.1757 (−0.1067; 0.4803)	0.1414	0.881
	$\lambda_i \exp(\beta x_{ij})$	0.1846 (−0.1001; 0.4626)	0.1730	0.950
	$\lambda u_i \exp(\beta x_{ij})$	0.1788 (−0.0691; 0.4376)	0.1536	0.944
	$h_{i0}(t) \exp(\beta x_{ij})$	0.1603 (−0.1201; 0.4895)	0.2010	0.962
Second setting	$\lambda \exp(\beta x_{ij})$	0.1817 (−0.1299; 0.5079)	0.1414	0.849
	$\lambda_i \exp(\beta x_{ij})$	0.1871 (−0.1268; 0.5117)	0.1930	0.949
	$\lambda u_i \exp(\beta x_{ij})$	0.1836 (−0.0723; 0.4540)	0.1601	0.947
	$h_{i0}(t) \exp(\beta x_{ij})$	0.2007 (−0.2007; 0.5645)	0.2247	0.952
Third setting	$\lambda \exp(\beta x_{ij})$	0.1666 (−0.0928; 0.4204)	0.1655	0.964
	$\lambda_i \exp(\beta x_{ij})$	0.2222 (−0.1523; 0.6007)	0.1975	0.906
	$\lambda u_i \exp(\beta x_{ij})$	0.1858 (−0.1004; 0.4663)	0.1724	0.951
	$h_{i0}(t) \exp(\beta x_{ij})$	0.1744 (−0.1691; 0.5288)	0.2132	0.952

We now estimate the effect of the time-varying ureum concentration on the hazard of first insemination using different types of semiparametric models.

The semiparametric model stratified for herd is given by

$$h_{ij}(t) = h_{i0}(t) \exp(x_{ij}(t)\beta) \tag{3.10}$$

where $h_{ij}(t)$ is the hazard of first insemination at time t for cow j from herd i having at time t ureum concentration equal to $x_{ij}(t)$ whereas β corresponds to the linear effect of the ureum concentration on the loghazard of first insemination.

The partial likelihood for this model is given by

$$\prod_{i=1}^{s} \prod_{j=1}^{n_i} \left[\frac{\exp(x_{ij}(y_{ij})\beta)}{\sum_{l \in R_i(y_{ij})} \exp(x_{il}(y_{ij})\beta)} \right]^{\delta_{ij}} \tag{3.11}$$

The risk set for cow j from herd i having a first insemination at time y_{ij}, $R_i(y_{ij})$, now contains only cows from herd i, namely, those cows from herd i that are still at risk at time y_{ij}.

Fitting this model leads to an estimate $\hat{\beta} = -0.0588$ with corresponding hazard ratio $\exp(-0.0588) = 0.943$ (see Table 3.6). There is a significant effect of the milk ureum concentration on the hazard of first insemination (p=0.003).

Table 3.6. Parameter estimates with standard errors (in parentheses) for the time to first insemination based on different semiparametric models.

Model	$\hat{\beta}$ (s.e.)	Hazard ratio	95% CI	p-value
Unadjusted	-0.0273 (0.0162)	0.973	[0.943; 1.005]	0.094
Fixed effects	-0.0562 (0.0189)	0.945	[0.911; 0.981]	0.003
Stratified	-0.0588 (0.0198)	0.943	[0.907; 0.980]	0.003

Within the context of semiparametric modelling, it is clear from Section 3.1 that this model can be simplified in two different ways. In the simplest model, we do not take into account the clustering and use the same baseline hazard for each cluster

$$h_{ij}(t) = h_0(t)\exp(x_{ij}(t)\beta) \tag{3.12}$$

The partial likelihood is the same as the partial likelihood in expression (3.11), except that we now work with the risk set $R(y_{ij})$ which contains all cows still at risk at time y_{ij}, regardless the herd.

For this simplified model, we obtain $\hat{\beta} = -0.0273$ and hazard ratio 0.973. The effect of the milk ureum concentration on the hazard of first insemination is no longer significant (p=0.094) at the 5% significance level.

A second alternative is a model that contains the same unspecified baseline hazard function, but with a fixed effect added for each herd:

$$h_{ij}(t) = h_0(t)\exp(x_{ij}(t)\beta + c_i) \tag{3.13}$$

The corresponding partial likelihood is

$$\prod_{i=1}^{s}\prod_{j=1}^{n_i}\left[\frac{\exp(x_{ij}(y_{ij})\beta + c_i)}{\sum_{kl \in R(y_{ij})}\exp(x_{kl}(y_{ij})\beta + c_k)}\right]^{\delta_{ij}} \tag{3.14}$$

where again the risk set $R(y_{ij})$ contains all cows still at risk at time y_{ij} regardless the herd. The effect of the milk ureum concentration on the hazard of first insemination is again significant in this model (p=0.003) with $\hat{\beta} =$ −0.0562 and corresponding hazard ratio equal to 0.945.

The estimate of the milk ureum concentration effect on the hazard of first insemination in the semiparametric unadjusted model (3.12) is quite different from the estimate in the semiparametric model with fixed cluster effects (3.13) and in the semiparametric stratified model (3.10). Although the unadjusted model has the smallest standard error for $\hat{\beta}$, it does not lead to a significant effect as its estimate $\hat{\beta}$ is much closer to zero. As in the parametric model, the standard error of the unadjusted model is too small and incorrect because the clustering is not taken into account. On the other hand, the two semiparametric models that are adjusted for the herd effect, whether by stratification or inclusion of a fixed herd effect, lead to a significant effect.

To understand the reason for the difference between the analysis based on the unadjusted model and the models that adjust for the herd effect, we obtain the estimated risk coefficients $\hat{\beta}_i$ for each herd separately. We then plot (Figure 3.1a) the $\hat{\beta}_i$'s against the estimated fixed herd effects $\hat{c}_i$'s obtained from (3.13).

There are several herds for which the fixed effect is substantially smaller than the average of the fixed herd effects. The logarithm of the hazard ratio of six of these herds is exactly equal to zero as no inseminations at all have taken place in these herds. Therefore, the logarithm of the hazard ratio is estimated to be zero (since all $\delta_{ij} = 0$).

For each specific herd, the mean ureum concentration is calculated as

$$\bar{x}_i = \frac{\sum\limits_{j=1}^{n_i} \sum\limits_{l=1}^{k_{ij}} x_{ij}(t_{ijl})}{\sum\limits_{j=1}^{n_i} k_{ij}}, \quad i = 1, \ldots, s$$

and compared to the average ureum concentration over the different herds

$$\bar{x} = \frac{\sum\limits_{i=1}^{s} \bar{x}_i}{s} \tag{3.15}$$

We note that the average in (3.15) is an average of the herd averages, so that each herd has the same contribution, regardless of how many times the ureum concentration was measured. In the overall mean with each measurement contributing equally, there would be an overrepresentation of cows with high ureum concentration as these cows need more time to be inseminated for the first time, thereby contributing more measurements.

The six herds with no inseminations have average values for the mean ureum concentration that are close or below the average ureum concentration over the different herds (Figure 3.1b). Both the unadjusted and adjusted

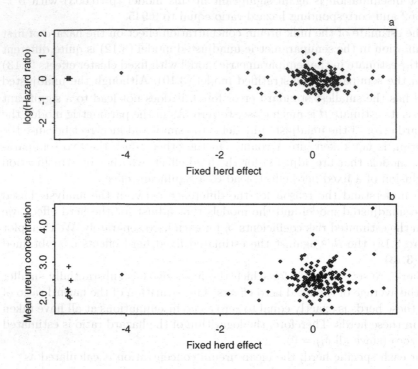

Fig. 3.1. Herd-specific estimates $\hat{\beta}_i$ representing the effect of milk ureum concentration on the loghazard of first insemination (a) and the average herd milk ureum concentration (b) as a function of the estimate of the fixed herd effect $\hat{c}_i$. Six herds in which no inseminations took place are denoted by a plus.

semiparametric models predict that cows with low ureum concentration have a higher hazard of first insemination but the herds with no inseminations at all and low to average mean ureum concentration contradict this global relationship. The semiparametric model with fixed herd effects corrects for this by assigning a large negative value for the herd effect and thus all cows of these herds have low hazard. This obviously does not happen in the unadjusted model, so that these cows will contradict the overall relationship between ureum concentration and hazard of first insemination. Because of this, the hazard ratio in the unadjusted model is closer to one and no longer significant. The adjusted model picks up this specific feature of the data while the unadjusted model is not flexible enough to capture this specific feature.

∎

3.3 The copula model

3.3.1 Notation and definitions for the conditional, joint, and population survival functions

We first introduce definitions and corresponding notation to denote the conditional, joint, and population survival, hazard, and density functions. Transparent notation is required to clearly see the differences and similarities between the copula model and the frailty model. We start from the (conditional) frailty model

$$h_{ij}(t) = u_i h_0(t) \exp\left(\mathbf{x}_{ij}^t \boldsymbol{\beta}\right) = u_i h_{ij,c}(t) \qquad (3.16)$$

with $h_{ij,c}(t)$ the conditional hazard function for subject j from cluster i assuming that the frailty term for that cluster equals one. This model is written alternatively as

$$h_{ij}(t) = u_i h_{\mathbf{x},c}(t) \qquad (3.17)$$

when the covariate information for subject j from cluster i, $\mathbf{x}_{ij}$, equals $\mathbf{x}$. This notation will be used if we want to stress the fact that this subject has particular covariate information $\mathbf{x}$. The subindex c is added to the hazard on the right side of (3.16) and (3.17) to denote that these hazard functions originate from the conditional model. We further define the conditional survival function for subject j from cluster i

$$S_{ij}(t) = \exp\left(-u_i H_{ij,c}(t)\right)$$

with $H_{ij,c}(t) = \int_0^t h_{ij,c}(v)dv$. For subject j from cluster i with covariate information $\mathbf{x}$ we write alternatively

$$S_{ij}(t) = \exp\left(-u_i H_{\mathbf{x},c}(t)\right)$$

The joint conditional survival function is

$$S_i(\mathbf{t}_{n_i}) = S_i(t_1, \ldots, t_{n_i}) = \exp\left(-u_i H_{i.,c}(\mathbf{t}_{n_i})\right)$$

with $\mathbf{t}_{n_i} = (t_1, \ldots, t_{n_i})$ and $H_{i.,c}(\mathbf{t}_{n_i}) = \sum_{j=1}^{n_i} H_{ij,c}(t_j)$ or alternatively

$$S_i(\mathbf{t}_{n_i}) = \exp\left(-u_i H_{\mathbf{x},c}(\mathbf{t}_{n_i})\right)$$

with $H_{\mathbf{x},c}(\mathbf{t}_{n_i})$ the sum of the cumulative hazards of the n_i subjects in cluster i. The vector $\mathbf{x}$ is the collection of the actual covariate values, say $\mathbf{x}_1, \ldots,$ $\mathbf{x}_{n_i}$, of the n_i subjects in cluster i, i.e., $\mathbf{x} = \left(\mathbf{x}_1^t, \ldots, \mathbf{x}_{n_i}^t\right)^t$. The joint survival function for a cluster of size n with covariate information $\mathbf{x} = (\mathbf{x}_1^t, \ldots, \mathbf{x}_n^t)^t$ is obtained from the joint conditional survival function by integrating out the frailty with respect to the frailty distribution. As notation for the joint survival function we use

$$S_{\mathbf{x},f}(\mathbf{t}_n) = S_{\mathbf{x},f}(t_1, \ldots, t_n)$$

The population survival function for subjects having covariate information $\mathbf{x}$ is obtained from $S_{ij}(t) = \exp(-u_i H_{\mathbf{x},c}(t))$ by integrating out the frailty with respect to the frailty distribution. As notation for the population survival function with covariate information $\mathbf{x}$ we write $S_{\mathbf{x},f}(t)$.

It is often the case that each cluster has the same number of observations (for each cluster the observations within that cluster can be collected in a vector and all vectors have the same length), and that the position of the observation in the vector also denotes the covariate information for that observation. Consider, for instance, the udder quarter infection data presented in Example 1.4. The cluster is the cow, and within each cow there are exactly four udder quarters. If the covariate of interest is the location of the udder quarter (right-left and front-rear), we can order all observations (front left, front right, rear left, rear right) in such a way that the first observation corresponds to the front left udder quarter, and the fourth observation to the rear right udder quarter. If we use the same ordering of the observations for each cow, then the order of the observation is also referring to the covariate information. In such setting, there is no need to use the x and $\mathbf{x}$ symbols to denote the covariate information, and the joint survival function is then denoted by the more simple expression $S_f(\mathbf{t}_n)$ and the population survival function for the jth observation by $S_{j,f}(t)$.

The joint survival function and the population survival function have a subindex f to denote that they are derived from a frailty model and to stress that the frailty distribution determines the particular form of the joint and population survival functions. The fact that the analytic form of the joint survival function and of the population survival function depends on the underlying frailty distribution is the germ for the difference between frailty models and copula models (see Sections 3.3.2–3.3.4 for a detailed discussion). Typical for copula models is that the joint survival function and the population survival function are not generated through the use of a frailty distribution. Therefore, in copula models, the population survival function with covariate information $\mathbf{x}$ is written as $S_{\mathbf{x},p}(t)$ and the joint survival function as $S_{\mathbf{x},p}(\mathbf{t}_n) = S_{\mathbf{x},p}(t_1, \ldots, t_n)$. If the covariate information follows immediately from the position of the subjects in the cluster, we rather use again the simplified expressions $S_p(\mathbf{t}_n)$ and $S_{j,p}(t)$. For hazard and density functions the same indexing system is used as for the survival functions.

3.3.2 Definition of the copula model

The copula model specification starts from the population survival functions of each subject in a cluster, the copula being the function that links the population survival functions to generate the joint survival function (Frees et al., 1996).

The population survival functions of the n subjects in the cluster with covariate information $\mathbf{x} = (\mathbf{x}_1^t, \ldots, \mathbf{x}_n^t)^t$ are denoted by $S_{\mathbf{x}_1, p}(t), \ldots, S_{\mathbf{x}_n, p}(t)$. These population survival functions are obtained from the marginal approach (see Section 3.4) not taking into consideration the clustering. The joint survival function is given by

$$S_{\mathbf{x}, p}(\mathbf{t}_n) = S_{\mathbf{x}, p}(t_1, \ldots, t_n) = C_{\boldsymbol{\theta}}(S_{\mathbf{x}_1, p}(t_1), \ldots, S_{\mathbf{x}_n, p}(t_n)) \qquad (3.18)$$

for a function $C_{\boldsymbol{\theta}}(v_1, \ldots, v_n)$ defined for $(v_1, \ldots, v_n) \in [0, 1]^n$ and taking values in $[0, 1]$. $C_{\boldsymbol{\theta}}$ is called a copula function with parameter vector $\boldsymbol{\theta}$. The existence of $C_{\boldsymbol{\theta}}$ follows from Sklar's theorem (Sklar, 1959). For continuous population survival functions there is a unique copula $C_{\boldsymbol{\theta}}$ that links the population survival functions and the joint survival function through (3.18). See Nelsen (2006) for precise definitions and for an in-depth discussion on copulas.

For survival data, copulas are often restricted to the family of Archimedean copulas (Genest and MacKay, 1986) defined by

$$S_{\mathbf{x}, p}(t_1, \ldots, t_n) = p\left[q\left(S_{\mathbf{x}_1, p}(t_1)\right) + \ldots + q\left(S_{\mathbf{x}_n, p}(t_n)\right)\right] \qquad (3.19)$$

with $p(.)$ a decreasing function defined on $[0, \infty]$ with values in $[0, 1]$ and satisfying $p(0) = 1$. Further, we assume that $p(.)$ has positive second derivative and we denote the inverse function of $p(.)$ as $q(.)$.

The copula approach is extensively used for bivariate data. Also here, we restrict the discussion to bivariate survival data. For bivariate survival data, we can distinguish between two different situations. In the first situation we assume that the population survival functions $S_{\mathbf{x}_1, p}(t)$ and $S_{\mathbf{x}_2, p}(t)$ are identical. Twin data are a typical example. In the second situation we consider the case of different population survival functions. Examples include bivariate data on event times for father ($S_{\mathbf{x}_1, p}(t)$ is the population survival function of all fathers) and son ($S_{\mathbf{x}_2, p}(t)$ is the population survival function of all sons); or matched pairs with one patient receiving a treatment and the other patient being the control.

At this stage, we simplify the notation by dropping the $\mathbf{x}$ and x symbols and denote the population survival functions by $S_{1, p}(t)$ and $S_{2, p}(t)$, where $S_{1, p}(t)$ stands for the population survival of the first component of the cluster (e.g., always the father), and $S_{2, p}(t)$ for the population survival of the second component of the cluster (e.g., always the son). We therefore assume that all

j^{th} components have the same covariate information, whatever the cluster. The joint survival function is then denoted by $S_p(\mathbf{t}_n) = S_p(t_1, t_2)$.

Also the time to diagnosis data set in Example 1.2 is an example of bivariate survival data with different population survival functions for the two event times. Each dog (the cluster) has been assessed with the two different techniques (RX and US).

Fitting the copula model is often based on a two-stage estimation approach (Shih and Louis, 1995a; Glidden, 2000; Andersen, 2005). In the first stage, the population survival functions are estimated. This can be done in different ways. Shih and Louis (1995a) discuss parametric as well as nonparametric (Kaplan–Meier) separate estimation of $S_{1,p}(t)$ and $S_{2,p}(t)$. Modelling the population survival functions through Cox models for the corresponding population hazard functions, Glidden (2000) and Andersen (2005) discuss extensions of the approach of Shih and Louis (1995a) for survival functions depending on covariates. They also include the situation where the population hazard is common for all the event times within a cluster as well as intermediate specifications. It will be shown in Section 3.4.2 that the (semi)parametric or nonparametric estimates of the population survival functions, obtained without taking the clustering into account, are consistent (Spiekerman and Lin, 1998) and can therefore be used in the second step of a two-stage estimation approach. In that second step we estimate the θ parameter.

We now discuss in detail how the two-stage approach can be applied in practice for parametric population survival functions. The parameters fully describing the population survival functions are first estimated using straightforward likelihood maximisation techniques. For instance, in the case of Weibull distributed event times and assuming different population survival functions $S_{1,p}(t)$ and $S_{2,p}(t)$, the parameters (λ_1, ρ_1) and (λ_2, ρ_2) are obtained, leading to the estimated population survival functions obtained by plugging in these parameter estimates in the population survival expressions.

The estimated population survival functions can be plugged into the likelihood expression

$$\prod_{i=1}^{s} (f_p(y_{i1}, y_{i2}))^{\delta_{i1}\delta_{i2}} \left(-\frac{\partial S_p(y_{i1}, y_{i2})}{\partial y_{i1}} \right)^{\delta_{i1}(1-\delta_{i2})}$$

$$\times \left(-\frac{\partial S_p(y_{i1}, y_{i2})}{\partial y_{i2}} \right)^{(1-\delta_{i1})\delta_{i2}} (S_p(y_{i1}, y_{i2}))^{(1-\delta_{i1})(1-\delta_{i2})} \quad (3.20)$$

So we have four different possible contributions, depending on the censoring status of the two subjects in the cluster. A cluster with two censored subjects has contribution $L_{i,(0,0)} = S_p(y_{i1}, y_{i2})$, a cluster with two event times has contribution $L_{i,(1,1)} = f_p(y_{i1}, y_{i2})$; the contribution of a cluster with one event time and one censored observation is $L_{i,(1,0)} = -\dfrac{\partial S_p(y_{i1}, y_{i2})}{\partial y_{i1}}$, respectively $L_{i,(0,1)} = -\dfrac{\partial S_p(y_{i1}, y_{i2})}{\partial y_{i2}}$, if we observe an event time for the first (second) subject and a censored observation for the second (first) subject.

As the estimated population survival functions are plugged into (3.20) and do therefore no longer contain unknown parameters, the only unknown parameters in (3.20) are related to the parameter vector θ of the copula function and the likelihood is therefore maximised with respect to the parameter vector θ.

Alternatively, the likelihood expressions can be maximised with respect to the parameters of the population survival functions and the parameter vector θ, which in most cases leads to similar results (Durrleman et al., 2000).

In the next section, we give explicit expressions for the likelihood contributions in the case of one particular copula, the Clayton copula.

3.3.3 The Clayton copula

A key paper in the use of the copula function to model bivariate survival data is due to Clayton (1978). The Clayton copula for bivariate survival data is given by

$$S_p(t_1, t_2) = \left(S_{1,p}^{-\theta}(t_1) + S_{2,p}^{-\theta}(t_2) - 1\right)^{-1/\theta} \tag{3.21}$$

with $\theta \geq 0$. This copula corresponds to an Archimedean copula with $p(s) = (1 + \theta s)^{-1/\theta}$ and $q(s) = \left(s^{-\theta} - 1\right)/\theta$. The likelihood contributions of the different clusters are given by

$$L_{i,(0,0)} = \left(S_{1,p}^{-\theta}(y_{i1}) + S_{2,p}^{-\theta}(y_{i2}) - 1\right)^{-1/\theta} \tag{3.22}$$

for clusters with two censored observations,

$$
\begin{aligned}
L_{i,(1,0)} = &\left(S_{1,p}^{-\theta}(y_{i1}) + S_{2,p}^{-\theta}(y_{i2}) - 1\right)^{-1/\theta-1} \\
&\times S_{1,p}^{-\theta-1}(y_{i1}) f_{1,p}(y_{i1})
\end{aligned} \tag{3.23}
$$

for clusters with an event for the first subject and a censored observation for the second subject,

$$
\begin{aligned}
L_{i,(0,1)} = &\left(S_{1,p}^{-\theta}(y_{i1}) + S_{2,p}^{-\theta}(y_{i2}) - 1\right)^{-1/\theta-1} \\
&\times S_{2,p}^{-\theta-1}(y_{i2}) f_{2,p}(y_{i2})
\end{aligned} \tag{3.24}
$$

for clusters with an event for the second subject and a censored observation for the first subject, and finally

$$L_{i,(1,1)} = (1 + \theta) \left(S_{1,p}^{-\theta}(y_{i1}) + S_{2,p}^{-\theta}(y_{i2}) - 1 \right)^{-1/\theta - 2}$$
$$S_{1,p}^{-\theta - 1}(y_{i1}) S_{2,p}^{-\theta - 1}(y_{i2}) f_{1,p}(y_{i1}) f_{2,p}(y_{i2}) \qquad (3.25)$$

for clusters with two events. Using in (3.20) the estimated population survival and density functions obtained in the first stage of the estimation procedure, the only unknown parameter that remains in (3.20) is θ.

Example 3.5 The Clayton copula for time to diagnosis of being healed

We consider the copula model for the time to diagnosis data set (Example 1.2). The time to diagnosis data are bivariate data with two diagnosis times within a cluster (Y_{i1}, Y_{i2}). Furthermore, the covariate of interest (RX versus US as diagnostic technique) is binary in such a way that one observation in the cluster has one covariate level (corresponding to the first measurement in the cluster, diagnostic technique is RX) and the other observation in the cluster has the other covariate level (corresponding to the second measurement in the cluster, diagnostic technique is US). We first consider the following model for the population hazard functions:

$$\text{RX: } h_{1,p}(t) = \lambda_1 \rho_1 t^{\rho_1 - 1}$$
$$\text{US: } h_{2,p}(t) = \lambda_2 \rho_2 t^{\rho_2 - 1} \qquad (3.26)$$

resulting in the population survival functions

$$\text{RX: } S_{1,p}(t) = \exp\left(-\lambda_1 t^{\rho_1}\right)$$
$$\text{US: } S_{2,p}(t) = \exp\left(-\lambda_2 t^{\rho_2}\right)$$

and the population density functions

$$\text{RX: } f_{1,p}(t) = \lambda_1 \rho_1 t^{\rho_1 - 1} \exp\left(-\lambda_1 t^{\rho_1}\right)$$
$$\text{US: } f_{2,p}(t) = \lambda_2 \rho_2 t^{\rho_2 - 1} \exp\left(-\lambda_2 t^{\rho_2}\right)$$

The joint survival function is

$$S_p\left(t_1, t_2\right) = \left(\exp\left(\lambda_1 \theta t_1^{\rho_1}\right) + \exp\left(\lambda_2 \theta t_2^{\rho_2}\right) - 1\right)^{-1/\theta}$$

Using the two-stage estimation approach, the parameter estimates are $\hat{\lambda}_1 = 0.106$, $\hat{\rho}_1 = 2.539$, $\hat{\lambda}_2 = 0.219$, and $\hat{\rho}_2 = 2.323$. These estimates are now used to obtain estimated values for $S_{1,p}\left(y_{i1}\right)$, $S_{2,p}\left(y_{i2}\right)$, $f_{1,p}\left(y_{i1}\right)$, and $f_{2,p}\left(y_{i2}\right)$ which are then used to obtain the required clusterwise likelihood contributions (3.22)–(3.25). Based on these clusterwise likelihood contributions we obtain (3.20) which then contains only θ as unknown parameter. Maximising (3.20) with respect to θ leads to $\hat{\theta} = 0.89$.

Alternatively, we can maximise (3.20) for the four parameters related to the population survival functions and θ simultaneously. This leads to parameter estimates $\hat{\lambda}_1 = 0.145$, $\hat{\rho}_1 = 2.341$, $\hat{\lambda}_2 = 0.233$, $\hat{\rho}_2 = 2.212$, and $\hat{\theta} = 1.066$.

We can also model the population hazard functions differently, assuming the same value for ρ in the two populations:

$$\text{RX:} \quad h_{1,p}\left(t\right) = \lambda \rho t^{\rho - 1}$$

$$\text{US:} \quad h_{2,p}\left(t\right) = \lambda \exp(\beta) \rho t^{\rho - 1} \tag{3.27}$$

The parameter estimates for this model are given by $\hat{\lambda} = 0.119$, $\hat{\rho} = 2.42$, $\hat{\beta} = 0.522$. Based on these parameter estimates, we can again estimate the population survival and density functions and use the estimated values in $L_{i(j_1, j_2)}$, $j_1 = 0, 1$ and $j_2 = 0, 1$ in (3.20). Maximising this expression with respect to θ gives the estimate $\hat{\theta} = 0.87$. For this particular data set with a restricted number of clusters, it appears that using a different model for the population survival functions (with one parameter less), has less impact on the resulting association parameters than switching the estimation technique from two-stage estimation to simultaneous estimation. The simultaneous estimation procedure is preferred. In the semiparametric case, however, simultaneous estimation is impossible, as the Kaplan–Meier estimates obtained in the first stage are introduced in the copula function. In such cases, Shih and Louis (1995a) demonstrate that the two-stage estimation procedure estimates θ in a consistent way, but with a small to moderate number of clusters the two-stage estimation procedure should be used with caution. ∎

3.3.4 The Clayton copula versus the gamma frailty model

It has been claimed that particular copula models can be deduced from shared frailty models by choosing the appropriate distribution for the frailty term

(Oakes, 1989; Manatunga and Oakes, 1999; Andersen, 2005). We show in this section, however, that the two models are only equivalent with respect to the copula function used. The Clayton copula is used as an example. In Chapter 4, we demonstrate nonequivalence for several other distributions. The claim arises from the fact that the joint survival function derived from a frailty model looks similar to the copula formulation, although it is not the same. To see the similarity, we first derive the joint survival function starting from the conditional frailty model for bivariate survival data with a binary covariate where we assume that the first (second) event time has the first (second) level of the covariate.

We start from the conditional frailty model

$$h_{ij}(t) = u_i h_{ij,c}(t)$$

with $h_{ij}(t)$ the hazard at time t for the subject with covariate level j in cluster i, $h_{ij,c}(t)$ the hazard function at time t for a subject with covariate information x_{ij} ($x_{ij} = j$ for the subject in position j, $j = 1, 2$) and frailty term equal to one, and u_i the frailty term for cluster i.

The joint conditional survival function is

$$S_i(t_1, t_2) = \exp\left[-u_i(H_{i1,c}(t_1) + H_{i2,c}(t_2))\right]$$

The joint survival function can be obtained by integrating out the frailties using the frailty distribution

$$S_f(t_1, t_2) = \int_0^\infty \exp\left[-u(H_{1,c}(t_1) + H_{2,c}(t_2))\right] f_U(u) du$$

The joint survival function has a subindex f to denote that it is derived from the frailty model. This subindex is needed because there is a difference between the joint survival function derived from the frailty model and the joint survival function defined through the copula model; see the discussion after (3.32) for details.

This integral can be solved analytically for the gamma distribution, resulting in

$$S_f(t_1, t_2) = \left[1 + \theta(H_{1,c}(t_1) + H_{2,c}(t_2))\right]^{-1/\theta} \tag{3.28}$$

On the other hand, the population survival function can be obtained from the conditional frailty model using a similar derivation as for the joint survival function

$$S_{1,f}(t) = \int_0^\infty \exp\left(-uH_{1,c}(t)\right) f_U(u)du$$

$$= (1 + \theta H_{1,c}(t))^{-1/\theta} \qquad (3.29)$$

and similarly

$$S_{2,f}(t) = (1 + \theta H_{2,c}(t))^{-1/\theta} \qquad (3.30)$$

It follows that

$$H_{1,c}(t) = \frac{S_{1,f}^{-\theta}(t) - 1}{\theta} \quad \text{and} \quad H_{2,c}(t) = \frac{S_{2,f}^{-\theta}(t) - 1}{\theta} \qquad (3.31)$$

Now use (3.31) in (3.28) to obtain

$$S_f(t_1, t_2) = \left(S_{1,f}^{-\theta}(t_1) + S_{2,f}^{-\theta}(t_2) - 1\right)^{-1/\theta} \qquad (3.32)$$

Although the functional forms of the joint survival functions in (3.21) and (3.32) are the same, $S_p(t_1, t_2)$ and $S_f(t_1, t_2)$ are different. Indeed the modelling of the population survival functions in (3.21) is not related to the modelling of the copula function C_θ. In (3.32) the choice of the frailty distribution determines the functional form of the copula as well as the functional form of the population survival functions $S_{j,f}(t)$, $j = 1, 2$. It is indeed clear from (3.29) and (3.30) that the population survival function arising from the conditional frailty model is also a function of θ, which is not the case for the model in (3.21). This has important consequences as is demonstrated in the next example.

Example 3.6 Shared gamma frailty models and the Clayton copulas for time to diagnosis of being healed

We model the time to diagnosis data set (Example 1.2) using two different shared gamma frailty models and compare this model to the copula model (3.21).

The shared gamma frailty models are generally given by

$$\text{RX: } h_{i1}(t) = u_i h_{i1,c}(t)$$

$$\text{US: } h_{i2}(t) = u_i h_{i2,c}(t)$$

Different choices for the hazard functions $h_{i1,c}(t)$ and $h_{i2,c}(t)$ are possible. We first consider the standard frailty model with Weibull baseline hazard, one-parameter gamma distributed frailties, and a binary covariate for diagnostic technique. With this approach we assume that the shape parameter ρ of the Weibull baseline hazard is the same for the two diagnostic techniques and we compare the results with the copula with corresponding population hazard functions given in (3.27).

Next, we extend this model and allow the shape parameter to differ between the two diagnostic techniques. This extended model, however, is no longer a proportional hazards model. Nevertheless, we use this modelling approach below to obtain parameter estimates that are comparable to the parameter estimates from the copula with corresponding population hazard functions given in (3.26).

The standard frailty model for the time to diagnosis data is given by

$$\text{RX: } h_{i1}(t) = u_i h_0(t)$$

$$\text{US: } h_{i2}(t) = u_i h_0(t) \exp(\beta) \tag{3.33}$$

This is a conditional model. The population survival functions are obtained by integrating out the frailties

$$\text{RX: } S_{1,f}(t) = (1 + \theta H_0(t))^{-1/\theta}$$

$$\text{US: } S_{2,f}(t) = (1 + \theta H_0(t) \exp(\beta))^{-1/\theta} \tag{3.34}$$

Assuming a Weibull baseline hazard $h_0(t) = \lambda \rho t^{\rho-1}$ ($H_0(t) = \lambda t^\rho$) we get

$$\text{RX: } S_{1,f}(t) = (1 + \theta \lambda t^\rho)^{-1/\theta}$$

$$\text{US: } S_{2,f}(t) = (1 + \theta \lambda \exp(\beta) t^\rho)^{-1/\theta}$$

and using (3.32)

$$S_f(t_1, t_2) = \left(S_{1,f}^{-\theta}(t_1) + S_{2,f}^{-\theta}(t_2) - 1\right)^{-1/\theta}$$

$$= [(1 + \theta\lambda t_1^\rho) + (1 + \theta\lambda \exp(\beta)t_2^\rho) - 1]^{-1/\theta}$$

$$= [\theta\lambda (t_1^\rho + \exp(\beta)t_2^\rho) + 1]^{-1/\theta}$$

Parameter estimates can be obtained easily by maximising the marginal loglikelihood (2.7) in which the baseline hazard assumption in (3.33) has been plugged in. The parameter estimates of this standard frailty model are $\hat{\lambda} = 0.094$, $\hat{\rho} = 3.620$, $\hat{\beta} = 0.7326$ and $\hat{\theta} = 0.905$. This model, therefore, gives $\hat{\lambda}_1 = 0.094$ as scale parameter for RX and $\hat{\lambda}_2 = \hat{\lambda}\exp(\hat{\beta}) = 0.195$ as scale parameter for US.

So the frailty model (3.33) and the two-stage estimation approach for the copula model based on hazard specifications (3.27) (see Example 3.5) do not lead to the same parameter estimates. This is not surprising, however, as the parameters in the frailty model approach correspond, up to the multiplicative factor u_i, to hazards in a conditional model. In the two-stage approach the parameter estimates correspond to the population hazards. Better insight can therefore be obtained by looking at the population hazard functions of the two models. It can easily be derived that the population hazard functions based on the frailty model are given by

$$h_{1,f}(t) = S_{1,f}^\theta(t)\lambda\rho t^{\rho-1}$$

$$h_{2,f}(t) = S_{2,f}^\theta(t)\lambda \exp(\beta)\rho t^{\rho-1}$$

The resulting population hazard functions are depicted in Figure 3.2a. Note that this type of population hazard function arising from the frailty model (first increasing and at later times decreasing) is not possible for the copula model (3.21) using the increasing population hazards ($\hat{\rho} > 1$) given by (3.27).

We now extend this frailty model to allow the shape parameter to differ between the two diagnostic techniques

$$\text{RX: } h_{i1}(t) = u_i\lambda_1\rho_1 t^{\rho_1-1}$$

$$\text{US: } h_{i2}(t) = u_i\lambda_2\rho_2 t^{\rho_2-1} \tag{3.35}$$

resulting in the population survival functions

$$\text{RX: } S_{1,f}(t) = (1 + \theta \lambda_1 t^{\rho_1})^{-1/\theta}$$

$$\text{US: } S_{2,f}(t) = (1 + \theta \lambda_2 t^{\rho_2})^{-1/\theta} \tag{3.36}$$

and the joint survival function

$$S_f(t_1, t_2) = (\theta (\lambda_1 t_1^{\rho_1} + \lambda_2 t_2^{\rho_2}) + 1)^{-1/\theta}$$

Note that this is no longer a proportional hazards model.

The parameter estimates of this extended frailty model are $\hat{\lambda}_1 = 0.079$, $\hat{\rho}_1 = 3.827$, $\hat{\lambda}_2 = 0.218$, $\hat{\rho}_2 = 3.456$, and $\hat{\theta} = 0.909$.

The resulting population hazard functions are depicted in Figure 3.2b and compared to the corresponding copula model. The pictures clearly demonstrate that the shapes of the population hazard functions derived from the frailty and copula model are very different. ■

3.4 The marginal model

3.4.1 Defining the marginal model

In the marginal model approach, we do not take the clustering into account and act as if the event times of the subjects are independent of each other, even if they belong to the same cluster. This results in an independent contribution of each subject to the likelihood. Therefore, this is called the likelihood of the Independence Working Model (IWM). When neglecting the clustering, we use the population distributions of the subjects.

To simplify the notation, we consider bivariate survival data with a binary covariate so that the first (second) event time has the first (second) level of the covariate. The population density and survival functions for the first and second event time are denoted by $f_{1,p}(t)$, $f_{2,p}(t)$, $S_{1,p}(t)$, and $S_{2,p}(t)$. Let η denote the vector containing all the parameters used in the (parametric) specification of $S_{1,p}(t)$ and $S_{2,p}(t)$.

There are two main issues with respect to the parameter estimates coming from the IWM approach. First, we demonstrate that under certain conditions the likelihood estimate $\hat{\eta}$ obtained from the IWM is a consistent estimate for the vector η in spite of the fact that observations are correlated. In the discussion that follows, we assume that the correlation structure is given by an Archimedean copula leading to the joint survival function

$$S_p(t_1, t_2) = p[q(S_{1,p}(t_1)) + q(S_{2,p}(t_2))]$$

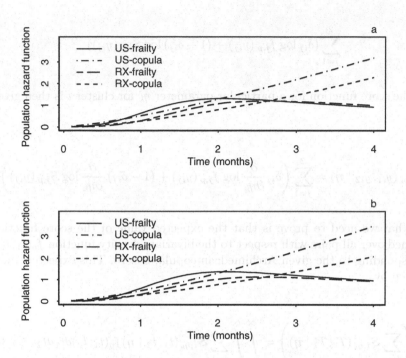

Fig. 3.2. The population hazard functions obtained from the frailty model and the copula model for the time to diagnosis of healing data assessed by either US or RX. For the frailty model the gamma frailty distribution is used in combination with a Weibull baseline hazard for the conditional hazard functions. In (a) the Weibull shape parameter is the same for US and RX (see also (3.27)). In (b) the shape parameters are different (see also (3.26)).

Second, we look at appropriate variance estimators of the parameter estimates. Indeed, we need to take into account the variance–covariance structure of the data (hence the clustering of the data) to arrive at good estimators for the variances of the estimated parameters.

3.4.2* Consistency of parameter estimates from marginal model

For the estimation of η the IWM does not take into account that observations are correlated within clusters. To show that the estimator $\hat{\eta}$ is consistent with respect to a specified distribution of the observations, it must be shown that the expected value of the score function of $\hat{\eta}$ with respect to the specified distribution is zero (Huster et al., 1989).

The loglikelihood contribution of the ith pair for the IWM is given by

$$\sum_{j=1}^{2} \left(\delta_{ij} \log f_{j,p}(y_{ij}) + (1 - \delta_{ij}) \log S_{j,p}(y_{ij}) \right)$$

The score function for a particular parameter η_k for cluster i is then given by

$$\boldsymbol{S}_{i,\eta_k}(y_{i1}, y_{i2} \mid \boldsymbol{\eta}) = \sum_{j=1}^{2} \left(\delta_{ij} \frac{\partial}{\partial \eta_k} \log f_{j,p}(y_{ij}) + (1 - \delta_{ij}) \frac{\partial}{\partial \eta_k} \log S_{j,p}(y_{ij}) \right)$$

What we need to prove is that the expected value of the score function summed over all pairs with respect to the bivariate density function $f_p(t_1, t_2)$, corresponding to the given Archimedean copula, is zero. This expected value is given by

$$\mathrm{E}\left(\sum_{i=1}^{s} \boldsymbol{S}_{i,\eta_k}(T_1, T_2 \mid \boldsymbol{\eta}) \right) = \int_0^\infty \int_0^\infty \sum_{i=1}^{s} \boldsymbol{S}_{i,\eta_k}(t_1, t_2 \mid \boldsymbol{\eta}) f_p(t_1, t_2) dt_1 dt_2 \quad (3.37)$$

This can be rewritten as

$$\sum_{i=1}^{s} \int_0^\infty \left(\delta_{i1} \frac{\partial \log f_{1,p}(t_1)}{\partial \eta_k} + (1 - \delta_{i1}) \frac{\partial \log S_{1,p}(t_1)}{\partial \eta_k} \right) \left(\int_0^\infty f_p(t_1, t_2) \, dt_2 \right) dt_1 +$$

$$\sum_{i=1}^{s} \int_0^\infty \left(\delta_{i2} \frac{\partial \log f_{2,p}(t_2)}{\partial \eta_k} + (1 - \delta_{i2}) \frac{\partial \log S_{2,p}(t_2)}{\partial \eta_k} \right) \left(\int_0^\infty f_p(t_1, t_2) \, dt_1 \right) dt_2$$

Due to the fact that the joint density function is derived from an Archimedean copula we have

$$\int_0^\infty f_p(t_1, t_2) \, dt_2 = f_{1,p}(t_1) \quad \text{and} \quad \int_0^\infty f_p(t_1, t_2) \, dt_1 = f_{2,p}(t_2)$$

Then we can write the expected value as

$$\sum_{i=1}^{s} \int_{0}^{\infty} \left(\delta_{i1} \frac{\partial \log f_{1,p}(t_1)}{\partial \eta_k} + (1 - \delta_{i1}) \frac{\partial \log S_{1,p}(t_1)}{\partial \eta_k} \right) f_{1,p}(t_1) \, dt_1 +$$

$$\sum_{i=1}^{s} \int_{0}^{\infty} \left(\delta_{i2} \frac{\partial \log f_{2,p}(t_2)}{\partial \eta_k} + (1 - \delta_{i2}) \frac{\partial \log S_{2,p}(t_2)}{\partial \eta_k} \right) f_{2,p}(t_2) \, dt_2$$

Since the IWM estimator $\hat{\eta}$ is a consistent estimator for the parameters of the distributions $S_{1,p}(t)$ and $S_{2,p}(t)$ under the assumption of independence, the expected value of the score for each subject with respect to the population density function equals zero, i.e., for $j = 1, 2$ and $i = 1, \ldots, s$,

$$\int_{0}^{\infty} \left(\delta_{ij} \frac{\partial \log f_{j,p}(t_j)}{\partial \eta_k} + (1 - \delta_{ij}) \frac{\partial \log S_{j,p}(t_j)}{\partial \eta_k} \right) f_{j,p}(t_j) \, dt_j = 0$$

and therefore the expected score in (3.37) is indeed equal to zero, and it follows that $\hat{\eta}$ is a consistent estimator even for paired observations clustered according to an Archimedean copula. Spiekerman and Lin (1998) also discuss consistency of the parameter estimates from the IWM in a more general context.

3.4.3 Variance of parameter estimates adjusted for correlation structure

Although the estimator $\hat{\eta}$ from the IWM is consistent under certain conditions, the inverse of the information matrix of $\hat{\eta}$ is not a consistent estimator of the asymptotic variance–covariance matrix because of the correlation between survival times.

In complex data problems where the variance of estimators cannot be easily obtained, the jackknife estimator of the variance has been proposed. The jackknife estimator is based on the following idea: leave out the ith observation and obtain $\hat{\eta}_{-i}$, the estimator of η based on the remaining $N-1$ observations. Do this for $i = 1, \ldots, N$, i.e., we have N data sets with $N - 1$ observations each and we obtain $\hat{\eta}_{-i}$ with $i = 1, \ldots, N$. One form of the jackknife estimator for the variance of $\hat{\eta}$ (Wu, 1986) is then given by

$$\left(\frac{N - a}{N} \right) \sum_{i=1}^{N} (\hat{\eta}_{-i} - \hat{\eta}) (\hat{\eta}_{-i} - \hat{\eta})^t \tag{3.38}$$

with a the dimension of the vector $\boldsymbol{\eta}$. An important aspect of the jackknife estimator is that the observations that are left out are independent of the observations left in. Therefore, in the situation of correlated data, the grouped jackknife technique has to be used, leaving out complete clusters of observations instead of a single observation.

The grouped jackknife technique provides an appropriate tool to estimate the variance of the components of $\hat{\boldsymbol{\eta}}$ where $\hat{\boldsymbol{\eta}}$ is estimated using the IWM. We merely have to fit the model s times, each time leaving out another cluster. However, this can become computationally intensive and therefore Lipsitz et al. (1994) and Lipsitz and Parzen (1996) proposed the following approximation. First consider the maximisation of the likelihood to find $\hat{\boldsymbol{\eta}}$. This is most often based on the Newton–Raphson technique, an iterative algorithm based on a Taylor series approximation. In step k, we have that

$$\hat{\boldsymbol{\eta}}^{(k+1)} = \hat{\boldsymbol{\eta}}^{(k)} + \left(\sum_{i=1}^{s} \mathbf{I}_i \left(y_{i1}, y_{i2} \mid \hat{\boldsymbol{\eta}}^{(k)} \right) \right)^{-1} \sum_{i=1}^{s} \boldsymbol{S}_i \left(y_{i1}, y_{i2} \mid \hat{\boldsymbol{\eta}}^{(k)} \right)$$

with $\boldsymbol{S}_i \left(y_{i1}, y_{i2} \mid \boldsymbol{\eta} \right)$ the contribution to the score vector from cluster i and $\mathbf{I}_i \left(y_{i1}, y_{i2} \mid \boldsymbol{\eta} \right)$ the contribution to the observed information matrix for cluster i, with the jth column given by $-\frac{\partial \boldsymbol{S}_i (y_{i1}, y_{i2} \mid \boldsymbol{\eta})}{\partial \eta_j}$. The iteration continues until $\left(\hat{\boldsymbol{\eta}}^{(k+1)} - \hat{\boldsymbol{\eta}}^{(k)} \right)$ is smaller than a preset value ϵ. To obtain $\hat{\boldsymbol{\eta}}_{-i}$, a good starting value is obviously $\hat{\boldsymbol{\eta}}$, and the first step of the Newton–Raphson algorithm is then given by

$$\hat{\boldsymbol{\eta}}_{-i}^{(1)} = \hat{\boldsymbol{\eta}} + \left(\sum_{j=1, j \neq i}^{s} \mathbf{I}_j \left(y_{i1}, y_{i2} \mid \hat{\boldsymbol{\eta}} \right) \right)^{-1} \sum_{j=1, j \neq i}^{s} \boldsymbol{S}_j \left(y_{i1}, y_{i2} \mid \hat{\boldsymbol{\eta}} \right)$$

but in this expression

$$\sum_{j=1, j \neq i}^{s} \boldsymbol{S}_j \left(y_{i1}, y_{i2} \mid \hat{\boldsymbol{\eta}} \right) = \left(\sum_{j=1}^{s} \boldsymbol{S}_j \left(y_{i1}, y_{i2} \mid \hat{\boldsymbol{\eta}} \right) \right) - \boldsymbol{S}_i \left(y_{i1}, y_{i2} \mid \hat{\boldsymbol{\eta}} \right)$$

$$= 0 - \boldsymbol{S}_i \left(y_{i1}, y_{i2} \mid \hat{\boldsymbol{\eta}} \right)$$

and thus

$$\left(\hat{\boldsymbol{\eta}}_{-i}^{(1)} - \hat{\boldsymbol{\eta}} \right) = - \left(\sum_{j=1, j \neq i}^{s} \mathbf{I}_j \left(y_{i1}, y_{i2} \mid \hat{\boldsymbol{\eta}} \right) \right)^{-1} \boldsymbol{S}_i \left(y_{i1}, y_{i2} \mid \hat{\boldsymbol{\eta}} \right) \qquad (3.39)$$

Plugging this into the grouped jackknife version of formula (3.38) leads to

$$\left(\frac{s-a}{s}\right)\sum_{i=1}^{s}\left[\left(\sum_{j=1,j\neq i}^{s}\mathbf{I}_j\left(y_{i1},y_{i2}\mid\hat{\eta}\right)\right)^{-1}\boldsymbol{S}_i\left(y_{i1},y_{i2}\mid\hat{\eta}\right)\right.$$

$$\left.\boldsymbol{S}_i^t\left(y_{i1},y_{i2}\mid\hat{\eta}\right)\left(\sum_{j=1,j\neq i}^{s}\mathbf{I}_j\left(y_{i1},y_{i2}\mid\hat{\eta}\right)\right)^{-1}\right]$$

This expression can be simplified further by first dropping the term $(s-a)/s$, assuming that there are far more clusters than parameters to estimate, so that this term goes to one. Furthermore, instead of deriving always a new information matrix upon deleting a cluster, the same information matrix based on all observations could be used, leading to the following expression for the robust variance estimator:

$$\mathbf{I}^{-1}\left(\hat{\eta}\right)\boldsymbol{S}\left(\hat{\eta}\right)\boldsymbol{S}^t\left(\hat{\eta}\right)\mathbf{I}^{-1}\left(\hat{\eta}\right)$$

with $\mathbf{I}(\hat{\eta}) = \sum_{i=1}^{s}\mathbf{I}_i\left(y_{i1},y_{i2}\mid\hat{\eta}\right)$ the information matrix of the IWM for all observations and $\boldsymbol{S}(\hat{\eta}) = \sum_{i=1}^{s}\boldsymbol{S}_i\left(y_{i1},y_{i2}\mid\hat{\eta}\right)$ the score vector of the IWM for all observations evaluated at $\hat{\eta}$. This corresponds to the sandwich estimator that was obtained by White (1982) starting from a completely different viewpoint.

Example 3.7 Marginal and conditional model for time to blood–milk barrier recovery

The IWM for the time to blood–milk barrier recovery was already fitted in Example 3.1 leading to parameter estimates $\hat{\lambda} = 0.216$ and $\hat{\beta} = 0.176$ with standard error equal to 0.162. The IWM does not take into account the clustering of the data in pairs, and therefore the variance estimate is incorrect. The grouped jackknife estimator of the variance of β is derived here in two different ways. We calculate the one-step grouped jackknife estimator as in (3.39) and compare it to the ordinary grouped jackknife estimator, fitting the model with each time one cluster deleted until convergence.

Both the one-step grouped jackknife estimator and the ordinary grouped jackknife estimator of the standard error are equal to 0.153. So both estimators are substantially lower than the standard error obtained from the IWM. It is important to realise that the grouped jackknife estimator of the standard error can be either smaller or larger than the standard error from the IWM. Huster et al. (1989) give some asymptotic efficiency results for the grouped jackknife estimator for paired observations. ∎

In the example above, we observe that the standard error of the IWM is larger than the grouped jackknife estimator. On the other hand, the simulation studies shown in Table 3.5 demonstrate that the coverage of the 95% confidence interval for the IWM is often substantially lower than 95%. Therefore, we run simulations using the same three settings as in Table 3.5 in order to evaluate the standard error and the coverage of the 95% confidence interval when using the grouped jackknife estimator (Table 3.7). In any of the three settings, the coverage based on the grouped jackknife is slightly smaller than 95% but certainly acceptable from a practical point of view. It is clear that the grouped jackknife estimator is capable of correcting for the dependence structure in the data whereas the IWM has often too small variance. The standard error in the IWM in the first two settings is the same for all simulated data sets, as it is only a function of the structure of the experiment (the clustering) and not of the observed outcomes; this is clear from (3.7) and (3.8). The grouped jackknife estimator, however, takes the actual outcome into account, leading to sometimes higher, sometimes lower standard error estimates than the constant value from the IWM, but the median value of the standard errors is larger than the corresponding median value when using the IWM.

Table 3.7. Simulation results for the Independence Working Model with the unadjusted and grouped jackknife estimator of the variance based on 2000 data sets each consisting of 100 pairs with exponentially distributed event times with $\lambda = 0.23$, $\beta = 0.18$, and $\theta = 0.3$. First setting: no censoring and covariates within pair different. Second setting: no censoring and only for 80% of the pairs covariates within pair different. Third setting: 20% censoring and covariates within pair different. The third column ($\hat{\beta}$) contains the median for $\hat{\beta}$ and the 5%-95% quantiles in brackets, the fourth column (s.e.($\hat{\beta}$)) contains the median for the standard error of $\hat{\beta}$, and the last column gives the actual coverage of the 95% confidence interval.

	Model	$\hat{\beta}$ Median (5%-95% quantile)	s.e. ($\hat{\beta}$) Median	Coverage 95% CI
First setting	IWM	0.1757 ($-0.1067; 0.4803$)	0.1414	0.881
	Grouped jackknife	0.1757 ($-0.1067; 0.4803$)	0.1698	0.946
Second setting	IWM	0.1817 ($-0.1299; 0.5079$)	0.1414	0.849
	Grouped jackknife	0.1817 ($-0.1299; 0.5079$)	0.1797	0.941
Third setting	IWM	0.1666 ($-0.0928; 0.4204$)	0.1655	0.964
	Grouped jackknife	0.1666 ($-0.0928; 0.4204$)	0.1730	0.947

3.5 Population hazards from conditional models

In the marginal model presented in the previous section, the hazard function specified in the model refers to the whole population. All subjects with the same covariate information have the same hazard function. In the conditional hazards model, however, the hazard model is only valid for the subjects within a cluster due to the specification of a frailty for each cluster. The baseline hazard function, given by $u_i h_0(t)$ for cluster i, behaves in a similar fashion over time for the different clusters: if the hazard increases (decreases) in a monotone way for one cluster, it will do so in any other cluster regardless what frailty term u_i the cluster has. This is, however, not necessarily true for the population hazard derived from the conditional model: where the conditional hazard increases, the population hazard might decrease. We will discuss the derivation of the population hazard for the univariate frailty model, as the first theoretical developments have been mostly based on this model (Aalen, 1988, 1992, 1994). In univariate frailty models, with each subject having its own frailty term, we model overdispersion rather than clustering. The theoretical development for univariate frailty models, however, extends to clusters of any size. For simplicity, we assume a gamma distribution for the frailties; other frailty distributions are discussed in Chapter 4. Furthermore, even if the proportional hazards assumption is true for the conditional model, it does not necessarily hold at the level of the population, as is demonstrated in this section for bivariate survival data.

3.5.1 Population versus conditional hazard from frailty models

It is important to understand that frailty models are conditional models and that the implied assumptions such as a particular parametric form and proportional hazards only hold conditionally. We demonstrate this for the univariate frailty model without covariates and with each individual ($i = 1, \ldots, s$) having a specific frailty u_i, assumed to have a gamma distribution

$$h_i(t) = u_i h_0(t)$$

where $h_0(t)$ is the conditional baseline hazard function for a subject with $u_i = 1$. The conditional survival function for subject i is then given by

$$S_i(t) = \exp\left(-u_i \int_0^t h_0(t)\right) = \exp\left(-u_i H_0(t)\right)$$

In order to know how the hazard evolves over time in the population, we need to derive the population survival function by integrating out the frailty

$$S_f(t) = \int\limits_0^\infty \exp\left(-uH_0(t)\right) f_U(u)du = (1 + \theta H_0(t))^{-1/\theta}$$

The population density function is then given by

$$f_f(t) = -\frac{\partial S_f(t)}{\partial t} = \frac{h_0(t)}{(1 + \theta H_0(t))^{1+1/\theta}}$$

and the population hazard function is

$$h_f(t) = \frac{f_f(t)}{S_f(t)} = \frac{h_0(t)}{1 + \theta H_0(t)} = h_0(t)S_f^\theta(t) \qquad (3.40)$$

It is clear from this expression that at time 0 the population hazard corresponds to $h_0(t)$, but after that $h_f(t)$ is always smaller than $h_0(t)$ as $H_0(t)$ is increasing with time. The larger the heterogeneity parameter θ, the faster the population hazard will deviate from $h_0(t)$. Furthermore, if the considered event is rare, then $H_0(t)$ will only increase slowly and the difference between the population hazard and $h_0(t)$ will also increase slowly. Since

$$f_U(u \mid T > t) = \frac{P\left(T > t \mid u\right) f_U(u)}{P(T > t)} = \frac{\exp\left(-uH_0(t)\right) f_U(u)}{(1 + \theta H_0(t))^{-1/\theta}}$$

it follows that the expected value is given by

$$E\left(U \mid T > t\right) = \int\limits_0^\infty \frac{u \exp\left(-uH_0(t)\right) f_U(u)}{(1 + \theta H_0(t))^{-1/\theta}} du = (1 + \theta H_0(t))^{-1}$$

We therefore can rewrite the expression for the population hazard as

$$h_f(t) = h_0(t)E\left(U \mid T > t\right) \qquad (3.41)$$

The interpretation of this expression is as follows. Obviously, the frailty term for a particular subject is fixed. Nevertheless, the frailty distribution changes over time, due to the fact that the more frail individuals drop out first, and therefore, the mean of the frailty distribution, which starts off at one at time zero, is becoming smaller and smaller as the less frail individuals remain.

We now consider what happens with the parametric form of a conditional hazard model at the population level. As an example, we consider the frailty model with Weibull parametric form

$$h_i(t) = \lambda u_i \rho t^{\rho - 1}$$

which corresponds to Weibull distributed event times $W(\lambda u_i, \rho)$. Note that the first parameter λu_i is changing with the frailty term, whereas the second parameter remains constant. This leads to different hazard functions when subjects are in different clusters. The population hazard is now given by

$$h_f(t) = \frac{\lambda \rho t^{\rho - 1}}{1 + \theta \lambda t^\rho}$$

It is obvious that this population hazard function no longer corresponds to Weibull distributed event times. The cumulative hazard λt^ρ increases over time, and therefore the population hazard will eventually go to zero.

Example 3.8 Population and conditional hazard for time to ECF contact

As an example, consider the time to East Coast Fever (ECF) contact data set explained in Example 1.1. We fit a univariate frailty model with each cow having its own frailty term which is assumed to be gamma distributed with mean one, and baseline hazard corresponding to Weibull distributed event times. The parameter estimates are given by $\hat{\lambda} = 0.0084$, $\hat{\rho} = 1.124$, and $\hat{\theta} = 0.666$.

In Figure 3.3, the conditional hazard function for a cluster with frailty term equal to one is shown as a fine solid line. Furthermore, the hazard function for a cluster with a small frailty value equal to 0.736, corresponding to the 25th percentile of the gamma frailty distribution with θ equal to the estimated value 0.666, is shown as a dotted line, whereas the hazard function for a cluster with a large frailty value equal to 1.216, corresponding to the 75th percentile of that same gamma frailty distribution, is shown as a dashed line. On the logarithmic scale these lines are parallel. All these functions clearly represent hazard functions for Weibull distributed event times with ρ the estimated value 1.124 and, as this value is above one, all hazard functions are increasing over time.

The population hazard function for the time to ECF contact data set is shown in Figure 3.3 as a bold solid line. The population hazard first increases and then decreases. ∎

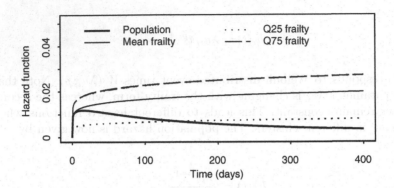

Fig. 3.3. The conditional and population hazard function for the time to ECF contact data set.

3.5.2 Population versus conditional hazard ratio from frailty models

We can also study the hazard ratio at the population level in the univariate frailty model with gamma frailty distribution. For simplicity consider just a binary (zero–one) covariate x_i leading to the conditional model

$$h_i(t) = u_i h_0(t) \exp(x_i \beta)$$

Based on the same derivations as before, the population hazards in the two treatment groups are given by

$$h_{\mathbf{x},f}(t) = \begin{cases} \dfrac{h_0(t)}{1 + \theta H_0(t)} & \text{for } \mathbf{x} = 0 \\[2ex] \dfrac{h_0(t) HR}{1 + \theta H_0(t) HR} & \text{for } \mathbf{x} = 1 \end{cases}$$

with $HR = \exp(\beta)$.

Therefore, the population hazard ratio is given by

$$HR_p(t) = \frac{(1 + \theta H_0(t)) HR}{1 + \theta H_0(t) HR} \tag{3.42}$$

From (3.42), it follows that $HR_p(t)$ goes to one as $H_0(t)$ goes to infinity if t goes to infinity. Taking the logarithm we get

$$\log\left(HR_p(t)\right) = \log\left(HR\right) + \log\left(1 + \theta H_0(t)\right) - \log\left(1 + \theta H_0(t)HR\right)$$

If $HR > 1$ ($HR < 1$), the last term of this expression is always larger (smaller) than the second term, and therefore $\log\left(HR_p(t)\right)$ is always smaller (larger) than $\log(HR)$ and thus less extreme and closer to zero.

Example 3.9 Population hazard ratio for time to ECF contact

We consider again the time to ECF contact data (Example 1.1) and study how the population hazard ratio for the breed effect evolves over time given the frailty model. Consider a parametric baseline hazard corresponding to Weibull distributed event times for the frailty model with the breed effect as binary covariate. Fitting this frailty model results in parameter estimates $\hat{\lambda} = 0.00734$, $\hat{\rho} = 1.138$, $\hat{\theta} = 0.697$, and $\hat{\beta} = 0.194$. The hazard ratio of cow i of breed 1 ($x_i = 1$) relative to cow j from breed 2 ($x_j = 0$) is given by

$$\frac{h_0(t)u_i \exp\left(\beta\right)}{h_0(t)u_j} = (u_i/u_j)\exp(0.194)$$

Although this hazard ratio differs according to which two cows are compared and is a function of the ratio of the two frailty terms, the hazard ratio is constant over time. The hazard ratio for two cows with the same frailty term, $u_i = u_j$, corresponds to $\exp(0.194) = 1.21$ which is shown in Figure 3.4 as the fine solid line. The hazard ratio of a cow of breed 1 with a small frailty value equal to 0.39 (the 25th percentile of the gamma frailty distribution) relative to a cow of breed 2 with a large frailty value equal to 1.37 (the 75th percentile of the gamma frailty distribution) equals 0.35 (dotted line in Figure 3.4). Alternatively, the hazard ratio of a cow of breed 1 with a large frailty value equal to 1.37 relative to a cow of breed 2 with a small frailty value equal to 0.39 equals 4.25 (dashed line in Figure 3.4). The population hazard ratio given by

$$\frac{\theta\lambda t^\rho + 1}{\theta\lambda t^\rho + 1/\exp(\beta)}$$

is no longer constant and is depicted in Figure 3.4 as a bold solid line. It decreases slightly at the start and then remains at a value slightly below the conditional hazard ratio of two subjects with the same frailty. ∎

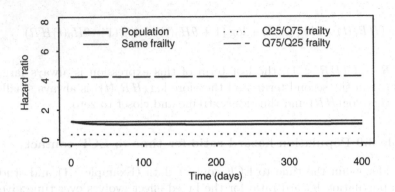

Fig. 3.4. The conditional and population hazard ratio for the time to ECF contact data set.

3.6 Further extensions and references

In this chapter we discussed alternatives for frailty models. Copula models and marginal models received considerable attention. A rich literature providing further applications and further extensions is available. We mention some important references for further reading.

Copulas have been used by many authors as alternatives to the frailty model mainly to model bivariate survival data (Andersen et al., 2005; Pipper and Martinussen, 2003; Roy and Mukherjee, 1998; Phelps and Weissfeld, 1997; Nelsen, 1997).

Marginal models have been used in different settings. Huang et al. (2004) study the marginal model in the context of recurrent events. Bjarnason and Hougaard (2000) study the Fisher information for a marginal distribution of Weibull form. Finally, semiparametric marginal models are studied by Vu (2004), Spiekerman and Lin (1998), Lin (1994), and Liang et al. (1993).

Adjustments of rank-based tests taking into account the correlation between subjects have also been considered by a number of authors (Jeong and Jung, 2006; Kosorok and Gangnon, 2006; Li et al., 2002). Li and Lagakos (2004) compare different adjustment techniques for testing covariate effects in correlated survival data.

4

Frailty distributions

Different distributions have been proposed for the frailty term. In Chapter 2 the gamma distribution was introduced. In this chapter we discuss different frailty distributions that are proposed in the literature. Although the discussion in this chapter is rather technical (most of the results appeared in methodological journals), it is important to collect what is available in a detailed way. Indeed, in practice mainly the gamma distribution and the lognormal distribution are used to model the frailty term and most of the software limits the choice of the frailty distribution to these cases. But the right choice of the frailty distribution is of crucial importance to arrive at a good description of the dependence structure present in the data. Therefore, the choice of the frailty distribution is even more important as the choice of the distribution of the random effect(s) in mixed models since, in frailty models, the dependence between correlated observations changes over time and the frailty distribution dictates how the dependence changes. Few results are available on comparing models with different frailty distributions; more research is needed in this area.

The general characteristics of frailty distributions are studied in detail in Section 4.1. We further discuss how the effect of particular frailty distributions on the survival and hazard function of individuals can be investigated by using the Laplace transform. Important global and local measures of dependence, such as Kendall's τ and the cross ratio function, are introduced in general terms. In Section 4.2 the gamma distribution is discussed in detail. The inverse Gaussian frailty distribution and the positive stable distribution are discussed in Sections 4.3 and 4.4, respectively. It is demonstrated that the positive stable distribution has specific and advantageous properties. For instance, the marginal model deduced from the conditional model still obeys the proportional hazards assumption. In Section 4.5, the power variance function family is discussed in general terms. This family contains the gamma, inverse Gaussian, and positive stable frailty. The compound Poisson distribution is discussed in Section 4.6. It allows a proportion of the population to be not susceptible for the event under consideration. This part of the population has frailty equal to zero, and thus hazard function equal to zero. In Section 4.7, the lognormal distribution is discussed. Its use in frailty models mainly originates from the link with generalised mixed models, where a standard assumption is that the random effects follow a normal distribution. This is the reason why, compared to the other choices of the frailty distribution, the status of the lognormal frailty distributions is different (see also Section 4.1).

4.1 General characteristics of frailty distributions

The frailty distributions that have been studied most belong to the power variance function family, a particular family of distributions introduced first by Tweedy (1984) and later independently studied by Hougaard (1986b). The gamma, inverse Gaussian, positive stable, and compound Poisson distribution are all members of this family. Before we study these particular distributions, we collect in this section a few results that hold for all these distributions. We demonstrate how the dependence induced by the frailty distributions can be expressed in terms of their Laplace transforms. We indeed see that the Laplace transform is the key ingredient for several measures of dependence. A further important frailty distribution is the lognormal distribution. This distribution is not a member of the power variance function family. The characteristics discussed here can generally not be obtained for this distribution because it does not have a simple expression for the Laplace transform.

The shared frailty model is given by

$$h_{ij}(t) = u_i h_0(t) \exp(\mathbf{x}_{ij}^t \boldsymbol{\beta}) = u_i h_{ij,c}(t)$$

where u_i is the common risk factor for all subjects in cluster i, $h_0(t)$ is the common baseline for all subjects, $\exp(\mathbf{x}_{ij}^t \boldsymbol{\beta})$ is the factor that gives the subject specific contribution to the hazard, and $h_{ij,c}(t)$ is the hazard for subject j from cluster i after the frailty effect of the cluster has been factored out. The u_i's, $i = 1, \ldots, s$, are the actual values of a sample from a density f_U.

This model induces correlation between event times of subjects within the same cluster. The effect of the frailty term can be studied at different levels. First, we investigate the joint survival function for a cluster. It is demonstrated that the Laplace transform is a useful mathematical tool in this context. Second, the frailty term has an effect on the population survival function. Due to the fact that more frail subjects experience on average the event earlier, the population structure changes over time with an obvious impact on the population survival function. Third, conditional on time the frailty distribution changes, although the frailty term itself for a particular cluster is fixed at the start. It is due to the fact that the clusters having large values for the frailty terms drop out earlier. Finally, we discuss several measures of dependence which will be useful to compare different frailty distributions.

4.1.1 Joint survival function and the Laplace transform

Assume $j = 1, \ldots, n_i$ (thus n_i subjects in cluster i), then the joint conditional survival function for cluster i is given by

$$S_i(\mathbf{t}_{n_i}) = \exp\left[-u_i\left(H_0(t_1)\exp(\mathbf{x}_{i1}^t\boldsymbol{\beta}) + \ldots + H_0(t_{n_i})\exp(\mathbf{x}_{in_i}^t\boldsymbol{\beta})\right)\right]$$

with $\mathbf{t}_{n_i} = (t_1, \ldots, t_{n_i})$ and $H_0(t) = \int_0^t h_0(v)dv$. Furthermore we use as notation $H_{ij,c}(t) = H_0(t)\exp(\mathbf{x}_{ij}^t\boldsymbol{\beta})$ and $H_{i.,c}(\mathbf{t}_{n_i}) = \sum_{j=1}^{n_i} H_{ij,c}(t_j)$.

Since the baseline hazard $h_0(t)$ is the same for all subjects, the hazard function differences between subjects are due to either the frailty term (the cluster they belong to) or the fixed effects.

Using the notation introduced in Section 3.3.1, the joint survival function for a cluster of size n with covariate information $\mathbf{x} = (\mathbf{x}_1^t, \ldots, \mathbf{x}_n^t)^t$ is obtained from the joint conditional survival function by integrating out the frailty with respect to the frailty distribution

$$S_{\mathbf{x},f}(\mathbf{t}_n) = \int_0^\infty \exp\left(-uH_{\mathbf{x},c}(\mathbf{t}_n)\right) f_U(u)du$$

$$= \mathrm{E}\left[\exp\left(-UH_{\mathbf{x},c}(\mathbf{t}_n)\right)\right]$$

with $U \sim f_U$. The last line of the equation above is the Laplace transform of U, $\mathcal{L}(s) = \mathrm{E}(\exp(-Us))$, evaluated at $s = H_{\mathbf{x},c}(\mathbf{t}_n)$, so we can write

$$S_{\mathbf{x},f}(\mathbf{t}_n) = \mathcal{L}(H_{\mathbf{x},c}(\mathbf{t}_n)) \tag{4.1}$$

The Laplace transform has an important role in the study of frailty models. For instance, the derivatives of the Laplace transform are used to obtain general results for the power variance function family. The kth derivative is given by

$$\mathcal{L}^{(k)}(s) = (-1)^k \mathrm{E}\left(U^k \exp(-Us)\right)$$

From the joint survival function, the joint density function for a cluster of size n with covariate information $\mathbf{x} = (\mathbf{x}_1^t, \ldots, \mathbf{x}_n^t)^t$ can be obtained as

$$f_{\mathbf{x},f}(\mathbf{t}_n) = (-1)^n \frac{\partial^n}{\partial t_1 \ldots \partial t_n} S_{\mathbf{x},f}(t_1, \ldots, t_n)$$

$$= (-1)^n \int_0^\infty \frac{\partial^n}{\partial t_1 \ldots \partial t_n} \exp\left[-u\left(H_{\mathbf{x}_1,c}(t_1) + \ldots + H_{\mathbf{x}_n,c}(t_n)\right)\right] f_U(u) du$$

$$= (-1)^n \prod_{j=1}^n h_{\mathbf{x}_j,c}(t_j) \int_0^\infty \exp\left(-u H_{\mathbf{x},c}(\mathbf{t}_n)\right)(-u)^n f_U(u) du$$

$$= (-1)^n \prod_{j=1}^n h_{\mathbf{x}_j,c}(t_j) \mathcal{L}^{(n)}\left(H_{\mathbf{x},c}(\mathbf{t}_n)\right) \qquad (4.2)$$

These expressions for the joint survival and density functions are useful in deriving the contribution of different clusters to the marginal likelihood. The likelihood contribution corresponds to the survival up to the time of censoring for censored subjects and the density at the event time for the subjects that experience the event. Therefore, the conditional likelihood contribution of cluster i is given by

$$\left(\prod_{j=1}^{n_i} h_{ij,c}^{\delta_{ij}}(y_{ij})\right) u_i^{d_i} \exp\left(-u_i \sum_{j=1}^{n_i} H_{ij,c}(y_{ij})\right)$$

with $d_i = \sum_{j=1}^{n_i} \delta_{ij}$. To obtain the marginal likelihood contribution for cluster i of size n_i with covariate information $\mathbf{x}_i = \left(\mathbf{x}_{i1}^t, \ldots, \mathbf{x}_{in_i}^t\right)^t$ and d_i the number of events, we take the expected value of this expression with respect to U_i

$$\left(\prod_{j=1}^{n_i} h_{\mathbf{x}_{ij},c}^{\delta_{ij}}(y_{ij})\right) \mathrm{E}\left[U_i^{d_i} \exp\left(-U_i \sum_{j=1}^{n_i} H_{\mathbf{x}_{ij},c}(y_{ij})\right)\right]$$

which can be written in terms of the Laplace transform as

$$\left(\prod_{j=1}^{n_i} h_{\mathbf{x}_{ij},c}^{\delta_{ij}}(y_{ij})\right)(-1)^{d_i} \mathcal{L}^{(d_i)}\left(\sum_{j=1}^{n_i} H_{\mathbf{x}_{ij},c}(y_{ij})\right)$$

4.1.2 Population survival function and the copula

The population survival function is also of interest as it tells how the survival function evolves over time for a randomly chosen individual with covariate information $\mathbf{x}$. Obviously, since the more frail subjects die sooner, the population itself changes over time, and this has an important impact on the population survival function. The population survival function for subjects having covariate information $\mathbf{x}$ is obtained from the conditional survival function $S_{ij}(t) = \exp\left(-u_i H_{\mathbf{x},c}(t)\right)$ by integrating out the frailty with respect to the frailty density function

$$S_{\mathbf{x},f}(t) = \int_0^\infty \exp\left(-u H_{\mathbf{x},c}(t)\right) f_U(u) du$$

It follows that

$$S_{\mathbf{x},f}(t) = \mathcal{L}(H_{\mathbf{x},c}(t)) \tag{4.3}$$

and for the density function we have

$$f_{\mathbf{x},f}(t) = \frac{d\left(1 - S_{\mathbf{x},f}(t)\right)}{dt} = -\mathcal{L}^{(1)}\left(H_{\mathbf{x},c}(t)\right) h_{\mathbf{x},c}(t) \tag{4.4}$$

The population hazard function is then obtained as the ratio of the population density and survival function

$$h_{\mathbf{x},f}(t) = \frac{-\mathcal{L}^{(1)}\left(H_{\mathbf{x},c}(t)\right)}{\mathcal{L}\left(H_{\mathbf{x},c}(t)\right)} h_{\mathbf{x},c}(t) \tag{4.5}$$

In the previous section, the joint survival function was expressed in terms of $H_{\mathbf{x},c}(t_n)$ which originates from the conditional model. Alternatively, the joint survival function can also be given in terms of the population survival functions for the subjects in a cluster (take as an example clusters of size n with covariate information $\mathbf{x}$). From (4.3), it follows that

$$H_{\mathbf{x},c}(t) = \mathcal{L}^{-1}\left(S_{\mathbf{x},f}(t)\right)$$

Using this expression for each subject $j = 1, \ldots, n$, the joint survival function (4.1) can be rewritten as

$$S_{\mathbf{x},f}(t_n) = \mathcal{L}\left[\mathcal{L}^{-1}\left(S_{\mathbf{x}_1,f}(t_1)\right) + \ldots + \mathcal{L}^{-1}\left(S_{\mathbf{x}_n,f}(t_n)\right)\right] \tag{4.6}$$

This is the copula representation of the joint survival function obtained from the frailty model; it links the joint survival function with the population survival functions. Note that the population survival functions in (4.6) are obtained from the conditional survival functions $S_{ij}(t)$ by integrating out the frailty with respect to the frailty density. Therefore, the population survival functions contain the frailty density parameter(s). This is different from the copula models discussed in Section 3.3.2. There the population survival functions are modelled in a marginal way, i.e., they do not contain the copula parameter. As a consequence the joint survival function obtained from the frailty model is not equivalent to the joint survival function from Section 3.3.2.

Many clustered data sets have the following structure: the cluster size is fixed, say n, and the order of the observations within a cluster denotes in fact the covariate information (e.g., the first observation is the observed value when the covariate takes level one, etc.). In such cases, the notation can often be simplified and (4.6) can be written as

$$S_f\left(\mathbf{t}_n\right) = \mathcal{L}\left[\mathcal{L}^{-1}\left(S_{1,f}(t_1)\right) + \ldots + \mathcal{L}^{-1}\left(S_{n,f}(t_n)\right)\right] \tag{4.7}$$

i.e., we drop the subindex x and $\mathbf{x}$ in the joint and population survival functions.

Up to now, we have introduced joint and population survival functions starting from the conditional survival function. Just like the survival function, the hazard ratio can also be considered at the conditional or at the population level. In frailty models, results are most often shown in terms of the conditional hazard ratio, corresponding to the ratio in hazards of subjects within the same cluster. It is also of interest to study the hazard ratio at the population level. The constant hazard ratio assumption at the conditional level does, in most cases, not lead to constant hazard ratio at the population level.

For simplicity, consider a binary covariate, for instance treatment and placebo. Assume a constant conditional hazard ratio $HR = \exp(\beta)$. The population hazard ratio $HR_p(t)$ for a treated versus a placebo subject then corresponds to

$$HR_p(t) = \frac{\mathcal{L}^{(1)}\left(H_0(t)\exp(\beta)\right)}{\mathcal{L}\left(H_0(t)\exp(\beta)\right)} \frac{\mathcal{L}\left(H_0(t)\right)}{\mathcal{L}^{(1)}\left(H_0(t)\right)} \exp(\beta) \tag{4.8}$$

Whether the population hazard ratio is constant over time depends on the frailty distribution (and corresponding Laplace transform) used.

4.1.3 Conditional frailty density changes over time

The frailty density f_U is fully characterized by its Laplace transform $\mathcal{L}(s) = \mathrm{E}\left(\exp(-Us)\right)$. If $\mathcal{L}(s)$ exists in a neighbourhood of zero, the expected value of U is minus the first derivative of the Laplace transform evaluated at zero:

$$\mathrm{E}\left(U\right) = -\mathcal{L}^{(1)}(0)$$

In general, we have that

$$\mathcal{L}^{(k)}(s) = (-1)^k \mathrm{E}\left(U^k \exp(-Us)\right)$$

and therefore

$$E\left(U^k\right) = (-1)^k \mathcal{L}^{(k)}(0) \tag{4.9}$$

The variance of the frailty term can therefore be expressed as

$$\mathrm{Var}(U) = E\left(U^2\right) - (E\left(U\right))^2 = \mathcal{L}^{(2)}(0) - \left(-\mathcal{L}^{(1)}(0)\right)^2$$

The frailty density f_U describes the population at the start. The population, however, changes over time, as on average more frail individuals drop out earlier. Due to this fact, the conditional (on $T > t$) frailty density will change over time. The change can be expressed in a general way. For simplicity, assume no covariate information (so that, see (4.3) and the notation in Section 1.5, $S_f(t) = \mathcal{L}(H_0(t))$). We first consider the frailty density for the survivors at time t

$$f_U(u \mid T > t) = \frac{\exp\left(-uH_0(t)\right) f_U(u)}{\mathcal{L}\left(H_0(t)\right)} \tag{4.10}$$

The expected value of the conditional frailty term equals one at time zero. It decreases with time as the remaining subjects tend to be more and more the subjects with small frailty values. Similarly, using (4.4), we can derive the frailty density for subjects that die at time t

$$f_U(u \mid T = t) = -\frac{u\exp\left(-uH_0(t)\right) f_U(u)}{\mathcal{L}^{(1)}\left(H_0(t)\right)}$$

When discussing the different frailty distributions in the next sections, we mainly focus on (4.10), the frailty density for the survivors at time t.

4.1.4 Measures of dependence

Since most dependence measures have been developed for bivariate data, we describe the measures for such data.

For two randomly chosen clusters i and k of size two, the event times are (T_{i1}, T_{i2}) and (T_{k1}, T_{k2}). As discussed in Section 3.3.2, a typical assumption for bivariate survival data (that we also adopt here) is that the covariate information is the same in each cluster, i.e., $\mathbf{x}_i = (\mathbf{x}_{i1}, \mathbf{x}_{i2}) = (\mathbf{x}_1, \mathbf{x}_2) = \mathbf{x}$, and again we therefore drop the subindex $\mathbf{x}$ and $\mathbf{x}$ in the joint and population survival functions.

Kendall's τ (Kendall, 1938) is defined as

$$\tau = E\left[\mathrm{sign}\left((T_{i1} - T_{k1})(T_{i2} - T_{k2})\right)\right]$$

where $\mathrm{sign}(x) = -1, 0, 1$ for $x < 0, x = 0, x > 0$. An alternative formulation for continuous distributions (Genest and MacKay, 1986) is given by

$$\tau = P\left((T_{i1} - T_{k1})(T_{i2} - T_{k2}) > 0\right) - P\left((T_{i1} - T_{k1})(T_{i2} - T_{k2}) < 0\right)$$

$$= 2P\left((T_{i1} - T_{k1})(T_{i2} - T_{k2}) > 0\right) - 1$$

$$= 2p - 1$$

Kendall's τ has a strong intuitive appeal as demonstrated in the following example.

Example 4.1 Kendall's τ in time to blood–milk barrier reconstitution

Consider the time to blood–milk barrier reconstitution in cows that had two udder quarters infected (Example 1.3). The times to reconstitution in the two udder quarters of a cow can be assumed to be correlated as it is mainly the general health status of the cow that determines the time needed to have reconstitution of the blood–milk barrier. The probability p is the probability that the left udder quarter of cow i is reconstituted before (after) the left udder quarter of cow k ($T_{i1} < T_{k1}$) and that the right udder quarter of cow i is reconstituted before (after) the right udder quarter of cow k ($T_{i2} < T_{k2}$). A value $p = 0.5$, or $\tau = 0$ corresponds to independence. ∎

We can express p in terms of the joint survival and density function

$$p = P\left((T_{i1} - T_{k1})(T_{i2} - T_{k2}) > 0\right)$$

$$= \int_0^\infty \int_0^\infty P\left((t_1 - T_{k1})(t_2 - T_{k2}) > 0\right) f_f(t_1, t_2) dt_1 dt_2$$

$$= \int_0^\infty \int_0^\infty P\left(T_{k1} > t_1, T_{k2} > t_2\right) f_f(t_1, t_2) dt_1 dt_2$$

$$+ \int_0^\infty \int_0^\infty P\left(T_{k1} < t_1, T_{k2} < t_2\right) f_f(t_1, t_2) dt_1 dt_2$$

$$= \int_0^\infty \int_0^\infty S_f(t_1, t_2) f_f(t_1, t_2) dt_1 dt_2$$

$$+ \int_0^\infty \int_0^\infty F_f(t_1, t_2) f_f(t_1, t_2) dt_1 dt_2$$

Note that $F_f(t_1, t_2) = S_f(t_1, t_2) + F_{1,f}(t_1) + F_{2,f}(t_2) - 1$ and thus

$$p = 2 \int_0^\infty \int_0^\infty S_f(t_1, t_2) f_f(t_1, t_2) dt_1 dt_2$$

$$+ \int_0^\infty F_{1,f}(t_1) \left(\int_0^\infty f_f(t_1, t_2) dt_2 \right) dt_1$$

$$+ \int_0^\infty F_{2,f}(t_2) \left(\int_0^\infty f_f(t_1, t_2) dt_1 \right) dt_2 - 1$$

The two middle terms in the previous equation are 0.5, therefore

$$p = 2 \int_0^\infty \int_0^\infty S_f(t_1, t_2) f_f(t_1, t_2) dt_1 dt_2$$

and

$$\tau = 4 \int_0^\infty \int_0^\infty S_f(t_1, t_2) f_f(t_1, t_2) dt_1 dt_2 - 1 \qquad (4.11)$$

In the case of frailty models, this equation can be reexpressed in terms of the Laplace transform as follows. Rewrite (4.11) as

$$\tau = 4 \int_0^\infty \int_0^\infty \mathcal{L}(x+y) \mathcal{L}^{(2)}(x+y) dx dy - 1$$

with $x = H_{1,c}(t_1)$ and $y = H_{2,c}(t_2)$. Using the transformation $s = x + y$ and $v = y$, we obtain

$$\tau = 4 \int_0^\infty \int_0^s \mathcal{L}(s) \mathcal{L}^{(2)}(s) dv ds - 1$$

$$= 4 \int_0^\infty s \mathcal{L}(s) \mathcal{L}^{(2)}(s) ds - 1 \qquad (4.12)$$

Kendall's τ is an overall measure of dependence. An important local measure of dependence is the cross ratio function (Clayton, 1978); it allows us to investigate how dependence changes over time. It is given by

$$\zeta(t_1, t_2) = \frac{h_{1,f}(t_1 \mid T_2 = t_2)}{h_{1,f}(t_1 \mid T_2 > t_2)}$$

Example 4.2 Cross ratio function in time to blood–milk barrier reconstitution

The cross ratio function also has a strong intuitive appeal. For the udder quarter data in Example 1.3, the rear udder quarters are infected and then treated (with a drug) or not treated (placebo or untreated). The cross ratio function corresponds to the ratio of the hazard of having reconstitution in the treated udder quarter at time t_1 given that, in the untreated udder quarter, reconstitution takes place at time t_2 over the hazard of having reconstitution in the treated udder quarter at time t_1 given that, in the untreated udder quarter, no reconstitution has yet taken place at time t_2. A positive (good) disease experience for the cow is to have reconstitution at time $T_2 = t_2$ in the untreated udder quarter, and a negative disease experience is to have reconstitution at a later time $T_2 > t_2$. For positively correlated data, we therefore expect the ratio of these two conditional hazards to be larger than one. ∎

The cross ratio function can also be written in terms of the joint survival function

$$\zeta(t_1, t_2) = \frac{f_{1,f}(t_1 \mid T_2 = t_2)/S_{1,f}(t_1 \mid T_2 = t_2)}{f_{1,f}(t_1 \mid T_2 > t_2)/S_{1,f}(t_1 \mid T_2 > t_2)}$$

$$= \frac{f_f(t_1, t_2) \Big/ \dfrac{\partial S_f(t_1, t_2)}{\partial t_2}}{\dfrac{\partial S_f(t_1, t_2)}{\partial t_1} \Big/ S_f(t_1, t_2)}$$

$$= \frac{S_f(t_1, t_2) f_f(t_1, t_2)}{\dfrac{\partial S_f(t_1, t_2)}{\partial t_1} \dfrac{\partial S_f(t_1, t_2)}{\partial t_2}} \tag{4.13}$$

This last expression leads to an alternative interpretation for the cross ratio function in terms of an odds ratio (Anderson et al., 1992). We use the time to reconstitution example to develop this odds ratio interpretation. We can construct a 2×2 contingency table for matched rear udder quarters (the same cow) conditional on having no reconstitution until the timepoint (t_1, t_2), with t_1 and t_2 denoting the reconstitution time of the treated and untreated udder quarter, respectively

Reconstitution		Treated Udder Quarter		
Status		0	1	
Untreated	0	P_{00}	P_{01}	P_{0+}
Udder Quarter	1	P_{10}	P_{11}	P_{1+}
		P_{+0}	P_{+1}	1

The row and column variables stand for the reconstitution status of the untreated and treated udder quarter of a cow conditional on not being reconstituted up to time (t_1, t_2). A zero for the treated (untreated) udder quarter means that, given no reconstitution up to time (t_1, t_2), the treated (untreated) udder quarter is not reconstituted in the interval $]t_1, t_1 + \delta]$ ($]t_2, t_2 + \delta]$) with $\delta > 0$. A one means that reconstitution of the treated (untreated) udder quarter does take place in $]t_1, t_1 + \delta]$ ($]t_2, t_2 + \delta]$).

The odds ratio of this 2×2 table is then given by

$$
\begin{aligned}
OR(t_1, t_2, \delta) &= \frac{P_{00} P_{11}}{P_{10} P_{01}} = \frac{P_{11}/P_{01}}{P_{10}/P_{00}} \\[2mm]
&= \frac{\dfrac{P(t_1 < T_1 \le t_1 + \delta, t_2 < T_2 < t_2 + \delta \mid T_1 > t_1, T_2 > t_2)}{P(T_1 > t_1 + \delta, t_2 < T_2 \le t_2 + \delta \mid T_1 > t_1, T_2 > t_2)}}{\dfrac{P(t_1 < T_1 \le t_1 + \delta, T_2 > t_2 + \delta \mid T_1 > t_1, T_2 > t_2)}{P(T_1 > t_1 + \delta, T_2 > t_2 + \delta \mid T_1 > t_1, T_2 > t_2)}} \\[2mm]
&= \frac{\dfrac{P(t_1 < T_1 \le t_1 + \delta \mid T_1 > t_1, t_2 < T_2 \le t_2 + \delta)}{1 - P(t_1 < T_1 \le t_1 + \delta \mid T_1 > t_1, t_2 < T_2 \le t_2 + \delta)}}{\dfrac{P(t_1 < T_1 \le t_1 + \delta \mid T_1 > t_1, T_2 > t_2 + \delta)}{1 - P(t_1 < T_1 \le t_1 + \delta \mid T_1 > t_1, T_2 > t_2 + \delta)}} \\[2mm]
&= \frac{\text{odds}\,(t_1 < T_1 \le t_1 + \delta \mid T_1 > t_1, t_2 < T_2 \le t_2 + \delta)}{\text{odds}\,(t_1 < T_1 \le t_1 + \delta \mid T_1 > t_1, T_2 > t_2 + \delta)}
\end{aligned}
$$

Anderson et al. (1992) show that the odds ratio of this 2×2 contingency table converges to the cross ratio function (4.13) as $\delta \to 0$.

The cross ratio function can also be interpreted as a local version of Kendall's τ.

With $\tau = 2p - 1$, we could have used as dependence measure

$$\frac{p}{1-p} = \frac{P\left((T_{i1} - T_{k1})\,(T_{i2} - T_{k2}) > 0\right)}{P\left((T_{i1} - T_{k1})\,(T_{i2} - T_{k2}) < 0\right)}$$

A local version of this measure is

$$\frac{p(t_1, t_2)}{1 - p(t_1, t_2)} = \frac{P\left((T_{i1} - T_{k1})\,(T_{i2} - T_{k2}) > 0 \mid T_{i1} \wedge T_{k1} = t_1, T_{i2} \wedge T_{k2} = t_2\right)}{P\left((T_{i1} - T_{k1})\,(T_{i2} - T_{k2}) < 0 \mid T_{i1} \wedge T_{k1} = t_1, T_{i2} \wedge T_{k2} = t_2\right)}$$

$$= \frac{P\left((T_{i1} - T_{k1})\,(T_{i2} - T_{k2}) > 0, T_{i1} \wedge T_{k1} = t_1, T_{i2} \wedge T_{k2} = t_2\right)}{P\left((T_{i1} - T_{k1})\,(T_{i2} - T_{k2}) < 0, T_{i1} \wedge T_{k1} = t_1, T_{i2} \wedge T_{k2} = t_2\right)} \quad (4.14)$$

The numerator can be written as

$$p(t_1, t_2) = P\left(T_{i1} = t_1, T_{k1} > t_1, T_{i2} = t_2, T_{k2} > t_2\right)$$
$$+ P\left(T_{i1} > t_1, T_{k1} = t_1, T_{i2} > t_2, T_{k2} = t_2\right)$$
$$= 2 f_f(t_1, t_2) S_f(t_1, t_2)$$

and for the denominator we have

$$1 - p(t_1, t_2) = P\left(T_{i1} = t_1, T_{k1} > t_1, T_{i2} > t_2, T_{k2} = t_2\right)$$
$$+ P\left(T_{i1} > t_1, T_{k1} = t_1, T_{i2} = t_2, T_{k2} > t_2\right)$$
$$= 2 \frac{\partial S_f(t_1, t_2)}{\partial t_1} \frac{\partial S_f(t_1, t_2)}{\partial t_2}$$

It easily follows that

$$\zeta(t_1, t_2) = \frac{p(t_1, t_2)}{1 - p(t_1, t_2)}$$

An important characteristic of the cross ratio function is that it depends on t_1 and t_2 only through the joint survival function $S_f(t_1, t_2)$. This characteristic follows easily using the Laplace transform representation. In general we have

$$S_f(t_1, t_2) = \mathcal{L}\left[\mathcal{L}^{-1}\left(S_{1,f}(t_1)\right) + \mathcal{L}^{-1}\left(S_{2,f}(t_2)\right)\right]$$

and therefore

$$\mathcal{L}^{-1}\left(S_f(t_1, t_2)\right) = \mathcal{L}^{-1}\left(S_{1,f}(t_1)\right) + \mathcal{L}^{-1}\left(S_{2,f}(t_2)\right)$$

The first and second derivatives of the joint survival function with respect to t_1 and t_2 are given by

$$\frac{\partial S_f(t_1, t_2)}{\partial t_j} = -\frac{\mathcal{L}^{(1)}\left[\mathcal{L}^{-1}\left(S_f(t_1, t_2)\right)\right]}{\mathcal{L}^{(1)}\left[\mathcal{L}^{-1}\left(S_{j,f}(t_j)\right)\right]} f_{j,f}(t_j)$$

$$\frac{\partial^2 S_f(t_1, t_2)}{\partial t_1 \partial t_2} = \frac{\mathcal{L}^{(2)}\left[\mathcal{L}^{-1}\left(S_f(t_1, t_2)\right)\right]}{\mathcal{L}^{(1)}\left[\mathcal{L}^{-1}\left(S_{1,f}(t_1)\right)\right]\mathcal{L}^{(1)}\left[\mathcal{L}^{-1}\left(S_{2,f}(t_2)\right)\right]} f_{1,f}(t_1) f_{2,f}(t_2)$$

Using these expressions in (4.13) and elementary calculus we obtain

$$\zeta(t_1, t_2) = S_f(t_1, t_2) \frac{\mathcal{L}^{(2)}\left[\mathcal{L}^{-1}\left(S_f(t_1, t_2)\right)\right]}{\left\{\mathcal{L}^{(1)}\left[\mathcal{L}^{-1}\left(S_f(t_1, t_2)\right)\right]\right\}^2}$$

$$= -S_f(t_1, t_2) \frac{\left(\mathcal{L}^{-1}\right)^{(2)}\left(S_f(t_1, t_2)\right)}{\left(\mathcal{L}^{-1}\right)^{(1)}\left(S_f(t_1, t_2)\right)}$$

For further reading on this representation of the cross ratio function, see Oakes (1989), Genest and MacKay (1986), and Chen and Bandeen-Roche (2005).

Another local dependence measure that we will consider is the ratio of the joint survival function and the product of the population survival functions of the two subjects in the cluster (Anderson et al., 1992) given by

$$\psi(t_1, t_2) = \frac{S_f(t_1, t_2)}{S_{1,f}(t_1) S_{2,f}(t_2)} \tag{4.15}$$

For interpretation, the following alternative form is helpful

$$\psi(t_1, t_2) = \frac{\mathrm{P}(T_1 > t_1 \mid T_2 > t_2)}{\mathrm{P}(T_1 > t_1)} \tag{4.16}$$

Example 4.3 Ratio of the joint survival function and the product of the population survival functions in time to blood–milk barrier reconstitution

In terms of Example 1.3, $\psi(t_1, t_2)$ is the ratio of the conditional probability that the time to reconstitution for the treated udder quarter is larger than t_1 given that the time to reconstitution for the untreated udder quarter is larger than t_2 and the probability that the the time to reconstitution for the treated udder quarter is larger than t_1. ∎

For visualisation of the local dependence measures, we will plot $\zeta(t_1, t_2)$, $\psi(t_1, t_2)$, and also the ratio of the joint density function over the product of the population density functions

$$\phi(t_1, t_2) = \frac{f_f(t_1, t_2)}{f_{1,f}(t_1) f_{2,f}(t_2)}$$

Under independence we have $\zeta(t_1, t_2) \equiv 1$, $\psi(t_1, t_2) \equiv 1$, and $\phi(t_1, t_2) \equiv 1$.

4.2 The gamma distribution

4.2.1 Definitions and basic properties

The two-parameter gamma density function is given by

$$f_U(u) = \frac{\gamma^\delta u^{\delta-1} \exp(-\gamma u)}{\Gamma(\delta)}$$

with $\delta > 0$ the shape parameter and $\gamma > 0$ the scale parameter. The Laplace transform is

$$\mathcal{L}(s) = \int_0^\infty \exp(-us) f_U(u) du$$
$$= \gamma^\delta (s + \gamma)^{-\delta} \tag{4.17}$$

Since $\mathcal{L}(s)$ exists in a neighbourhood of zero, the mean and the variance can be obtained by using the first and second derivatives of the Laplace transform

$$\mathcal{L}^{(1)}(s) = -\delta\gamma^\delta(s+\gamma)^{-\delta-1}$$
$$\mathcal{L}^{(2)}(s) = \delta(\delta+1)\gamma^\delta(s+\gamma)^{-\delta-2}$$

Evaluating these derivatives at $s = 0$ we find

$$\mathrm{E}(U) = (-1)\mathcal{L}^{(1)}(0) = \delta/\gamma$$
$$\mathrm{Var}(U) = \mathcal{L}^{(2)}(0) - \left(-\mathcal{L}^{(1)}(0)\right)^2 = \delta/\gamma^2$$

In frailty modelling the typical choice of the parameters of the gamma distribution is $\delta = \gamma$. Using θ as notation for the variance of U, we then have $E(U) = 1$, $\mathrm{Var}(U) = \theta = 1/\gamma$. This distribution with parameters $(1/\theta, 1/\theta)$ is called a one-parameter gamma distribution with variance parameter θ. The density is given by

$$f_U(u) = \frac{u^{1/\theta-1}\exp(-u/\theta)}{\Gamma(1/\theta)\theta^{1/\theta}}$$

with corresponding Laplace transform

$$\mathcal{L}(s) = (1 + \theta s)^{-1/\theta}$$

One-parameter gamma distributions with different variances (or equivalently different values for Kendall's τ (see 4.28)) are depicted in Figure 4.1.

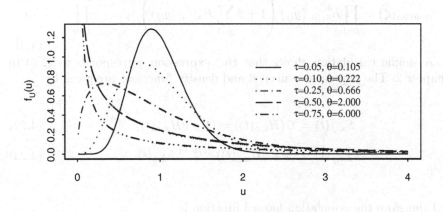

Fig. 4.1. Gamma density functions.

4.2.2 Joint and population survival function

The joint survival function is given by

$$S_{x,f}(t_n) = (1 + \theta H_{x,c}(t_n))^{-1/\theta} \qquad (4.18)$$

The joint density function can be expressed in terms of the nth derivative of the Laplace transform. The kth derivative is given by

$$\mathcal{L}^{(k)}(s) = (-1)^k (1 + \theta s)^{-1/\theta - k} \prod_{l=0}^{k-1} (1 + l\theta) \tag{4.19}$$

and therefore the joint density function is

$$f_{\mathbf{x},f}(\mathbf{t}_n) = (1 + \theta H_{\mathbf{x},c}(\mathbf{t}_n))^{-1/\theta - n} \prod_{l=0}^{n-1} (1 + l\theta) \prod_{j=1}^{n} h_{\mathbf{x}_j,c}(t_j) \tag{4.20}$$

Using the d_i^{th} derivative of the Laplace transform we can write the contribution to the marginal likelihood of cluster i of size n_i with covariate information $\mathbf{x}_i$ as (set $\prod_{l=0}^{d_i-1} (1 + l\theta) = 1$ for $d_i = 0$)

$$L_{marg,i}(\zeta) = \prod_{j=1}^{n_i} h_{\mathbf{x}_{ij},c}^{\delta_{ij}}(y_{ij}) \left(1 + \theta \sum_{j=1}^{n_i} H_{\mathbf{x}_{ij},c}(y_{ij}) \right)^{-1/\theta - d_i} \prod_{l=0}^{d_i-1} (1 + l\theta) \tag{4.21}$$

A simple calculation shows that this expression corresponds to (2.6) in Chapter 2. The population survival and density functions are given by

$$S_{\mathbf{x},f}(t) = \mathcal{L}(H_{\mathbf{x},c}(t)) = (1 + \theta H_{\mathbf{x},c}(t))^{-1/\theta} \tag{4.22}$$

$$f_{\mathbf{x},f}(t) = (1 + \theta H_{\mathbf{x},c}(t))^{-1/\theta - 1} h_{\mathbf{x},c}(t) \tag{4.23}$$

and therefore the population hazard function is

$$h_{\mathbf{x},f}(t) = (1 + \theta H_{\mathbf{x},c}(t))^{-1} h_{\mathbf{x},c}(t) = S_{\mathbf{x},f}^{\theta}(t) h_{\mathbf{x},c}(t) \tag{4.24}$$

The ratio of the population and the conditional hazard is

$$\frac{h_{\mathbf{x},f}(t)}{h_{\mathbf{x},c}(t)} = S_{\mathbf{x},f}^{\theta}(t) \tag{4.25}$$

The time evolution of this ratio is given in Figure 4.2 for different values of θ. Clearly, the ratio starts at one (both hazards are equal at time zero since $S_{\mathbf{x},f}(0) = 1$) and decreases with time (the population survival function decreases in time), with a steeper decrease for higher values of θ. For instance,

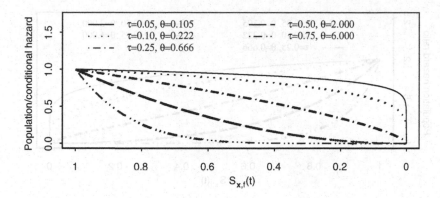

Fig. 4.2. The ratio of the population and the conditional hazard function for the gamma frailty distribution for different values of θ.

for $\theta = 2$, the ratio drops to 0.2 when approximately 60% of the subjects in the population are dead.

We now compare the conditional and the population hazard ratio for a binary covariate. With $HR = \exp(\beta)$ the constant conditional hazard ratio, the population hazard ratio is given by

$$HR_p(t) = \frac{(1 + \theta H_0(t) \exp(\beta))^{-1} h_0(t) \exp(\beta)}{(1 + \theta H_0(t))^{-1} h_0(t)}$$

$$= \frac{1 + \theta H_0(t)}{1 + \theta H_0(t) \exp(\beta)} \exp(\beta) \qquad (4.26)$$

In the conditional model the within-cluster hazard ratio for a binary covariate is constant over time. From (4.26) it is clear that the population hazard ratio is decreasing over time whenever $\beta > 0$ (shown in Figure 4.3).

For high values of θ (e.g., $\theta = 6$) we see that for $S_{\mathbf{x},f}(t)$ values smaller than 0.6 ($S_{\mathbf{x},f}(t) = 0.6$ means that 40% of the population died) the population hazard ratio is approximately one. If we ignore the presence of clustering (i.e., if we look at the population hazard ratio as if it is a hazard ratio that is obtained from independent data), we will conclude that the proportional hazards assumption does not hold, as demonstrated in Figure 4.3, whereas the hazard ratio is constant at the conditional level. Moreover we will conclude that there is no longer a treatment effect for patients that survived the

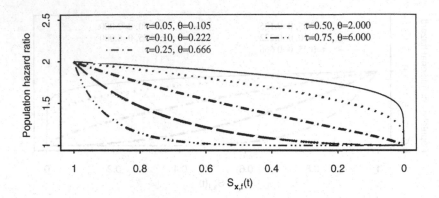

Fig. 4.3. The evolution of the population hazard ratio as a function of the population survival function for the conditional hazard ratio equal to two for the gamma frailty distribution for different values of θ.

timepoint $S_{x,f}^{-1}(0.6)$. This means that early in the study, with still 60% of the patients at risk, we conclude no further treatment effect. This is in conflict with the constant hazard ratio for the conditional model showing that, within a cluster, the beneficial effect of the treatment is constant over time.

4.2.3 Updating

An important property of the gamma distribution is that the conditional frailty density (conditional on $T > t$ or $T = t$) is still a gamma density. Assuming for simplicity no covariate information we indeed have

$$
\begin{aligned}
f_U(u \mid T > t) &= \frac{\exp\left(-uH_0(t)\right) f_U(u)}{\mathcal{L}\left(H_0(t)\right)} \\[2mm]
&= \frac{\exp\left(-uH_0(t)\right) f_U(u)}{(1 + \theta H_0(t))^{-1/\theta}} \\[2mm]
&= \frac{(1/\theta + H_0(t))^{1/\theta}\, u^{1/\theta - 1} \exp\left[-(1/\theta + H_0(t))u\right]}{\Gamma(1/\theta)}
\end{aligned}
$$

This is a two-parameter gamma density function with shape parameter $\delta = 1/\theta$ and scale parameter $1/\theta + H_0(t)$.

From this it follows that

$$E\left(U \mid T > t\right) = \frac{1/\theta}{1/\theta + H_0(t)} = (1 + \theta H_0(t))^{-1} = S_f^\theta(t)$$

and thus $E(U \mid T > t) \leq 1$. This is due to the fact that the frailer subjects (high values for the frailty term) experience on average the event earlier. Therefore, when proceeding in time, the population of subjects will contain less and less weaker subjects with high frailty values. As we start from $E(U) = 1$, the mean will therefore decrease over time and will thus be smaller than one. Note that the ratio at time t of the population and the conditional hazard function in (4.25) is exactly the same as the conditional mean of the frailty U given that the survival time is larger than t. Furthermore,

$$\text{Var}\left(U \mid T > t\right) = \frac{1/\theta}{\left(1/\theta + H_0(t)\right)^2}$$

hence the variance gets smaller with time. It is intuitively clear why the variability diminishes: the frailer individuals drop out and the remaining are more alike. How the variance changes over time is presented in Figure 4.4 for different values of θ.

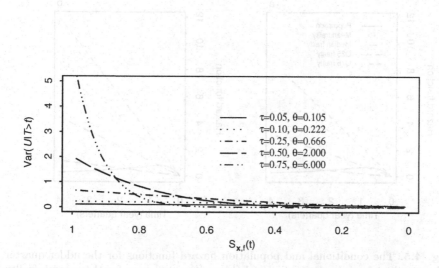

Fig. 4.4. The conditional variance of U given the survival time exceeds t for the gamma frailty distribution.

Example 4.4 The gamma frailty model for the udder quarter infection data

To demonstrate some of the characteristics of the gamma frailty model, we fit the gamma frailty model with Weibull baseline hazard to the udder quarter infection data in Example 1.4 including the binary variable heifer (primiparous versus multiparous) in the model. We obtain as parameter estimates $\hat{\lambda} = 0.838$ (s.e. $= 0.214$), $\hat{\rho} = 1.979$ (s.e. $= 0.106$), $\hat{\beta} = 0.317$ (s.e. $= 0.328$), and $\hat{\theta} = 1.793$ (s.e. $= 0.304$). The conditional hazard functions for the three different frailty values corresponding to the 25th, 50th, and 75th quantiles of the frailty distribution and the population hazard function are depicted in Figure 4.5 for primiparous and multiparous cows. It is clear that the conditional hazard in both groups is increasing over time and at a faster rate for cows with a high frailty value. On the contrary, the population hazard first increases but after approximately a quarter of a year the hazard decreases. The same evolution is observed in primiparous and multiparous cows, with the multiparous cows having a higher hazard. The evolution of the population hazard ratio of primiparous versus multiparous cows is depicted in Figure 4.6 and is contrasted with the constant conditional hazard ratio. With time, the population hazard ratio goes to one. Finally, the evolution of the expected value and variance of the frailties over time is depicted in Figure 4.7. ∎

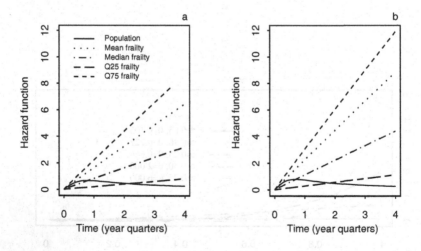

Fig. 4.5. The conditional and population hazard functions for the udder quarter infection data for (a) primiparous and (b) multiparous cows for the gamma frailty distribution with $\hat{\theta} = 1.793$.

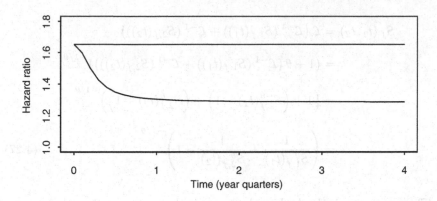

Fig. 4.6. The conditional hazard ratio (constant) and the population hazard ratio of primiparous versus multiparous cows for the udder quarter infection data for the gamma frailty distribution with $\hat{\theta} = 1.793$.

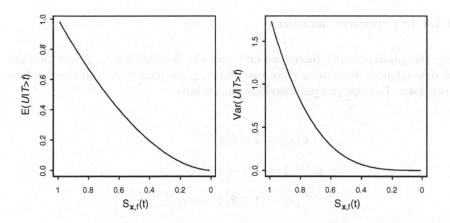

Fig. 4.7. The conditional mean and variance of U given the survival time exceeds t for the udder quarter infection data with the gamma frailty distribution with $\hat{\theta} = 1.793$.

4.2.4 Copula form representation

The joint survival function can also be written in terms of the population survival functions of the different subjects in the cluster. We work out this representation for bivariate data, but it can easily be extended to clusters with more subjects. From (4.6) we have, since $\mathcal{L}^{-1}(s) = \theta^{-1}\left(s^{-\theta} - 1\right)$,

$$
\begin{aligned}
S_f(t_1, t_2) &= \mathcal{L}\left(\mathcal{L}^{-1}\left(S_{1,f}(t_1)\right) + \mathcal{L}^{-1}\left(S_{2,f}(t_2)\right)\right) \\
&= \left(1 + \theta\left(\mathcal{L}^{-1}\left(S_{1,f}(t_1)\right) + \mathcal{L}^{-1}\left(S_{2,f}(t_2)\right)\right)\right)^{-1/\theta} \\
&= \left(1 + \left(S_{1,f}^{-\theta}(t_1) - 1\right) + \left(S_{2,f}^{-\theta}(t_2) - 1\right)\right)^{-1/\theta} \\
&= \left(\frac{1}{S_{1,f}^{\theta}(t_1)} + \frac{1}{S_{2,f}^{\theta}(t_2)} - 1\right)^{-1/\theta}
\end{aligned}
\tag{4.27}
$$

This expression is the Archimedean copula that corresponds with a gamma frailty distribution and is called the Clayton copula (Clayton, 1978). Note, however, the difference between (4.27) and the Clayton copula formulation given in, e.g., Shih and Louis (1995a). Although the functional form of the copula in Shih and Louis (1995a) and in (4.27) is the same, there is a clear difference in the way the population survival functions are modelled (see Sections 3.3.3 and 3.3.4, formulas (3.21) and (3.32)).

4.2.5 Dependence measures

For the gamma frailty model we first consider Kendall's τ, a global measure of dependence. To obtain τ we use (4.12), a formula based on the Laplace transform. For the gamma distribution, we have

$$
\mathcal{L}(s) = (1 + \theta s)^{-1/\theta}
$$

$$
\mathcal{L}^{(1)}(s) = -(1 + \theta s)^{-1/\theta - 1}
$$

$$
\mathcal{L}^{(2)}(s) = (1 + \theta)(1 + \theta s)^{-1/\theta - 2}
$$

so that using (4.12) we obtain

$$
\int_0^\infty s\mathcal{L}(s)\mathcal{L}^{(2)}(s)ds = \int_0^\infty \frac{1}{\theta}\left((1 + \theta s) - 1\right)(1 + \theta s)^{-1/\theta}
$$

$$
\times (1 + \theta)(1 + \theta s)^{-1/\theta - 2}\, ds
$$

which simplifies to

$$\int_0^\infty s\mathcal{L}(s)\mathcal{L}^{(2)}(s)ds = \frac{\theta+1}{\theta}\int_0^\infty (1+\theta s)^{-2/\theta-1}ds$$

$$-\int_0^\infty \frac{\theta+1}{\theta}(1+\theta s)^{-2/\theta-2}ds$$

$$= \frac{\theta+1}{\theta}\left(\frac{1}{2}-\frac{1}{\theta+2}\right)$$

and thus we have

$$\tau = 4\left(\frac{\theta+1}{\theta}\left(\frac{1}{2}-\frac{1}{\theta+2}\right)\right)-1$$

$$= \frac{\theta}{\theta+2} \tag{4.28}$$

In event time data, however, the dependence can evolve over time. The dependence over time can be depicted in several ways. First we can use survival functions. Note that in case of independence, i.e., for $\theta \to 0$, the logarithm of the (bivariate) joint survival function tends to the logarithm of the product of the two population survival functions. Indeed, using l'Hôpital's rule, we have

$$\lim_{\theta\to 0}\log S_f(t_1,t_2) = -\lim_{\theta\to 0}\frac{\log\left(S_{1,f}^{-\theta}(t_1)+S_{2,f}^{-\theta}(t_2)-1\right)}{\theta}$$

$$= -\lim_{\theta\to 0}\frac{S_{1,f}^{-\theta}(t_1)\log\left(1/S_{1,f}(t_1)\right)+S_{2,f}^{-\theta}(t_2)\log\left(1/S_{2,f}(t_2)\right)}{S_{1,f}^{-\theta}(t_1)+S_{2,f}^{-\theta}(t_2)-1}$$

$$= -\left[\log\left(1/S_{1,f}(t_1)\right)+\log\left(1/S_{2,f}(t_2)\right)\right]$$

$$= \log\left(S_{1,f}(t_1)S_{2,f}(t_2)\right)$$

To depict, for $\theta > 0$, the dependence in a graphical way we can make a contour plot (Figure 4.8a) or a three-dimensional plot (Figure 4.8b) of the ratio

$$\psi(t_1,t_2) = \frac{S_f(t_1,t_2)}{S_{1,f}(t_1)S_{2,f}(t_2)}$$

and see how the surface deviates from the horizontal plane at height one (which is the surface in case of independence).

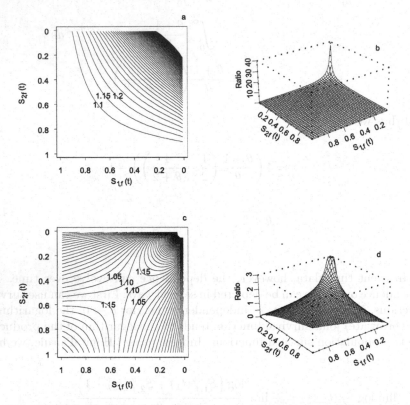

Fig. 4.8. The ratio of the joint survival function and the product of the population survival functions (a,b) and the ratio of the joint density function and the product of the population density functions (c,d) for the gamma frailty distribution with $\tau = 0.25$.

The contour lines in Figure 4.8a have 0.05 as span. It is clear that large values for $\psi(t_1, t_2)$ appear for large values of the time (or equivalently small values of the survival function), and that the contour lines are coming closer together with increasing time, so that the gamma distribution typically models late dependence.

Also, density functions can be used to show this late dependence. The joint density function can be obtained by differentiating the joint survival function with respect to t_1 and t_2 (see (4.2)).

Starting from (4.27) we easily obtain

$$f_f(t_1, t_2) = \frac{(\theta + 1) f_{1,f}(t_1) f_{2,f}(t_2)}{S_{1,f}^{\theta+1}(t_1) S_{2,f}^{\theta+1}(t_2) \left(S_{1,f}^{-\theta}(t_1) + S_{2,f}^{-\theta}(t_2) - 1 \right)^{2+1/\theta}}$$

Independence can then be studied in a graphical way by looking at the ratio

$$\frac{f_f(t_1, t_2)}{f_{1,f}(t_1) f_{2,f}(t_2)} = \frac{\theta + 1}{S_{1,f}^{\theta+1}(t_1) S_{2,f}^{\theta+1}(t_2) \left(S_{1,f}^{-\theta}(t_1) + S_{2,f}^{-\theta}(t_2) - 1 \right)^{2+1/\theta}}$$

For $\theta = 2/3$ ($\tau = 0.25$) a contour plot for this ratio is given in Figure 4.8c and a three-dimensional plot in Figure 4.8d. For small values of the survival functions (or large values of the survival time) the ratio moves away from one (late dependence). The contour lines have 0.05 as span. The ratio also moves away from one early in time, but to a lesser extent than later in time, which is demonstrated by the larger spread of the contour lines in the lower left corner compared to the upper right corner.

A further local dependence measure is the cross ratio function $\zeta(t_1, t_2)$ defined in (4.13). The expressions needed for (4.13) are given in (3.22)–(3.25) but with $S_{j,p}$ replaced by $S_{j,f}$, $j = 1, 2$. It follows immediately that the cross ratio function takes the constant value $\theta + 1$.

4.2.6 Diagnostics

Most research on diagnostics tests for the frailty distribution has been undertaken for the bivariate gamma frailty model. However in the first part of this section we describe a diagnostic test proposed by Shih and Louis (1995b) for the multivariate gamma frailty model (clusters of arbitrary size) which is based on the evolution of the conditional posterior mean of the frailties over time. Next, we discuss a diagnostic test for bivariate survival data with gamma frailty distribution which is based on the cross ratio function (Oakes, 1989; Viswanathan and Manatunga, 2001).

Posterior mean frailty as diagnostic tool

The use of the parametric proportional hazards model with gamma frailty distribution to fit multivariate survival data relies on the following assumptions:

the parametric form of the baseline hazard has been correctly specified, the covariates have a multiplicative effect (through the exponential $\exp\left(\mathbf{x}_{ij}^t\boldsymbol{\beta}\right)$), the frailty has a multiplicative effect on the hazard, and the frailty distribution is gamma. Assuming that the first three assumptions are satisfied, Shih and Louis (1995b) give a method to assess the adequacy of the gamma distribution assumption. Their technique uses the posterior frailty mean given the data at time t. For a precise definition we need the vector $\mathbf{z}(t)$ containing the data information at time t, i.e., for all $j = 1, \ldots, n_i$ and $i = 1, \ldots, s$ we need $y_{ij}(t) = y_{ij} \wedge t$ and the censoring indicator $\delta_{ij}(t) = \delta_{ij}I\left(y_{ij} \leq t\right)$. To obtain $\mathrm{E}\left(U \mid \mathbf{z}(t), \boldsymbol{\zeta}\right)$, the conditional frailty mean given $\mathbf{z}(t)$ or, for short, the posterior frailty mean, we first calculate for cluster i, $i = 1, \ldots, s$, the conditional density of U_i given $\mathbf{z}(t)$.

Therefore, with $\boldsymbol{\zeta} = (\boldsymbol{\xi}, \theta, \boldsymbol{\beta})$ and $\boldsymbol{\xi}$ the parameters of the baseline hazard (see Section 2.2), let $L_i\left(\boldsymbol{\xi}, \boldsymbol{\beta} \mid \mathbf{z}(t), u_i\right)$ and $L_{marg,i}\left(\boldsymbol{\zeta} \mid \mathbf{z}(t)\right)$ denote the conditional likelihood and the marginal likelihood defined in (2.4) and (2.6) but now evaluated at $\mathbf{y}_{n_i}(t) = (y_{i1}(t), \ldots, y_{in_i}(t))$ and $\boldsymbol{\delta}_{n_i}(t) = (\delta_{i1}(t), \ldots, \delta_{in_i}(t))$. In the further discussion we will use $l_i(.)$ and $l_{marg,i}(.)$ as notation for $\log L_i(.)$ and $\log L_{marg,i}(.)$. A further remark is that $L_{marg,i}(\boldsymbol{\zeta} \mid \mathbf{z}(\infty)) \equiv L_{marg,i}(\boldsymbol{\zeta})$ and $l_{marg,i}(\boldsymbol{\zeta} \mid \mathbf{z}(\infty)) \equiv l_{marg,i}(\boldsymbol{\zeta})$.

Now apply the Bayes theorem to obtain

$$
\begin{aligned}
f_U\left(u_i \mid \mathbf{z}(t), \boldsymbol{\zeta}\right) &= \frac{L_i\left(\boldsymbol{\xi}, \boldsymbol{\beta} \mid \mathbf{z}(t), u_i\right) f_U\left(u_i\right)}{L_{marg,i}\left(\boldsymbol{\zeta} \mid \mathbf{z}(t)\right)} \\[2mm]
&= u_i^{d_i(t)+1/\theta-1} \exp\left\{-u_i\left[1/\theta + \sum_{j=1}^{n_i} H_{ij,c}\left(y_{ij}(t)\right)\right]\right\} \\[2mm]
&\quad \times \frac{\left[1/\theta + \sum_{j=1}^{n_i} H_{ij,c}\left(y_{ij}(t)\right)\right]^{d_i(t)+1/\theta}}{\Gamma\left(d_i(t) + 1/\theta\right)}
\end{aligned}
\tag{4.29}
$$

with $d_i(t) = \sum_{j=1}^{n_i} \delta_{ij}(t)$. This expression corresponds to a gamma density with shape parameter $d_i(t)+1/\theta$ and scale parameter $\sum_{j=1}^{n_i} H_{ij,c}\left(y_{ij}(t)\right)+1/\theta$ and therefore the expected value is

$$
\mathrm{E}\left(U_i \mid \mathbf{z}(t), \boldsymbol{\zeta}\right) = \frac{d_i(t) + 1/\theta}{\sum_{j=1}^{n_i} H_{ij,c}\left(y_{ij}(t)\right) + 1/\theta}
\tag{4.30}
$$

Shih and Louis (1995b) propose the average of the posterior frailty means as diagnostic measure.

They show that

$$\bar{U}\left(\mathbf{z}(t),\boldsymbol{\zeta}\right) = \frac{1}{s}\sum_{i=1}^{s} \mathrm{E}\left(U_i \mid \mathbf{z}(t),\boldsymbol{\zeta}\right) \tag{4.31}$$

takes constant value one for all timepoints if the gamma distribution assumption for the frailty is correct. In fact, they obtain, under maximum likelihood regularity conditions and assuming boundedness of cluster sizes, a central limit result for $\sqrt{s}\left[\bar{U}\left(\mathbf{z}(t),\hat{\boldsymbol{\zeta}}\right) - 1\right]$ as $s \to \infty$ where $\hat{\boldsymbol{\zeta}}$ is the estimator for $\boldsymbol{\zeta}$. To formulate the precise result we need an expression for the asymptotic variance. We therefore define the quantities $\boldsymbol{S}(\boldsymbol{\zeta})$, $V(\boldsymbol{\zeta})$, $C(t,\boldsymbol{\zeta})$ and $B(t,\boldsymbol{\zeta})$: as in (2.8) we assume that the $\boldsymbol{\zeta} = (\boldsymbol{\xi},\theta,\boldsymbol{\beta})$ vector has q components. For $k = 1,\ldots,q$ we define

$$\boldsymbol{S}_k(\boldsymbol{\zeta}) = \frac{1}{\sqrt{s}}\frac{\partial}{\partial\zeta_k}l_{marg}(\boldsymbol{\zeta}) = \frac{1}{\sqrt{s}}\sum_{i=1}^{s}\frac{\partial l_{marg,i}(\boldsymbol{\zeta})}{\partial\zeta_k}$$

and

$$\boldsymbol{S}(\boldsymbol{\zeta}) = (\boldsymbol{S}_1(\boldsymbol{\zeta}),\ldots,\boldsymbol{S}_q(\boldsymbol{\zeta}))^t$$

Using the Hessian matrix in (2.8)

$$\mathbf{H}(\boldsymbol{\zeta}) = \left(\frac{\partial^2 l_{marg}(\boldsymbol{\zeta})}{\partial\zeta_a\partial\zeta_b}\right) = \left(\sum_{i=1}^{s}\frac{\partial^2 l_{marg,i}(\boldsymbol{\zeta})}{\partial\zeta_a\partial\zeta_b}\right)$$

we define

$$V(\boldsymbol{\zeta}) = \lim_{s\to\infty}\left(-\frac{1}{s}\mathbf{H}(\boldsymbol{\zeta})\right) \tag{4.32}$$

We finally need

$$C(t,\boldsymbol{\zeta}) = \lim_{s\to\infty} s\mathrm{Var}\left[\bar{U}\left(\mathbf{z}(t),\boldsymbol{\zeta}\right)\right] \tag{4.33}$$

and

$$B(t,\boldsymbol{\zeta}) = \mathrm{Cov}\left[\sqrt{s}\left(\bar{U}\left(\mathbf{z}(t),\boldsymbol{\zeta}\right) - 1,\boldsymbol{S}(\boldsymbol{\zeta})\right)\right] \tag{4.34}$$

In terms of (4.32)–(4.34) the precise formulation of the asymptotic normality result reads as follows: under regularity conditions we have distributional convergence, i.e., as $s \to \infty$,

$$\sqrt{s}\left[\bar{U}\left(\mathbf{z}(t),\hat{\boldsymbol{\zeta}}\right) - 1\right] \xrightarrow{D} N\left(0, C(t,\boldsymbol{\zeta}) - B^t(t,\boldsymbol{\zeta})V^{-1}(\boldsymbol{\zeta})B(t,\boldsymbol{\zeta})\right) \tag{4.35}$$

Consistent estimates of $C(t, \varsigma)$, $B(t, \varsigma)$, and $V(\varsigma)$ are given by

$$\hat{C}(t, \varsigma) = \frac{1}{s} \sum_{i=1}^{s} \left[\mathrm{E}\left(U_i \mid \mathbf{z}(t), \varsigma\right) - \bar{U}\left(\mathbf{z}(t), \varsigma\right) \right]^2 \qquad (4.36)$$

$$\hat{B}(t, \varsigma) = s^{-1} \sum_{i=1}^{s} \left[\mathrm{E}\left(U_i \mid \mathbf{z}(t), \varsigma\right) - \bar{U}\left(\mathbf{z}(t), \varsigma\right) \right] \begin{pmatrix} \dfrac{\partial l_{marg,i}(\varsigma)}{\partial \varsigma_1} \\ \cdots \\ \dfrac{\partial l_{marg,i}(\varsigma)}{\partial \varsigma_q} \end{pmatrix} \qquad (4.37)$$

$$\hat{V}(\varsigma) = -\frac{1}{s} \mathbf{H}(\varsigma) \qquad (4.38)$$

The partial derivatives of the marginal loglikelihood are given in Section 2.2. In concrete applications ς in (4.36)–(4.38) is replaced by $\hat{\varsigma}$.

Example 4.5 Diagnostics for the udder quarter infection data based on the conditional posterior mean frailty

We consider the udder quarter infection data (Example 1.4) to illustrate the use of the diagnostic test. The evolution of $\bar{U}\left(\mathbf{z}(t), \hat{\varsigma}\right) - 1$ over time is depicted in Figure 4.9, together with the 95% confidence limits for the statistic $\mathrm{E}\left(U_i \mid \mathbf{z}(t), \theta\right) - 1$. There seems to be a certain pattern in the evolution of the statistic, with a decrease at the start, followed by an increase to finally evolve towards zero. At the start, the test statistic crosses the lower limit of the confidence band. Therefore, the gamma frailty distribution assumption is questionable. ∎

Cross ratio function as diagnostic tool

In this section, we will discuss the cross ratio function as a diagnostic tool for bivariate survival data, assuming for simplicity that there is no censoring (extensions of this technique for censored data are discussed at the end of this section). We further assume for each data point that the two components have a specific meaning (e.g., for the diagnostic data set (Example 1.2) the first component has diagnosis=RX and the second component has diagnosis=US) so that for between-cluster comparison it is clear which components (observations) go together. The cross ratio function has not been extended yet to

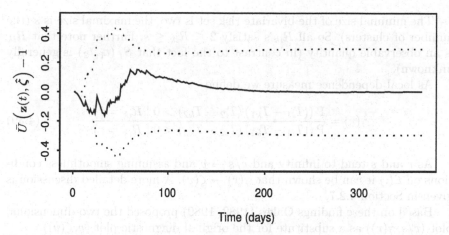

Fig. 4.9. The time evolution of the average of the conditional posterior means (minus one) of the 100 frailties of the udder quarter infection data.

clusters of larger size, and therefore this diagnostic tool is only available for bivariate survival data.

We already demonstrated that the cross ratio function is constant and equal to $\theta + 1$ in case of the gamma frailty distribution. Oakes (1982, 1989) proposed a nonparametric estimator for the cross ratio function for bivariate data without censoring which can be used as a diagnostic tool. If the nonparametric estimate deviates substantially from the constant value $\theta + 1$, the gamma frailty distribution assumption is questionable.

In Section 4.1.4 we showed that the cross ratio function depends on t_1 and t_2 only through the joint survival function $S_f(t_1, t_2)$:

$$\zeta(t_1, t_2) \equiv \zeta(S_f(t_1, t_2)) \equiv \zeta(v)$$

with $v = S_f(t_1, t_2)$. We therefore can use the two-dimensional plot $(v, \zeta(v))$ as a diagnostic tool. However, since $S_f(t_1, t_2)$ is generally unknown, the practical value of this idea is, at first sight, limited. To save this appealing idea, we define a new local dependence measure $\gamma(r)$ (see (4.39)) which is directly related to the cross ratio function. The details are as follows. For two pairs (T_{i1}, T_{i2}) and (T_{k1}, T_{k2}) consider the pair $(T_{i1} \wedge T_{k1}, T_{i2} \wedge T_{k2})$ and define the corresponding bivariate risk set as

$$R_{ik} = \{l : T_{l1} \geq T_{i1} \wedge T_{k1}, T_{l2} \geq T_{i2} \wedge T_{k2}\}$$

The minimal size of the bivariate risk set is two, the maximal size is s (the number of clusters). So all R_{ik}'s satisfy $2 \leq R_{ik} \leq s$. Further note that R_{ik} is an observable quantity (in contrast to the fact that $S_f(t_1, t_2)$ is generally unknown).

As local dependence measure we define

$$\gamma(r) = \frac{P\left((T_{i1} - T_{k1})(T_{i2} - T_{k2}) > 0 \mid R_{ik} = r\right)}{P\left((T_{i1} - T_{k1})(T_{i2} - T_{k2}) < 0 \mid R_{ik} = r\right)} \tag{4.39}$$

As r and s tend to infinity and $r/s \to v$ and assuming smoothness conditions on $\mathcal{L}(.)$ it can be shown that $\gamma(r) \to \zeta(v)$. A more detailed discussion is given in Section 4.2.7.

Based on these findings Oakes (1982, 1989) proposed the two-dimensional plot $(r/s, \gamma(r))$ as a substitute for the original diagnostic plot $(v, \zeta(v))$.

To obtain an estimate for $\gamma(r)$, we first need to determine the different risk set sizes. This can be done by considering all possible pairs of clusters and determining for each such pair, say (T_{i1}, T_{i2}) and (T_{k1}, T_{k2}), the size of the bivariate risk set R_{ik}. Denote the number of risk set sizes by q and order the risk set sizes according to size, i.e., $r_1, \ldots, r_a, \ldots, r_q$.

For each pair of clusters (T_{i1}, T_{i2}), (T_{k1}, T_{k2}) the size of the corresponding bivariate risk set R_{ik} takes one of the values $r_1, \ldots, r_q$. Note that there are $\binom{s}{2}$ bivariate risk sets. Let n_a denote the number of bivariate risk sets of size r_a. An estimate for $\gamma(r_a)$ is then given by the ratio of the number of concordant pairs over the number of discordant pairs.

For a particular bivariate risk set of size r_a the number n_a might be very small, moreover it might not contain any concordant pair, leading to a zero estimate for $\gamma(r_a)$, or any discordant pair, leading to ∞ as estimate. To circumvent these problems, Oakes (1982) proposed to combine bivariate risk sets with adjacent r_a values. A disadvantage of this approach is that the cross ratio function is estimated only for a small number of v values; this can make its use as diagnostic tool problematic.

A better approach is proposed by Viswanathan and Manatunga (2001). They first estimate $\gamma(r_a)$ for each bivariate risk set size r_a, $a = 1, \ldots, q$, and then use kernel regression estimation techniques to obtain a smooth estimator for the cross ratio. Additionally they use a bivariate analogue of the Kaplan–Meier estimate (Dabrowska, 1988) to estimate the survivor function in the presence of censoring.

Example 4.6 Diagnostics for the gamma frailty distribution for time to diagnosis of being healed based on the cross ratio function

In the example, we consider the original method proposed by Oakes (1982) and apply it to the time to diagnosis data (Example 1.2). To demonstrate the method, which has been discussed above for complete data (i.e., no censoring) we only consider dogs for which we observe event times for both RX and US. Therefore, we do not use 7 out of 106 dogs as these dogs have a censored RX time (US times were available for all dogs). The risk set size varies between 2 and 99. We combine adjacent r_a values in groups 1–10, 11–20, ..., 91–100, and use the average of the r_a values within each group. As demonstrated in Figure 4.10, the estimate of $\gamma(r)$, which itself is an estimate of the cross ratio function, deviates substantially from the time-constant cross ratio function estimated from the gamma distribution frailty model early in the study (corresponding with high values for the survival function). Note that $\gamma(r)$ is asymptotically equivalent to the cross ratio function if r and s tend to infinity and therefore r/s tends to $S_f(t_1, t_2)$ (see Section 4.2.7 for a proof of the asymptotic equivalence). ■

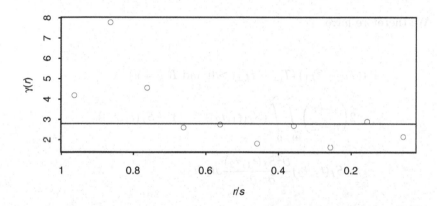

Fig. 4.10. The estimate of $\gamma(r)$ plotted against r/s for the time to diagnosis data. Adjacent r_a values are combined in groups 1–10, 11–20, ..., 91–100, and the average of the r_a values within each group, divided by s, is used as value to be plotted on the x-axis. The solid line is the time-constant cross ratio function estimated from the gamma distribution frailty model.

4.2.7* Estimation of the cross ratio function: some theoretical considerations

In the previous section we argued that for $r/s \to v$, the local dependence measure $\gamma(r)$ is asymptotically equivalent to $\zeta(v)$. A more detailed discussion on this relation is the subject of this section and is mainly based on the results presented by Oakes (1989). First note that

$$\gamma(r) = \frac{P\left((T_{i1} - T_{k1})(T_{i2} - T_{k2}) > 0 \text{ and } R_{ik} = r\right)}{P\left((T_{i1} - T_{k1})(T_{i2} - T_{k2}) < 0 \text{ and } R_{ik} = r\right)}$$

We discuss the asymptotic behaviour of the numerator. If $T_{i1} \wedge T_{k1} = t_1$ and $T_{i2} \wedge T_{k2} = t_2$, then the two pairs (T_{i1}, T_{i2}), (T_{k1}, T_{k2}) are concordant if and only if $T_{i1} = t_1$, $T_{k1} > t_1$, $T_{i2} = t_2$, $T_{k2} > t_2$ or $T_{i1} > t_1$, $T_{k1} = t_1$, $T_{i2} > t_2$, $T_{k2} = t_2$. The "probability" for this event is

$$2 S_f(t_1, t_2) \frac{\partial^2 S_f(t_1, t_2)}{\partial t_1 \partial t_2}$$

If $R_{ik} = r$, $r - 2$ of the remaining $s - 2$ clusters (of size two) should satisfy $T_{l1} > t_1$ and $T_{l2} > t_2$, the $s - r$ other clusters do not satisfy $T_{l1} > t_1$ and $T_{l2} > t_2$ simultaneously. The probability for this event is

$$\binom{s - r}{r - 2} \left(S_f(t_1, t_2) \right)^{r-2} \left(1 - S_f(t_1, t_2) \right)^{s-r}$$

We therefore have

$$P \left((T_{i1} - T_{k1}) (T_{i2} - T_{k2}) > 0 \text{ and } R_{ik} = r \right)$$

$$= 2 \binom{s - r}{r - 2} \int_0^\infty \int_0^\infty \left(S_f(t_1, t_2) \right)^{r-2} \left(1 - S_f(t_1, t_2) \right)^{s-r}$$

$$\times S_f(t_1, t_2) \frac{\partial^2 S_f(t_1, t_2)}{\partial t_1 \partial t_2} dt_1 dt_2$$

Using the transformation

$$u = \mathcal{L}^{-1} \left(S_{1,f}(t_1) \right) + \mathcal{L}^{-1} \left(S_{2,f}(t_2) \right)$$

$$w = \mathcal{L}^{-1} \left(S_{2,f}(t_2) \right)$$

we have

$$S_f(t_1, t_2) = \mathcal{L} \left[\mathcal{L}^{-1} \left(S_{1,f}(t_1) \right) + \mathcal{L}^{-1} \left(S_{2,f}(t_2) \right) \right]$$

$$= \mathcal{L} (u)$$

and

$$\frac{\partial^2 S_f(t_1, t_2)}{\partial t_1 \partial t_2} dt_1 dt_2$$

$$= \mathcal{L}^{(2)}(u) \frac{d}{dt_1} \mathcal{L}^{-1}(S_{1,f}(t_1)) \frac{d}{dt_2} \mathcal{L}^{-1}(S_{2,f}(t_2)) dt_1 dt_2$$

$$= \mathcal{L}^{(2)}(u) \frac{d}{dt_1} \left[\mathcal{L}^{-1}(S_{1,f}(t_1)) + \mathcal{L}^{-1}(S_{2,f}(t_2)) \right] \frac{d}{dt_2} \mathcal{L}^{-1}(S_{2,f}(t_2)) dt_1 dt_2$$

$$= \mathcal{L}^{(2)}(u) du dw$$

Using these findings we can write (note that $0 < w < u$)

$$P\left((T_{i1} - T_{k1})(T_{i2} - T_{k2}) > 0 \text{ and } R_{ik} = r\right)$$

$$= 2 \binom{s-r}{r-2} \int_0^\infty \int_0^u (\mathcal{L}(u))^{r-2} (1 - \mathcal{L}(u))^{s-r} \mathcal{L}(u) \mathcal{L}^{(2)}(u) dw du$$

$$= 2 \binom{s-r}{r-2} \int_0^\infty u (\mathcal{L}(u))^{r-1} (1 - \mathcal{L}(u))^{s-r} \mathcal{L}^{(2)}(u) du$$

$$= 2 \binom{s-r}{r-2} \int_0^1 \mathcal{L}^{-1}(y) y^{r-2} (1-y)^{s-r} \frac{y \left(\mathcal{L}^{-1}\right)^{(2)}(y)}{\left(\left(\mathcal{L}^{-1}\right)^{(1)}(y)\right)^2} dy$$

$$= 2 \binom{s-r}{r-2} B(r-1, s-r+1)$$

$$\times \int_0^1 \frac{y^{r-2}(1-y)^{s-r}}{B(r-1, s-r+1)} \frac{y \left(\mathcal{L}^{-1}\right)^{(2)}(y) \mathcal{L}^{-1}(y)}{\left(\left(\mathcal{L}^{-1}\right)^{(1)}(y)\right)^2} dy$$

$$= \frac{2}{s-1} \int_0^1 b(y; r-1, s-r+1) \frac{y \left(\mathcal{L}^{-1}\right)^{(2)}(y) \mathcal{L}^{-1}(y)}{\left(\left(\mathcal{L}^{-1}\right)^{(1)}(y)\right)^2} dy$$

$$\equiv \frac{2I(r, s)}{s-1}$$

where $b(y; r-1, s-r+1)$ is a beta density with parameters $r-1$ and $s-r+1$.

We now show that, if $r/s \to v$,

$$I(r, s) \to \frac{v\left(\mathcal{L}^{-1}\right)^{(2)}(v)\mathcal{L}^{-1}(v)}{\left(\left(\mathcal{L}^{-1}\right)^{(1)}(v)\right)^2}$$

This follows by an application of the Helly–Bray theorem provided we can show that the moment generating function of the beta distribution tends to a distribution that takes point mass one at v (a degenerate distribution at v) if $r/s \to v$.

The moment generating function of a beta distribution with parameters $r - 1$ and $s - r + 1$ is (Johnson et al., 1994)

$$M(t) = 1 + \sum_{k=1}^{\infty} \left(\prod_{l=0}^{k-1}\left(\frac{r-1+l}{s+l}\right)\right)\frac{t^k}{k!}$$

For $r/s \to v$ we have for a fixed l that $\dfrac{r-1+l}{s+l} \to v$; we therefore have

$$M(t) \approx 1 + \sum_{k=1}^{\infty}\frac{(vt)^k}{k!} = \exp(vt)$$

which is the moment generating function of a distribution that puts point mass one at v.

A similar discussion can be given for the denominator. Combining these results gives the asymptotic equivalence between $\gamma(r)$ and $\zeta(v)$ for $r/s \to v$.

4.3 The inverse Gaussian distribution

4.3.1 Definitions and basic properties

The inverse Gaussian density function is given by

$$f_U(u) = (\alpha/2\pi)^{1/2}u^{-3/2}\exp\left(\frac{-\alpha}{2u\mu^2}(u-\mu)^2\right) \tag{4.40}$$

with $\mu > 0$ and $\alpha > 0$. A reparameterisation from an exponential family point of view is given by

$$f_U(u) = (2\pi)^{-1/2}u^{-3/2}\psi^{1/2}\exp\left(\psi^{1/2}\phi^{1/2}\right)\exp\left(-\phi u/2 - \psi/2u\right) \tag{4.41}$$

with $\psi = \alpha$ and $\phi = \alpha/\mu^2$ (see, e.g., Hougaard (2000), Section A.3.2).

The Laplace transform is

$$\mathcal{L}(s) = \int_0^\infty \exp(-su) \left(\frac{\alpha}{2\pi}\right)^{1/2} u^{-3/2} \exp\left(\frac{-\alpha}{2u\mu^2}(u-\mu)^2\right) du$$

$$= \left(\frac{\alpha}{2\pi}\right)^{1/2} \exp\left(\frac{\alpha}{\mu}\right) \int_0^\infty u^{-3/2} \exp\left(-\left(\frac{\alpha}{2\mu^2}+s\right)u\right) \exp\left(-\frac{\alpha}{2u}\right) du$$

$$= \exp\left(\frac{\alpha}{\mu}\right) \exp\left(-2\left(\frac{\alpha}{2}\right)^{1/2}\left(\frac{\alpha}{2\mu^2}+s\right)^{1/2}\right)$$

$$= \exp\left(\frac{\alpha}{\mu} - \left(\frac{\alpha^2}{\mu^2}+2\alpha s\right)^{1/2}\right) \tag{4.42}$$

the third equality in (4.42) follows by rewriting the integrand as a density function of form (4.41). The first and second derivatives of the Laplace transform are given by

$$\mathcal{L}^{(1)}(s) = -\alpha \exp\left(\frac{\alpha}{\mu}\right) \exp\left(-\left(\frac{\alpha^2}{\mu^2}+2\alpha s\right)^{1/2}\right)\left(\frac{\alpha^2}{\mu^2}+2\alpha s\right)^{-1/2} \tag{4.43}$$

$$\mathcal{L}^{(2)}(s) = \alpha^2 \exp\left(\frac{\alpha}{\mu}\right) \exp\left(-\left(\frac{\alpha^2}{\mu^2}+2\alpha s\right)^{1/2}\right)\left(\frac{\alpha^2}{\mu^2}+2\alpha s\right)^{-1}$$

$$+ \alpha^2 \exp\left(\frac{\alpha}{\mu}\right) \exp\left(-\left(\frac{\alpha^2}{\mu^2}+2\alpha s\right)^{1/2}\right)\left(\frac{\alpha^2}{\mu^2}+2\alpha s\right)^{-3/2}$$

Evaluating the derivatives at $s = 0$ we find

$$E(U) = -\mathcal{L}^{(1)}(0) = \mu$$

$$\text{Var}(U) = \mathcal{L}^{(2)}(0) - \left(-\mathcal{L}^{(1)}(0)\right)^2 = \mu^3/\alpha$$

Taking $\mu = 1$ we obtain the following simplified Laplace transform

$$\mathcal{L}(s) = \exp\left[\alpha\left(1 - (1+2\alpha^{-1}s)^{1/2}\right)\right]$$

For $\mu = 1$ we have that $\theta = \text{Var}(U) = 1/\alpha$ (so $\alpha = +\infty$ corresponds with no heterogeneity ($\theta = 0$)).

A number of inverse Gaussian density functions with mean one are shown in Figure 4.11 (see (4.58) for a definition of τ).

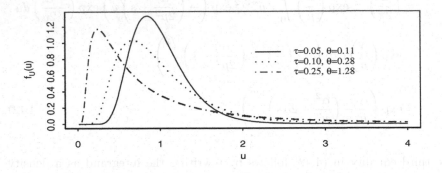

Fig. 4.11. Inverse Gaussian density functions.

4.3.2 Joint and population survival function

The joint survival function is given by

$$S_{x,f}\left(\mathbf{t}_n\right) = \exp\left\{\alpha\left[1 - \left(1 + 2\alpha^{-1}H_{x,c}\left(\mathbf{t}_n\right)\right)^{1/2}\right]\right\}$$

The joint density function can be obtained from the nth derivative of the Laplace transform, but no simple expression is obtained. We derive the first four derivatives as an example to be able to derive the marginal likelihood for the case of clusters of four observations (the situation of Example 1.4). With $z = \left(1 + 2\alpha^{-1}s\right)$, the first four derivatives of the Laplace transform are given by

$$\mathcal{L}^{(1)}(s) = -\exp\left(\alpha(1 - \sqrt{z})\right)z^{-1/2} \tag{4.44}$$

$$\mathcal{L}^{(2)}(s) = \exp\left(\alpha(1 - \sqrt{z})\right)z^{-1}\left(1 + \alpha^{-1}z^{-1/2}\right) \tag{4.45}$$

$$\mathcal{L}^{(3)}(s) = -\exp\left(\alpha(1 - \sqrt{z})\right)z^{-3/2}\left(1 + 3\alpha^{-1}z^{-1/2} + 3\alpha^{-2}z^{-1}\right) \tag{4.46}$$

$$\mathcal{L}^{(4)}(s) = \exp\left(\alpha(1 - \sqrt{z})\right)z^{-2}$$

$$\left(1 + 6\alpha^{-1}z^{-1/2} + 15\alpha^{-2}z^{-1} + 15\alpha^{-3}z^{-3/2}\right) \tag{4.47}$$

To demonstrate the use of the derivatives of the Laplace transform in the construction of the marginal loglikelihood we consider the specific situation of clusters of size four with right-censored observations. With

$$H_{\mathbf{x},c}(t_1, t_2, t_3, t_4) = \sum_{j=1}^{4} H_0(t_j) \exp\left(\mathbf{x}_j^t \boldsymbol{\beta}\right)$$

we have that

$$S_{\mathbf{x},f}(t_1, t_2, t_3, t_4) = \mathcal{L}\left(H_{\mathbf{x},c}(t_1, t_2, t_3, t_4)\right)$$

From (4.44)–(4.47) we can obtain explicit expressions for the marginal log-likelihood. The contribution of a specific cluster i depends on d_i, the number of events in that cluster. For clusters of size four, d_i varies from zero to four. For cluster i with $d_i = 0$ and covariate information $\mathbf{x}_i$, the contribution to the marginal loglikelihood is

$$\log S_{\mathbf{x}_i, f}(\mathbf{y}_i) = \log \mathcal{L}\left(H_{\mathbf{x}_i, c}(\mathbf{y}_i)\right)$$

$$= \alpha \left[1 - \left(1 + 2\alpha^{-1} H_{\mathbf{x}_i, c}(\mathbf{y}_i)\right)^{1/2}\right]$$

with $\mathbf{y}_i = (y_{i1}, y_{i2}, y_{i3}, y_{i4})^t$ and $H_{\mathbf{x}_i, c}(\mathbf{y}_i) = \sum_{j=1}^{4} H_{\mathbf{x}_{ij}, c}(y_{ij})$.

We order the subjects according to whether they experienced the event or not, starting from the uncensored subjects. For $d_i = 1, 2, 3, 4$ the generic terms in the marginal likelihood are of form

$$(-1)^l \frac{\partial^l}{\partial t_1 \ldots \partial t_l} S_{\mathbf{x}_i, f}(\mathbf{y}_i) = (-1)^l \mathcal{L}^{(l)}\left(H_{\mathbf{x}_i, c}(\mathbf{y}_i)\right)$$

$$\times \prod_{j=1}^{l} h_0(y_{ij}) \exp\left(\mathbf{x}_{ij}^t \boldsymbol{\beta}\right)$$

with $l = 1, 2, 3, 4$. The contribution of cluster i with covariate information $\mathbf{x}_i$ to the marginal loglikelihood can be written as

$$\sum_{j=1}^{4} \delta_{ij} \log\left(h_0(y_{ij}) \exp\left(\mathbf{x}_{ij}^t \boldsymbol{\beta}\right)\right) + \alpha \left[1 - \left(1 + 2H_{\mathbf{x}_i, c}(\mathbf{y}_i)/\alpha\right)^{1/2}\right]$$

$$- \frac{d_i}{2} \log\left(1 + 2H_{\mathbf{x}_i, c}(\mathbf{y}_i)/\alpha\right) + C_{i, d_i} \qquad (4.48)$$

where C_{i,d_i} is a term that depends on the number of events in the cluster. For clusters of size four we have

$$C_{i,0} = C_{i,1} = 0$$

$$C_{i,2} = \log\left(1 + \frac{\left(1 + 2H_{\mathbf{x}_i,c}\left(\mathbf{y}_i\right)/\alpha\right)^{-1/2}}{\alpha}\right)$$

$$C_{i,3} = \log\left(1 + \frac{3\left(1 + 2H_{\mathbf{x}_i,c}\left(\mathbf{y}_i\right)/\alpha\right)^{-1/2}}{\alpha} + \frac{3\left(1 + 2H_{\mathbf{x}_i,c}\left(\mathbf{y}_i\right)/\alpha\right)^{-1}}{\alpha^2}\right)$$

$$C_{i,4} = \log\left(1 + \frac{6\left(1 + 2H_{\mathbf{x}_i,c}\left(\mathbf{y}_i\right)/\alpha\right)^{-1/2}}{\alpha} + \frac{15\left(1 + 2H_{\mathbf{x}_i,c}\left(\mathbf{y}_i\right)/\alpha\right)^{-1}}{\alpha^2}\right.$$
$$\left. + \frac{15\left(1 + 2H_{\mathbf{x}_i,c}\left(\mathbf{y}_i\right)/\alpha\right)^{-3/2}}{\alpha^3}\right)$$

The population survival, density, and hazard function for a subject with covariate information $\mathbf{x}$ are easily obtained from (4.3)–(4.5):

$$S_{\mathbf{x},f}(t) = \mathcal{L}\left(H_{\mathbf{x},c}(t)\right) = \exp\left\{\alpha\left[1 - \left(1 + 2\alpha^{-1}H_{\mathbf{x},c}(t)\right)^{1/2}\right]\right\} \qquad (4.49)$$

$$f_{\mathbf{x},f}(t) = -\mathcal{L}^{(1)}\left(H_{\mathbf{x},c}(t)\right) h_{\mathbf{x},c}(t)$$

$$= \mathcal{L}\left(H_{\mathbf{x},c}(t)\right)\left(1 + 2\alpha^{-1}H_{\mathbf{x},c}(t)\right)^{-1/2} h_{\mathbf{x},c}(t)$$

$$= S_{\mathbf{x},f}(t)\left(1 + 2\alpha^{-1}H_{\mathbf{x},c}(t)\right)^{-1/2} h_{\mathbf{x},c}(t)$$

and

$$h_{\mathbf{x},f}(t) = \frac{-\mathcal{L}^{(1)}\left(H_{\mathbf{x},c}(t)\right) h_{\mathbf{x},c}(t)}{\mathcal{L}\left(H_{\mathbf{x},c}(t)\right)}$$

$$= \left(1 + 2\alpha^{-1}H_{\mathbf{x},c}(t)\right)^{-1/2} h_{\mathbf{x},c}(t) \qquad (4.50)$$

The ratio of the population hazard and the conditional hazard is

$$\frac{h_{\mathbf{x},f}(t)}{h_{\mathbf{x},c}(t)} = \left(1 + 2\alpha^{-1} H_{\mathbf{x},c}(t)\right)^{-1/2}$$

or, in terms of the population survival function,

$$\frac{h_{\mathbf{x},f}(t)}{h_{\mathbf{x},c}(t)} = \left\{1 + \frac{\log\left(S_{\mathbf{x},f}(t)\right)}{\alpha}\left[\frac{\log\left(S_{\mathbf{x},f}(t)\right)}{\alpha} - 2\right]\right\}^{-1/2}$$

The time evolution of this ratio is presented in Figure 4.12 for different values of θ. Clearly, the ratio starts at one (both hazards are equal at time zero, i.e., at $S_{\mathbf{x},f}(0) = 1$) and decreases when time increases (or decreasing population survival function $S_{\mathbf{x},f}(t)$), with a steeper decrease for higher values of θ.

The population hazard ratio for a binary covariate is given by

$$HR_p(t) = \frac{\left(1 + 2\alpha^{-1} H_0(t)\right)^{1/2}}{\left(1 + 2\alpha^{-1} H_0(t)\exp(\beta)\right)^{1/2}} \exp(\beta)$$

So also in the case of an inverse Gaussian frailty distribution, the population hazard ratio is not constant over time although the hazard ratio in the conditional model is. The case with constant hazard ratio equal to two in the conditional model is presented in Figure 4.13 for different values of θ.

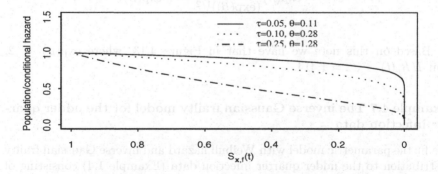

Fig. 4.12. The ratio of the population and the conditional hazard function for the inverse Gaussian frailty distribution for different values of θ.

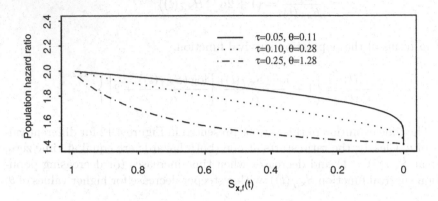

Fig. 4.13. The evolution of the population hazard ratio as a function of the population survival function for the conditional hazard ratio equal to two for the inverse Gaussian frailty distribution for different values of θ.

Note that

$$\lim_{t \to \infty} HR_p(t) = \exp(\beta) \lim_{t \to \infty} \left(\frac{1 + 2\alpha^{-1}H_0(t)}{1 + 2\alpha^{-1}H_0(t)\exp(\beta)} \right)^{1/2}$$

$$= \exp(\beta) \frac{1}{(\exp(\beta))^{1/2}} = \sqrt{\exp(\beta)}$$

Based on this note we have that in Figure 4.13, where $\exp(\beta) = 2$, $\lim_{t \to \infty} HR_p(t) = \sqrt{2} = 1.414$.

Example 4.7 The inverse Gaussian frailty model for the udder quarter infection data

We fit the parametric model with Weibull hazard and inverse Gaussian frailty distribution to the udder quarter infection data (Example 1.4) consisting of four units per cluster. We include the binary variable heifer as covariate. We maximise the marginal likelihood, which is the summation of (4.48) over the clusters. This leads to the parameter estimates $\hat{\lambda} = 0.903$ (s.e. $= 0.315$), $\hat{\rho} = 2.059$ (s.e. $= 0.109$), $\hat{\beta} = 0.502$ (s.e. $= 0.322$), and $\hat{\alpha} = 0.135$ resulting in $\hat{\theta} = 7.407$ (s.e. $= 3.166$).

The conditional hazard functions for three different frailties corresponding to the 25th, 50th, and 75th quantiles of the frailty distribution with $\hat{\alpha} = 0.135$ and the population hazard function are depicted in Figure 4.14 for primiparous and multiparous cows. It is clear that the conditional hazard in both groups is increasing over time and at a faster rate for cows with a high frailty value. On the contrary, the population hazard increases mainly in the first two months, after that the population hazard increases very little. The same evolution is observed in primiparous and multiparous cows, with the multiparous cows having a higher hazard. The evolution of the population hazard ratio is depicted in Figure 4.15 and contrasted with $\exp(\hat{\beta}) = 1.652$, the constant conditional hazard ratio. ■

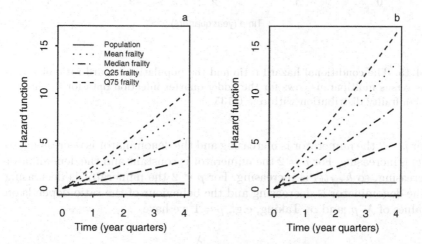

Fig. 4.14. The conditional and population hazard functions for the udder quarter infection for (a) primiparous and (b) multiparous cows for the inverse Gaussian frailty distribution with $\hat{\alpha} = 0.135$.

To understand the shape of the population hazard function in Figure 4.14, note that, for a Weibull baseline and for covariate information $\mathbf{x} = \mathbf{0}$, we obtain from (4.50) that the population hazard takes the form

$$h_{\mathbf{x},f}(t) = \left(1 + 2\alpha^{-1}\lambda t^{\rho}\right)^{-1/2} \lambda\rho t^{\rho-1}$$

$$= \frac{\lambda\rho t^{\rho-1}}{t^{\rho/2}\left(t^{-\rho} + 2\alpha^{-1}\lambda\right)^{1/2}}$$

$$= \frac{\lambda\rho t^{\rho/2-1}}{\left(t^{-\rho} + 2\alpha^{-1}\lambda\right)^{1/2}} \tag{4.51}$$

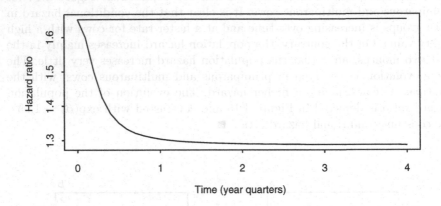

Fig. 4.15. The conditional hazard ratio and the population hazard ratio of primiparous versus multiparous cows for the udder quarter infection data for the inverse Gaussian frailty distribution with $\hat{\alpha} = 0.135$.

For $\rho > 2$ the numerator is increasing and the denominator is decreasing, so $h_{\mathbf{x},f}(t)$ is increasing. For $\rho = 2$ the numerator is constant and the denominator is decreasing, so $h_{\mathbf{x},f}(t)$ is increasing. For $\rho < 2$ the numerator is decreasing and the denominator is decreasing and the behaviour of the ratio depends on the values of λ, ρ, and α. Taking, e.g., $\rho = 1$ we have

$$h_{\mathbf{x},f}(t) = \frac{\lambda}{(1 + 2\alpha^{-1}\lambda t)^{1/2}} \tag{4.52}$$

which is decreasing in t.

4.3.3 Updating

The frailty density conditional on having survived until time t does not belong to the family of inverse Gaussian distributions, but still to the extended family of generalised inverse Gaussian distributions. More details are given in Hougaard (2000).

4.3.4 Copula form representation

The joint survival function can be rewritten as a copula.

Since $\mathcal{L}^{-1}(s) = \dfrac{\log s}{2}\left(\dfrac{\log s}{\alpha} - 2\right)$, we obtain from (4.6) for bivariate data without covariates

$$S_f(t_1, t_2) = \mathcal{L}\left[\mathcal{L}^{-1}(S_{1,f}(t_1)) + \mathcal{L}^{-1}(S_{2,f}(t_2))\right]$$

$$= \exp\left\{\alpha - \alpha\{1 + \alpha^{-2}\left[\log S_{1,f}(t_1)(\log S_{1,f}(t_1) - 2\alpha)\right.\right.$$

$$\left.\left. + \log S_{2,f}(t_2)(\log S_{2,f}(t_2) - 2\alpha)\right]\}^{1/2}\right\}$$

$$= \exp\left\{\alpha - \left[\alpha^2 + \log S_{1,f}(t_1)(\log S_{1,f}(t_1) - 2\alpha)\right.\right.$$

$$\left.\left. + \log S_{2,f}(t_2)(\log S_{2,f}(t_2) - 2\alpha)\right]^{1/2}\right\} \tag{4.53}$$

With

$$y = \alpha^2 + \log S_{1,f}(t_1)(\log S_{1,f}(t_1) - 2\alpha) + \log S_{2,f}(t_2)(\log S_{2,f}(t_2) - 2\alpha) \tag{4.54}$$

we have $S_f(t_1, t_2) = \exp(\alpha - y^{1/2})$. We use this shorthand notation to derive the joint density function

$$\frac{\partial}{\partial t_j} S_f(t_1, t_2) = S_f(t_1, t_2)\left(-0.5 y^{-1/2}\right)\left[-\frac{f_{j,f}(t_j)}{S_{j,f}(t_j)}(\log S_{j,f}(t_j) - 2\alpha)\right.$$

$$\left. + \log S_{j,f}(t_j)\left(-\frac{f_{j,f}(t_j)}{S_{j,f}(t_j)}\right)\right]$$

$$= S_f(t_1, t_2) y^{-1/2} h_{j,f}(t_j)(\log S_{j,f}(t_j) - \alpha) \tag{4.55}$$

and therefore $f_f(t_1, t_2)$ corresponds to

$$\frac{\partial^2}{\partial t_1 \partial t_2} S_f(t_1, t_2) = S_f(t_1, t_2) h_{1,f}(t_1) h_{2,f}(t_2)\left(y^{-1} + y^{-3/2}\right)$$

$$\times (\log S_{1,f}(t_1) - \alpha)(\log S_{2,f}(t_2) - \alpha) \tag{4.56}$$

The copula-based likelihood (3.20) can be given in an explicit way using (4.53)–(4.56) and can then be maximised to obtain parameter estimates starting from the copula formulation.

Example 4.8 Inverse Gaussian frailty models and copulas for time to diagnosis of being healed

The time to diagnosis data (Example 1.2) are now analysed using the frailty model (3.35) with different Weibull parameters for the US and RX diagnosis time but now assuming the inverse Gaussian frailty distribution. Parameter estimates can be obtained by maximising the sum of the loglikelihood contributions (4.48) over the different clusters. This leads to estimates $\hat{\lambda}_1 = 0.152$ (s.e. = 0.067), $\hat{\rho}_1 = 4.53$ (s.e. = 0.352) for RX, $\hat{\lambda}_2 = 0.438$ (s.e. = 0.192), $\hat{\rho}_2 = 4.205$ (s.e. = 0.337) for US, and finally $\hat{\theta} = 11.76$ (s.e. = 7.33) (and thus $\hat{\alpha} = 1/11.76 = 0.085$).

Alternatively, the two-stage estimation approach can be used. First, we ignore the correlation in the data and estimate the parameters for the Weibull models of the time to diagnosis data separately for the ultrasound (US) and radiography (RX) data. These parameter estimates are already presented in Example 3.5. Next we use the copula function presented in (4.53), where we replace the population survival functions obtained from the inverse Gaussian frailty model, $S_{1,f}(t_1)$ and $S_{2,f}(t_2)$, by the population survival functions $S_{1,p}(t_1)$ and $S_{2,p}(t_2)$ obtained from the marginal approach, i.e., we use

$$S_p(t_1, t_2) = \exp\Big\{\tilde{\alpha} - \big[\tilde{\alpha}^2 + \log S_{1,p}(t_1)(\log S_{1,p}(t_1) - 2\tilde{\alpha})$$

$$+ \log S_{2,p}(t_2)(\log S_{2,p}(t_2) - 2\tilde{\alpha})\big]^{1/2}\Big\} \tag{4.57}$$

We use $\tilde{\alpha}$ in (4.57) to stress that the meaning of the parameter is different from the meaning of α in (4.53). In Step 1 of the two-stage estimation approach we obtain estimates $\hat{S}_{j,p}(t)$ for $S_{j,p}(t)$, $j = 1, 2$, and we use these estimates in (4.57); in Step 2 the likelihood is then maximized with respect to the copula parameters. The copula form is essentially the same, but the population survival functions used in (4.57) are different from the population survival functions used in (4.53). In a similar way, the population hazard and density functions in (4.55) and (4.56) can be replaced by the estimates obtained from the marginal estimation approach. From these expressions the likelihood contribution for each cluster can be obtained and the sum of the loglikelihood contributions over the different clusters can then be maximised to obtain a parameter estimate for the only unknown parameter $\tilde{\alpha}$. This leads to an estimate for $\tilde{\alpha}$ equal to 0.062, and thus an estimate for $\tilde{\theta} = 1/\tilde{\alpha}$ equal to 16.21 (s.e. = 13.56). So the two techniques do not lead to the same parameter estimates. The resulting population hazard functions are depicted in Figure 4.16. ∎

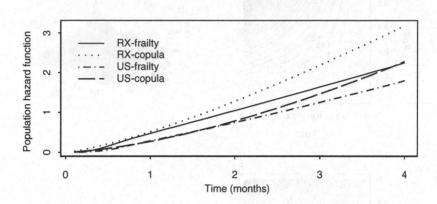

Fig. 4.16. The population hazard functions from the frailty model and the copula model with inverse Gaussian frailty distribution for the time to diagnosis of healing data assessed by either US or RX.

4.3.5 Dependence measures

In Section 4.5 we will show that the inverse Gaussian distribution is a member of the family of the power variance function distributions. For this family, (4.87) gives a general expression for Kendall's τ. For the inverse Gaussian distribution (take (4.87) with parameter $\nu = 0.5$ and $\alpha = 1/\theta$) we obtain

$$\tau = 0.5 - \alpha + 2\alpha^2 \exp(2\alpha) \int\limits_{2\alpha}^{\infty} u^{-1} \exp(-u)du \qquad (4.58)$$

Since

$$\int\limits_{2\alpha}^{\infty} u^{-1} \exp(-u)du \leq \frac{1}{2\alpha} \int\limits_{2\alpha}^{\infty} \exp(-u)du = \frac{1}{2\alpha} \exp(-2\alpha)$$

we easily obtain that $\tau \leq 1/2$.

To depict the evolution of the dependence in time, we can either use a contour plot (Figure 4.17a) or a three-dimensional plot (Figure 4.17b) of $\psi(t_1, t_2)$, the ratio of the joint survival function (4.53) and the product of the population survival functions (4.49).

Using (4.56) it is straightforward that, with y as in (4.54), the ratio of the joint density function and the product of the population density functions is

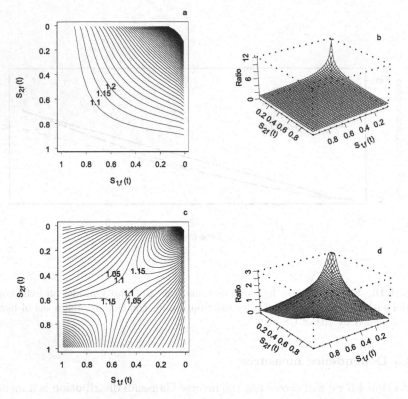

Fig. 4.17. The ratio of the joint survival function and the product of the population survival functions (a,b) and the ratio of the joint density function and the product of the population density functions (c,d) for the inverse Gaussian frailty distribution with $\tau=0.25$.

given by

$$\phi(t_1, t_2) = \frac{f_f(t_1, t_2)}{f_{1,f}(t_1) f_{2,f}(t_2)}$$

$$= \frac{S_f(t_1, t_2)}{S_{1,f}(t_1) S_{2,f}(t_2)} \left(\log S_{1,f}(t_1) - \alpha\right) \left(\log S_{2,f}(t_2) - \alpha\right)$$

$$\times \left(y^{-1} + y^{-3/2}\right)$$

and a graphical representation of this relationship is given in Figures 4.17c and 4.17d. The relationships presented in Figure 4.17 for the inverse Gaussian frailty distribution are similar to those of the gamma frailty distribution presented in Figure 4.8. The main difference is that the contour lines for the joint density function are closer together early in time (left lower corner) for the inverse Gaussian implying that, compared to the gamma frailty distribution, the dependence is stronger early in time for the inverse Gaussian frailty distribution. Additionally, the contour lines for the joint density function are closer together late in time (right upper corner) for the gamma distribution implying that dependence is stronger late in time for the gamma frailty distribution.

Using (4.53)–(4.56) in the general form for the cross ratio function (4.13) it follows that

$$\zeta(t_1, t_2) = 1 + y^{-1/2}$$

Note that $S_f(t_1, t_2) = \exp\left(\alpha - y^{1/2}\right)$, therefore, $y^{1/2} = \alpha - \log S_f(t_1, t_2)$ and

$$\zeta(t_1, t_2) = 1 + \frac{1}{\alpha - \log\left(S_f(t_1, t_2)\right)}$$

This relationship is shown in Figure 4.18. The highest value is obtained at the start and equals $1 + 1/\alpha$, and goes to one as the survival function goes to zero.

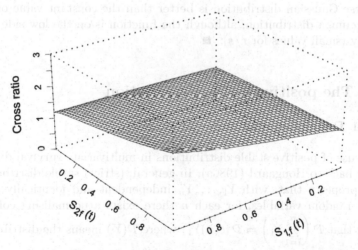

Fig. 4.18. Cross ratio function for the inverse Gaussian frailty distribution with $\tau = 0.25$.

4.3.6 Diagnostics

We can make use of the estimate of $\gamma(r)$ which is asymptotically equivalent to the cross ratio function proposed in Section 4.2.6 and compare it to the estimate based on the frailty model with inverse Gaussian frailty distribution, as is demonstrated in Example 4.9.

Example 4.9 Diagnostics for the inverse Gaussian frailty distribution for time to diagnosis of being healed based on the cross ratio function

In Example 4.6 the nonparametric estimate of $\gamma(r)$ of the cross ratio function was plotted for the time to diagnosis data (Example 1.2), together with the time-constant cross ratio function estimated from the gamma distribution. We now replace the cross ratio function estimate from the gamma distribution with that of the inverse Gaussian distribution, which is given by

$$\zeta\left(S_f\left(t_1, t_2\right)\right) = 1 + \frac{1}{\alpha - \log\left(S_f\left(t_1, t_2\right)\right)}$$

with $\alpha = 0.085$. As discussed previously in Section 4.2.7, $\gamma(r)$ is asymptotically equivalent to $\zeta\left(S_f\left(t_1, t_2\right)\right)$ if $r/s \to S_f\left(t_1, t_2\right)$. The relationship is depicted in Figure 4.19. It is obvious that the cross ratio function estimated from the inverse Gaussian distribution is better than the constant value obtained for the gamma distribution, although the function is on the low side late in the study (small values for r/s). ∎

4.4 The positive stable distribution

4.4.1 Definitions and basic properties

The use of positive stable distributions in multivariate survival data analysis goes back to Hougaard (1986a). In general, (strict) stable distributions have the property that, with $Y_1, \ldots, Y_n$ independent and identically distributed (iid) random variables, for each n there exists a normalising constant $c(n)$ such that $\mathcal{D}\left(\sum_{i=1}^{n} Y_i\right) = \mathcal{D}\left(c(n)Y_1\right)$ where $\mathcal{D}(Y)$ means the distribution (law) of Y. The constant $c(n)$ takes form $n^{1/\theta}$ with $\theta \in (0, 2]$, θ being called the characteristic exponent (see Feller (1971), Chapter 6.1).

The standard normal density function is a stable density. Indeed, for iid standard normal distributed random variables $Y_1, \ldots, Y_n$ we have $\mathcal{D}\left(\sum_{i=1}^{n} Y_i\right) = \mathcal{D}\left(n^{1/2}Y_1\right)$, i.e., $\theta = 2$. The stable distributions on the positive half line have $\theta \in (0, 1]$ ($\theta = 1$ corresponds to the degenerate distribution) and are called the

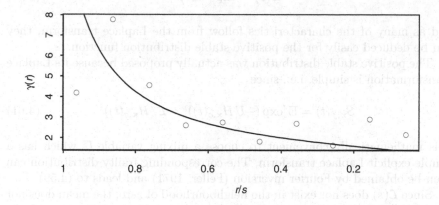

Fig. 4.19. The estimate of $\gamma(r)$ plotted against r/s for the time to diagnosis data. Adjacent r_a values are combined in groups 1–10, 11–20, ..., 91–100, and the average of the r_a values within each group, divided by s, is used as value to be plotted on the x-axis. The solid line is the cross ratio function estimated from the inverse Gaussian distribution frailty model.

positive stable distributions. For a detailed discussion we refer to Chapters 13.6 and 17.6 in Feller (1971). To link this with frailty distributions we set $U = Y_1$; the density function is then given by

$$f_U(u) = -\frac{1}{\pi u} \sum_{k=1}^{\infty} \frac{\Gamma(k\theta+1)}{k!} \left(-u^{-\theta}\right)^k \sin(\theta k\pi) \qquad (4.59)$$

with $0 < \theta < 1$. This density function has infinite mean and the variance is therefore also undetermined. At first sight, an infinite mean is more difficult to work with but the infinite mean is actually one of the main reasons why this density function was proposed. Only density functions with infinite mean have the property that the heterogeneity parameter is independent from the covariate information as shown by Hougaard (1986b). Furthermore, it is often stated as an attractive property of the positive stable frailty distribution that the proportionality property for the conditional hazard is inherited by the population hazard (with another proportionality constant (see (4.73) for a proof)). In our opinion, however, this is only an advantage if it is supported by the data information; it is rather the data that should guide the choice of the frailty distribution and not an attractive mathematical model property.

The Laplace transform has the simple form

$$\mathcal{L}(s) = \exp\left(-s^\theta\right) \tag{4.60}$$

and as many of the characteristics follow from the Laplace transform, they can be deduced easily for the positive stable distribution function.

The positive stable distribution was actually proposed because its Laplace transformation is simple, i.e., since

$$S_{\mathbf{x},f}(t) = \mathrm{E}\left[\exp\left(-U H_{\mathbf{x},c}(t)\right)\right] = \mathcal{L}\left(H_{\mathbf{x},c}(t)\right) \tag{4.61}$$

it is mathematically convenient to choose a mixing variable U which has a simple explicit Laplace transform. The corresponding frailty distribution can then be obtained by Fourier inversion (Feller, 1971) and leads to (4.59).

Since $\mathcal{L}(s)$ does not exist in the neighbourhood of zero, the mean does not exist; by taking the right limit of $\mathcal{L}(s)$ for $s \to 0$ we, indeed, do get evidence for the fact that the mean is infinite:

$$\lim_{\substack{s \to 0 \\ >}} \mathcal{L}^{(1)}(s) = -\theta \lim_{\substack{s \to 0 \\ >}} \frac{\exp\left(-s^\theta\right)}{s^{1-\theta}} = -\infty$$

Some specific density functions are given in Figure 4.20. For values of θ equal to or above 0.9, the probability of finding a frailty value below or equal to 4 is small (these cases are not shown in the figure).

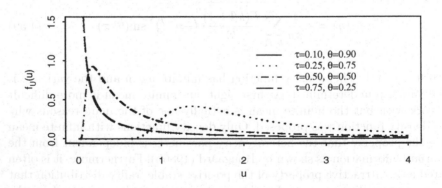

Fig. 4.20. Positive stable density functions.

4.4.2 Joint and population survival function

The joint survival function is given by

$$S_{x,f}(t_n) = \exp\left(-H_{x,c}^\theta(t_n)\right) \tag{4.62}$$

The joint density function can be obtained from the nth derivative of the Laplace transform, but as for the inverse Gaussian distribution, no simple expression exists, and therefore we will again only compute the first four derivatives and derive the marginal likelihood for clusters of size four.

The first four derivatives of the Laplace transform are given by

$$\mathcal{L}^{(1)}(s) = -\theta\mathcal{L}(s)s^{\theta-1} \tag{4.63}$$

$$\mathcal{L}^{(2)}(s) = \theta^2\mathcal{L}(s)s^{2(\theta-1)}\left(1 + \theta^{-1}(1-\theta)s^{-\theta}\right) \tag{4.64}$$

$$\mathcal{L}^{(3)}(s) = -\theta^3\mathcal{L}(s)s^{3(\theta-1)}\left(1 + 3\theta^{-1}(1-\theta)s^{-\theta}\right.$$
$$\left. + \theta^{-2}(1-\theta)(2-\theta)s^{-2\theta}\right) \tag{4.65}$$

$$\mathcal{L}^{(4)}(s) = \theta^4\mathcal{L}(s)s^{4(\theta-1)}\left(1 + 6\theta^{-1}(1-\theta)s^{-\theta} + \theta^{-2}(1-\theta)(11-7\theta)s^{-2\theta}\right.$$
$$\left. + \theta^{-3}(1-\theta)(2-\theta)(3-\theta)s^{-3\theta}\right) \tag{4.66}$$

As we did in Section 4.3.2 for the inverse Gaussian we will demonstrate the use of these derivatives in the construction of the marginal likelihood. Again we consider the specific situation of clusters of size four with right-censored observations. From (4.63)–(4.66) it easily follows that the contribution of the ith cluster with covariate information x_i to the marginal loglikelihood is, with $y_i = (y_{i1}, y_{i2}, y_{i3}, y_{i4})^t$,

$$\sum_{j=1}^{4} \delta_{ij}\log\left(h_0(y_{ij})\exp\left(x_{ij}^t\beta\right)\right) - H_{x_i,c}^\theta(y_i) + d_i\log\theta$$
$$+ d_i(\theta-1)\log H_{x_i,c}(y_i) + C_{i,d_i} \tag{4.67}$$

where C_{i,d_i} is a term that depends on the number of events in the cluster.

Below we give this term for up to four events per cluster:

$$C_{i,0} = C_{i,1} = 0$$

$$C_{i,2} = \log\left(1 + \theta^{-1}(1-\theta)H_{\mathbf{x}_i,c}^{-\theta}(\mathbf{y}_i)\right)$$

$$C_{i,3} = \log\left(1 + 3\theta^{-1}(1-\theta)H_{\mathbf{x}_i,c}^{-\theta}(\mathbf{y}_i) + \theta^{-2}(2-\theta)(1-\theta)H_{\mathbf{x}_i,c}^{-2\theta}(\mathbf{y}_i)\right)$$

$$C_{i,4} = \log\left(1 + 6\theta^{-1}(1-\theta)H_{\mathbf{x}_i,c}^{-\theta}(\mathbf{y}_i) + \theta^{-2}(1-\theta)(11-7\theta)H_{\mathbf{x}_i,c}^{-2\theta}(\mathbf{y}_i)\right.$$
$$\left. + \theta^{-3}(3-\theta)(2-\theta)(1-\theta)H_{\mathbf{x}_i,c}^{-3\theta}(\mathbf{y}_i)\right)$$

The population survival and density functions are given by

$$S_{\mathbf{x},f}(t) = \exp\left(-H_{\mathbf{x},c}^{\theta}(t)\right) \tag{4.68}$$

$$f_{\mathbf{x},f}(t) = S_{\mathbf{x},f}(t)\theta H_{\mathbf{x},c}^{\theta-1}(t)h_{\mathbf{x},c}(t) \tag{4.69}$$

and therefore the population hazard function is

$$h_{\mathbf{x},f}(t) = \theta H_{\mathbf{x},c}^{\theta-1}(t)h_{\mathbf{x},c}(t) \tag{4.70}$$

The ratio of the population and the conditional hazard is

$$\frac{h_{\mathbf{x},f}(t)}{h_{\mathbf{x},c}(t)} = \theta H_{\mathbf{x},c}^{\theta-1}(t) \tag{4.71}$$

or in terms of the population survival function,

$$\frac{h_{\mathbf{x},f}(t)}{h_{\mathbf{x},c}(t)} = \theta\left(-\log S_{\mathbf{x},f}(t)\right)^{1-1/\theta} \tag{4.72}$$

The time evolution of this ratio is presented in Figure 4.21 for different values of θ. We note, however, that these curves do not make much sense in the setting of the positive stable frailty distribution. The population hazard function is compared with the conditional hazard function for a subject with frailty equal to one. Setting the frailty equal to one makes sense for frailty distributions which have mean equal one. This is the case for all the frailty distributions studied in this chapter, except for the lognormal distribution (see Section 4.7) and the positive stable distribution. The mean for the positive stable distribution is equal to infinity, therefore the population hazard function cannot be compared to the conditional hazard function.

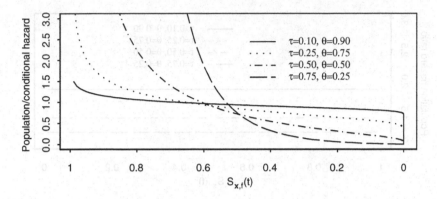

Fig. 4.21. The ratio of the population and the conditional hazard function for the positive stable frailty distribution for different values of θ.

One of the reasons why Hougaard (1986b) advocated the distribution was due to the fact that also marginally the hazard ratio is constant over time if that is the case for the conditional model. This can be shown as follows. The population hazard ratio for a binary covariate is given by

$$HR_p(t) = \frac{\theta H_0^{\theta-1}(t)\exp((\theta-1)\beta)h_0(t)\exp(\beta)}{\theta H_0^{\theta-1}(t)h_0(t)} = \exp(\theta\beta) \qquad (4.73)$$

This shows that the proportionality property for the conditional hazard is inherited by the population hazard (but with a different proportionality constant: $\theta\beta$ instead of β). Since $0 < \theta < 1$ the population hazard ratio will typically be closer to one, and the more $\theta\beta$ deviates from β (i.e., the more θ deviates from one) the more the population hazard ratio will deviate from the conditional hazard ratio.

The case with the hazard ratio in the conditional model equal to two is presented in Figure 4.22 for different values of θ.

Example 4.10 The positive stable frailty model for the udder quarter infection data

We fit the parametric model with Weibull hazard and positive stable frailty distribution to the udder quarter infection data (Example 1.4) having four units per cluster. We include the binary variable heifer as covariate. We maximise the marginal likelihood (4.67). This leads to the parameter estimates

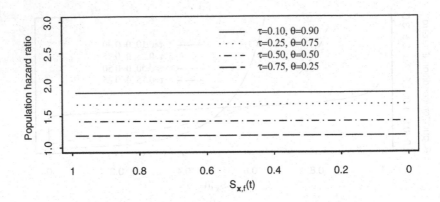

Fig. 4.22. The evolution of the population hazard ratio as a function of the population survival function for the conditional hazard ratio equal to two for the positive stable frailty distribution for different values of θ.

$\hat{\lambda} = 0.177$ (s.e. $= 0.052$), $\hat{\rho} = 2.129$ (s.e. $= 0.114$), $\hat{\beta} = 0.537$ (s.e. $= 0.351$) and $\hat{\theta} = 0.529$ (s.e. $= 0.039$).

Note that the parameter estimate $\hat{\lambda}$ is quite different from the parameter estimate obtained from either the gamma or the inverse Gaussian frailty distribution. This is due to the fact that the mean of the positive stable frailty distribution is infinite (for the frailty distributions considered so far the mean was one).

The conditional hazard functions for three different frailties corresponding to the 25th, 50th, and 75th quantiles of the frailty distribution and the population hazard function are depicted in Figure 4.23 for primiparous and multiparous cows. It is clear that the conditional hazard in both groups is increasing over time and at a faster rate for cows with a high frailty value. On the contrary, the population hazard increases mainly in the first two months, after that the population hazard increases very little. The same evolution is observed in primiparous and multiparous cows, with the multiparous cows having a higher hazard.

The estimated population hazard ratio is constant over time and equal to $\exp(\hat{\theta}\hat{\beta}) = 1.33$ compared to the estimate of the constant hazard ratio within a cluster which is equal to $\exp(\hat{\beta}) = 1.71$. ∎

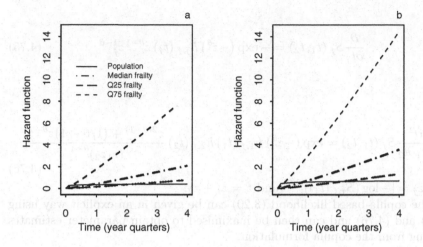

Fig. 4.23. The conditional and population hazard functions for the udder quarter infection for (a) primiparous and (b) multiparous cows for the positive stable frailty distribution.

4.4.3 Updating

Conditional on $T > t$, i.e., survival beyond time t, the frailty density takes the form (see (4.10))

$$f_U(u \mid T > t) = \frac{\exp\left(-uH_0(t)\right) f_U(u)}{\exp\left(-H_0^\theta(t)\right)}$$

$$= \exp\left(-H_0(t)\left(u - H_0^{\theta-1}(t)\right)\right) f_U(u)$$

This density function does no longer belong to the family of positive stable distributions, but is still a member of the extended class of the power variance function family discussed in Section 4.5.

4.4.4 Copula form representation

Since $\mathcal{L}^{-1}(s) = (-\log s)^{1/\theta}$ we easily obtain from (4.6) the bivariate survival function (copula version)

$$S_f(t_1, t_2) = \exp\left\{-\left[(-\log S_{1,f}(t_1))^{1/\theta} + (-\log S_{2,f}(t_2))^{1/\theta}\right]^\theta\right\} \qquad (4.74)$$

The first and second derivatives of this bivariate survival function are given by

$$\frac{\partial}{\partial t_j} S_f (t_1, t_2) = - \exp \left(-z^\theta \right) h_{j,f} (t_j) \, z^{\theta-1} z_j^{1-\theta} \tag{4.75}$$

and

$$\frac{\partial^2}{\partial t_1 \partial t_2} S_f (t_1, t_2) = \exp \left(-z^\theta \right) h_{1,f} (t_1) \, h_{2,f} (t_2) \, \frac{z^{2(\theta-1)} + (1/\theta - 1) z^{\theta-2}}{(z_1 z_2)^{\theta-1}} \tag{4.76}$$

with $z_j = [- \log (S_{j,f} (t_j))]^{1/\theta}$ and $z = z_1 + z_2$.

The copula-based likelihood (3.20) can be given in an explicit way using (4.75) and (4.76) and can then be maximised to obtain parameter estimates starting from the copula formulation.

Example 4.11 Positive stable frailty models and copulas for time to diagnosis of being healed

The time to diagnosis data (Example 1.2) are now analysed using the frailty model (3.35) with different Weibull parameters for the US and RX diagnosis time but now assuming the positive stable frailty distribution. This leads to estimates $\hat{\lambda}_1 = 0.0200$ (s.e. $= 0.009$), $\hat{\rho}_1 = 4.56$ (s.e. $= 0.438$) for RX, $\hat{\lambda}_2 = 0.0586$ (s.e. $= 0.021$), $\hat{\rho}_2 = 4.24$ (s.e. $= 0.411$) for US, and finally $\hat{\theta} = 0.546$ (s.e. $= 0.053$).

Alternatively, the two-stage estimation approach can be used. As for the gamma and inverse Gaussian copula, we first ignore the correlation in the data and estimate the parameters for the Weibull models separately for the ultrasound (US) and radiography (RX) data. These parameter estimates were obtained in Example 3.5. Next we use the copula function presented in (4.74), where we replace the population survival functions obtained from the positive stable frailty model, $S_{1,f}(t_1)$ and $S_{2,f}(t_2)$, by the population survival functions $S_{1,p}(t_1)$ and $S_{2,p}(t_2)$ obtained from the marginal approach, i.e., we use

$$S_p (t_1, t_2) = \exp \left\{ - \left[(- \log S_{1,p}(t_1))^{1/\tilde{\theta}} + (- \log S_{2,p}(t_2))^{1/\tilde{\theta}} \right]^{\tilde{\theta}} \right\} \tag{4.77}$$

We use $\tilde{\theta}$ in (4.77) to stress that the meaning of the parameter is different from the meaning of θ in (4.74). In Step 1 of the two-stage estimation approach we obtain estimates $\hat{S}_{j,p}(t)$ for $S_{j,p}(t)$, $j = 1, 2$, and we use these estimates in (4.77); in Step 2 the likelihood is then maximized with respect to the copula parameters. The copula form is essentially the same as in (4.74), but the population survival functions used in (4.77) are different from the population survival functions used in (4.74). In a similar way, the population hazard and density functions in (4.75) and (4.76) can be replaced by the estimates obtained from the marginal estimation approach. From these expressions the likelihood contribution for each cluster can be obtained and the sum of the loglikelihood contributions over the different clusters can then be maximised to obtain a parameter estimate for the only unknown parameter $\tilde{\theta}$. The estimate for $\tilde{\theta}$ equals 0.563 (s.e. = 0.045). So the two techniques do not lead to the same parameter estimates. The combined set of parameters, however, leads to essentially the same population hazard functions, as depicted in Figure 4.24. This is not surprising as there exists a one-to-one transformation between the parameters used in (4.74) and (4.77). Denoting the Weibull parameters from the marginal approach by $\tilde{\lambda}_1$, $\tilde{\lambda}_2$, $\tilde{\rho}_1$, $\tilde{\rho}_2$, and $\tilde{\theta}$, we can make the population survival functions equal by taking

$$\tilde{\theta} = \theta, \tilde{\lambda}_j = \lambda_j^\theta \text{ and } \tilde{\rho}_j = \theta\rho_j \tag{4.78}$$

Therefore, from a modelling point of view, the positive stable copula with marginally estimated population survival functions and the frailty model with positive stable frailty distribution result in the same population survival functions, and therefore joint survival functions, given that the parameters relate according to (4.78). However, the loglikelihood expressions that need to be maximised in the two approaches are not the same, and therefore estimated population survival functions from the two approaches are not necessarily exactly the same. ■

4.4.5 Dependence measures

Kendall's τ for the positive stable distribution can be derived using (4.12):

$$\tau = 4 \int_0^\infty s\mathcal{L}(s)\mathcal{L}^{(2)}(s)ds - 1$$

$$= 4 \int_0^\infty s\theta^2 \exp(-s^\theta)s^{2(\theta-1)} \exp(-s^\theta)ds$$

$$+ 4 \int_0^\infty s\theta^2 \exp(-s^\theta)s^{2(\theta-1)}\theta^{-1}(1-\theta)s^{-\theta} \exp(-s^\theta)ds - 1$$

$$= 4\frac{\theta}{4} + 4\left(\frac{1-\theta}{2}\right) - 1 = 1 - \theta$$

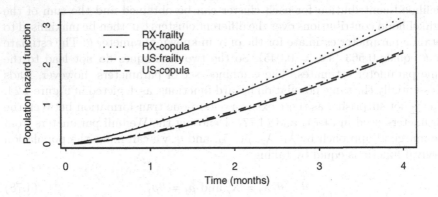

Fig. 4.24. The population hazard functions from the frailty model and the copula model with positive stable frailty distribution for the time to diagnosis of healing data assessed by either US or RX.

To depict the evolution of the dependence in time, we can use either a contour plot (Figure 4.25a) or a three-dimensional plot (Figure 4.25b) of $\psi(t_1, t_2)$, the ratio of the joint survival function (4.62), and the product of the population survival functions (4.68).

Using (4.76) it is straightforward that the ratio of the joint density function and the product of the population density functions is given by

$$\phi(t_1, t_2) = \frac{S_f(t_1, t_2)}{S_{1,f}(t_1) S_{2,f}(t_2)} \frac{z^{2(\theta-1)} + (1/\theta - 1)z^{\theta-2}}{(z_1 z_2)^{1/\theta - 1}}$$

and a graphical representation of this relationship is given in Figures 4.25c and 4.25d.

The relationships presented in Figure 4.25 for the positive stable distribution are similar to those of the gamma frailty distribution in Figure 4.8 and the inverse Gaussian frailty distribution in Figure 4.17. The main difference is that the contour lines indicating positive correlation (e.g., 1.1) for the joint density function appear earlier in time for the positive stable distribution compared to the gamma and inverse Gaussian frailty distribution, implying that the dependence is stronger earlier in time for the positive stable frailty distribution. The positive stable distribution and the gamma distribution are characterised by early and late dependence respectively, with the inverse Gaussian distribution taking a position in between the two.

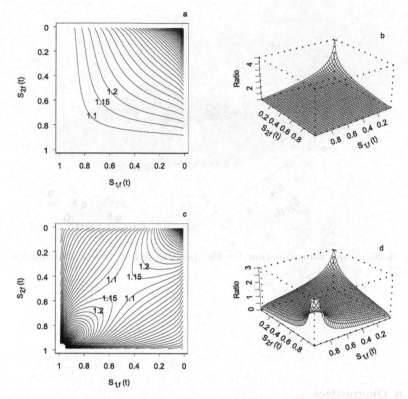

Fig. 4.25. The ratio of the joint survival function and the product of the population survival functions (a,b) and the ratio of the joint density function and the product of the population density functions (c,d) for the positive stable frailty distribution with τ=0.25.

Using (4.75) and (4.76) in the general expression for the cross ratio function (4.13) it follows that

$$\zeta(t_1, t_2) = 1 + \frac{\theta - 1}{\theta \log S_f(t_1, t_2)} \tag{4.79}$$

This relationship is shown in Figure 4.26.

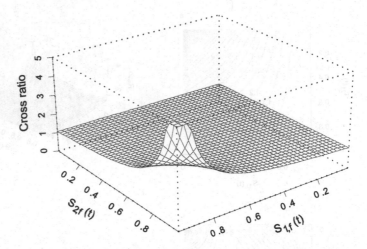

Fig. 4.26. Cross ratio function for the positive stable frailty distribution with $\tau=0.25$.

4.4.6 Diagnostics

We can make use of the estimate of $\gamma(r)$ which is asymptotically equivalent to the cross ratio function given in (4.79) and compare it to the estimate based on the frailty model with positive stable frailty distribution, as is demonstrated in Example 4.12.

Example 4.12 Diagnostics for the positive stable frailty distribution for time to diagnosis of being healed based on the cross ratio function

In Examples 4.6 and 4.9 the estimate of $\gamma(r)$ which is asymptotically equivalent to the cross ratio function was plotted for the time to diagnosis data (Example 1.2), together with the time-constant cross ratio function estimated from the gamma distribution and the estimated cross ratio function for the inverse Gaussian distribution. We now consider the cross ratio function estimate from the positive stable frailty distribution.

Comparing Figures 4.10, 4.19, and 4.27 it is clear that assuming a gamma frailty distribution is not a good choice. Based on the pictures, choosing between the inverse Gaussian and the positive stable frailty distribution is not easy. More formal approaches, e.g., likelihood ratio tests, might be an option (see, e.g., Andersen (2005)). ∎

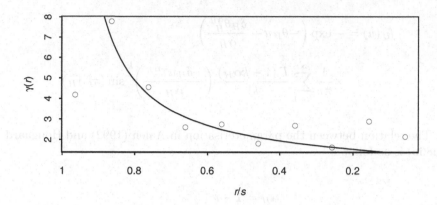

Fig. 4.27. The estimate of $\gamma(r)$ plotted against r/s for the time to diagnosis data. Adjacent r_a values are combined in groups 1–10, 11–20, ..., 91–100, and the average of the r_a values within each group, divided by s, is used as value to be plotted on the x-axis. The solid line is the cross ratio function estimated from the positive stable distribution frailty model.

4.5 The power variance function distribution

4.5.1 Definitions and basic properties

The family of the power variance function distributions was introduced as an extension of the positive stable distribution by Hougaard (1986b). It contains the gamma, inverse Gaussian, and positive stable distributions; they are obtained for choices of the parameters at the boundary of the parameter space. For that reason asymptotic arguments are needed to show that these distributions are members of the power variance function family.

The density function is given by

$$f_U(u) = \exp\left(-\frac{\nu}{\theta}\left(\frac{u}{\mu} + \frac{1}{\nu - 1}\right)\right)$$

$$\times \frac{1}{\pi u}\sum_{k=1}^{\infty}\frac{(\nu/\theta)^{k\nu}(u/\mu)^{k(\nu-1)}\,\Gamma(1 - k(\nu - 1))\sin(\pi k(\nu - 1))}{k!\,(\nu - 1)^k}$$

with $\mu > 0, \theta > 0$, and $0 < \nu \leq 1$. This definition is given in Aalen (1992). Hougaard (1986b) gives an excellent discussion on how, starting from the positive stable distribution, one can build the power variance function family. He gives the following alternative expression:

$$f_U(u) = -\exp\left(-\theta_H u + \frac{\delta_H \theta_H^{\alpha_H}}{\alpha_H}\right)$$

$$\times \frac{1}{\pi u} \sum_{k=1}^{\infty} \frac{\Gamma(1 + k\alpha_H)}{k!} \left(\frac{-\delta_H u^{-\alpha_H}}{\alpha_H}\right)^k \sin(\pi k\alpha_H)$$

The relation between the parameterisation in Aalen (1992) and Hougaard (1986b) is as follows:

$$\alpha_H = 1 - \nu$$

$$\delta_H = \mu^{1-\nu}\left(\frac{\nu}{\theta}\right)^{\nu}$$

$$\theta_H = \frac{\nu}{\mu\theta}$$

The Laplace transform is given by (Aalen, 1992)

$$\mathcal{L}(s) = \exp\left[\frac{\nu}{\theta(1-\nu)}\left(1 - \left(1 + \frac{\theta\mu s}{\nu}\right)^{1-\nu}\right)\right] \qquad (4.80)$$

with first and second derivatives given by

$$\mathcal{L}^{(1)}(s) = -\mathcal{L}(s)\mu\left(1 + \frac{\theta\mu s}{\nu}\right)^{-\nu}$$

$$\mathcal{L}^{(2)}(s) = \mathcal{L}(s)\mu^2\left(\left(1 + \frac{\theta\mu s}{\nu}\right)^{-2\nu} + \theta\left(1 + \frac{\theta\mu s}{\nu}\right)^{-\nu-1}\right)$$

Assuming that the derivatives above exist in the neighbourhood of zero (not the case for the positive stable distribution, for instance), we can evaluate them at $s = 0$ to find

$$E(U) = (-1)\mathcal{L}^{(1)}(0) = \mu$$

$$\text{Var}(U) = \mathcal{L}^{(2)}(0) - \left(-\mathcal{L}^{(1)}(0)\right)^2 = \theta\mu^2$$

Thus, the parameter μ corresponds to the mean and on the other hand

$$\theta = \frac{\text{Var}(U)}{(\text{E}(U))^2}$$

is the squared coefficient of variation. We will typically set $\mu = 1$ so that θ corresponds to the variance of the frailty. Finally, the parameter ν determines the type of dependence. For instance, for $\nu = 0.5$ (and $\mu = 1$) the Laplace transform (4.80) reduces to the Laplace transform of the inverse Gaussian frailty distribution given by (4.42) with $\alpha = 1/\theta$. With lower values for ν, the dependence is earlier in time; with values above 0.5, the dependence is later in time (see Section 4.5.5 for a more detailed discussion).

To obtain the positive stable distribution we need that the mean μ and the variance $\mu^2\theta$ tend to infinity in an appropriate way (Hougaard, 1986b). To obtain the Laplace transform of the positive stable distribution we take

$$1 - \nu = \frac{\mu^{1-\nu}\nu^\nu}{\theta^\nu} \tag{4.81}$$

or equivalently

$$\theta = \frac{\nu}{(1-\nu)^{1/\nu}}\mu^{1/\nu-1} \tag{4.82}$$

For $0 < \nu < 1$, (4.82) implies that if $\theta \to \infty$, then also $\mu \to \infty$. Moreover, we then have

$$\frac{\nu}{\mu\theta} \to 0 \tag{4.83}$$

Using (4.81)–(4.83), the Laplace transform (4.80) can be rewritten as

$$\mathcal{L}(s) = \exp\left[\frac{\nu}{\theta(1-\nu)}\left(1 - \left(1 + \frac{\theta\mu s}{\nu}\right)^{1-\nu}\right)\right]$$

$$= \exp\left[\frac{\nu\theta^\nu}{\theta\mu^{1-\nu}\nu^\nu}\left(1 - \left(\frac{\theta\mu}{\nu}\right)^{1-\nu}\left(\frac{\nu}{\theta\mu} + s\right)^{1-\nu}\right)\right]$$

$$= \exp\left[\frac{\nu\theta^\nu}{\theta\mu^{1-\nu}\nu^\nu}\left(\frac{\theta\mu}{\nu}\right)^{1-\nu}\left(\left(\frac{\nu}{\theta\mu}\right)^{1-\nu} - \left(\frac{\nu}{\theta\mu} + s\right)^{1-\nu}\right)\right]$$

$$= \exp\left(\left(\frac{\nu}{\theta\mu}\right)^{1-\nu} - \left(\frac{\nu}{\theta\mu} + s\right)^{1-\nu}\right)$$

Therefore, if (4.83) holds,

$$\lim_{\theta \to \infty} \mathcal{L}(s) = \exp\left(-s^{1-\nu}\right)$$

which corresponds to the Laplace transform (4.60) of the positive stable distribution with $1 - \nu$ in the role of θ in (4.60) (which is different from θ in (4.80)).

To obtain the gamma distribution, we restrict our attention to distributions with mean one, i.e., $\mu = 1$ with simplified power variance function Laplace transform

$$\mathcal{L}(s) = \exp\left[\frac{\nu}{\theta(1-\nu)}\left(1 - \left(1 + \frac{\theta s}{\nu}\right)^{1-\nu}\right)\right]$$

We will show that

$$\lim_{\nu \to 1} \mathcal{L}(s) = (1 + \theta s)^{-1/\theta}$$

which is the Laplace transform (4.17) of the one-parameter gamma distribution with $\theta = \text{Var}(U)$. We need to show that

$$\lim_{\nu \to 1} \frac{\nu}{\theta(1-\nu)}\left(1 - \left(1 + \frac{\theta s}{\nu}\right)^{1-\nu}\right) = -\frac{1}{\theta}\log(1 + \theta s)$$

or equivalently

$$\lim_{\nu \to 1} \frac{\nu\left(1 - \left(1 + \frac{\theta s}{\nu}\right)^{1-\nu}\right)}{1-\nu} = -\log(1 + \theta s)$$

Since the limit leads to $0/0$ we apply l'Hôpital's rule

$$\lim_{\nu \to 1} \frac{\nu\left(1 - (1 + \theta\nu^{-1}s)^{1-\nu}\right)}{1-\nu} = \lim_{\nu \to 1} \frac{\frac{d}{d\nu}\nu\left(1 - (1 + \theta\nu^{-1}s)^{1-\nu}\right)}{-1}$$

$$= \lim_{\nu \to 1}\left[-\left(1 - (1 + \theta\nu^{-1}s)^{1-\nu}\right) + \nu\left(1 + \theta\nu^{-1}s\right)^{1-\nu}\right.$$

$$\left. \times \left(-\log\left(1 + \theta\nu^{-1}s\right) + (1 - \nu)\left(1 + \theta\nu^{-1}s\right)^{-1}\left(-\theta\nu^{-2}s\right)\right)\right]$$

$$= -\log(1 + \theta s)$$

4.5.2 Joint and population survival function

The joint survival function is given by

$$S_{x,f}(t_n) = \exp\left\{\frac{\nu}{\theta(1-\nu)}\left[1 - \left(1 + \frac{\theta H_{x,c}(t_n)}{\nu}\right)^{1-\nu}\right]\right\} \qquad (4.84)$$

To obtain the marginal likelihood function we require, for clusters of size four, the first four derivatives of the Laplace transform. For the calculations below we assume $\mu = 1$, i.e., we consider frailty distributions with mean one (which excludes the stable distributions):

$$\mathcal{L}^{(1)}(s) = -\mathcal{L}(s)z^{-\nu}$$

$$\mathcal{L}^{(2)}(s) = \mathcal{L}(s)\left(z^{-2\nu} + \theta z^{-\nu-1}\right)$$

$$\mathcal{L}^{(3)}(s) = -\mathcal{L}(s)\left(z^{-3\nu} + 3\theta z^{-2\nu-1} + \theta^2(1+1/\nu)z^{-\nu-2}\right)$$

$$\mathcal{L}^{(4)}(s) = \mathcal{L}(s)\left(z^{-4\nu} + 6\theta z^{-3\nu-1} + \theta^2(7+4/\nu)z^{-2\nu-2}\right.$$
$$\left. + \theta^3(1+1/\nu)(1+2/\nu)z^{-\nu-3}\right)$$

with $z = z(s) = 1 + \theta s/\nu$. The contribution of cluster i with covariate information x_i to the marginal loglikelihood can now be written using the d_i^{th} derivative of the Laplace transform:

$$\sum_{j=1}^{4}\delta_{ij}\log\left(h_0\left(y_{ij}\right)\exp\left(x_j^t\beta\right)\right) + \left\{\frac{\nu}{\theta(1-\nu)}\left[1 - \left(1 + \frac{\theta H_{x_i,c}(y_i)}{\nu}\right)^{1-\nu}\right]\right\}$$
$$- d_i\nu\log\left(1 + \theta H_{x_i,c}(y_i)/\nu\right) + C_{i,d_i} \qquad (4.85)$$

where C_{i,d_i} is a term that depends on the number of events in the cluster:

$$C_{i,0} = C_{i,1} = 0$$

$$C_{i,2} = \log\left(1 + \theta a_{x_i}^{\nu-1}\right)$$

$$C_{i,3} = \log\left(1 + 3\theta a_{x_i}^{\nu-1} + \theta^2(1+1/\nu)a_{x_i}^{2\nu-2}\right)$$

$$C_{i,4} = \log\left(1 + 6\theta a_{x_i}^{\nu-1} + \theta^2(7+4/\nu)a_{x_i}^{2\nu-2}\right.$$
$$\left. + \theta^3(1+1/\nu)(1+2/\nu)a_{x_i}^{3\nu-3}\right)$$

with $a_{x_i} = (1 + \theta H_{x_i,c}(y_i)/\nu)$.

The population survival and density functions are given by

$$S_{\mathbf{x},f}(t) = \exp\left\{\frac{\nu}{\theta(1-\nu)}\left[1 - \left(1 + \frac{\theta H_{\mathbf{x},c}(t)}{\nu}\right)^{1-\nu}\right]\right\}$$

$$f_{\mathbf{x},f}(t) = S_{\mathbf{x},f}(t)\left(1 + \theta H_{\mathbf{x},c}(t)/\nu\right)^{-\nu} h_{\mathbf{x},c}(t)$$

and from this follows the population hazard function

$$h_{\mathbf{x},f}(t) = (1 + \theta H_{\mathbf{x},c}(t)/\nu)^{-\nu} h_{\mathbf{x},c}(t)$$

and the ratio of the population hazard and the conditional hazard is

$$\frac{h_{\mathbf{x},f}(t)}{h_{\mathbf{x},c}(t)} = (1 + \theta H_{\mathbf{x},c}(t)/\nu)^{-\nu}$$

or alternatively, in terms of the population survival function,

$$\frac{h_{\mathbf{x},f}(t)}{h_{\mathbf{x},c}(t)} = (1 + \theta(1 - 1/\nu)\log S_{\mathbf{x},f}(t))^{-\nu/(1-\nu)}$$

The time evolution of this ratio is presented in Figure 4.28a for $\nu = 0.25$ and in Figure 4.28b for $\nu = 0.75$ for different values of θ.

The hazard ratio is not constant over time and the evolution over time is a function of θ but also to a large extent of ν. The population hazard ratio for a binary covariate is given by

$$HR_p(t) = \left(\frac{1 + \nu^{-1}\theta H_0(t)}{1 + \nu^{-1}\theta \exp(\beta) H_0(t)}\right)^{\nu} \exp(\beta)$$

or in terms of the population survival function, we have, with $\mathbf{x} = 0$,

$$HR_p(t) = \left[\frac{1 + (\theta(1-1/\nu)\log S_{\mathbf{x},f}(t))^{1/(1-\nu)}}{1 + \exp(\beta)(\theta(1-1/\nu)\log S_{\mathbf{x},f}(t))^{1/(1-\nu)}}\right]^{\nu} \exp(\beta)$$

The case with the hazard ratio in the conditional model equal to two is presented in Figure 4.29a for $\nu = 0.25$ and in Figure 4.29b for $\nu = 0.75$ for different values of θ. Note that $\lim_{t\to\infty} HR_p(t) = (\exp(\beta))^{1-\nu}$. With $\exp(\beta) = 2$ and $\nu = 0.25$, resp. $\nu = 0.75$, this limit is 1.68, resp. 1.18.

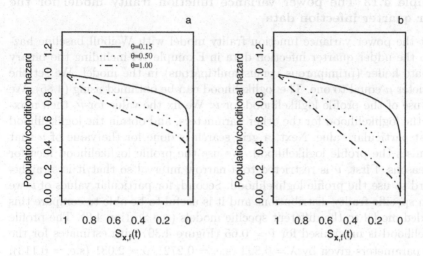

Fig. 4.28. The ratio of the population and the conditional hazard function for the power variance function frailty distribution with (a) $\nu = 0.25$ and (b) $\nu = 0.75$ for different values of θ.

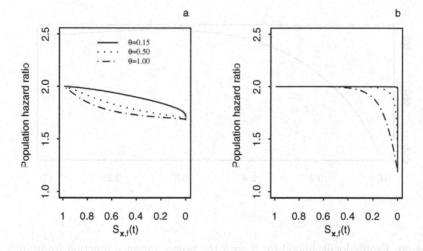

Fig. 4.29. The evolution of the population hazard ratio as a function of the population survival function for the conditional hazard ratio equal to two for the power variance function frailty distribution with (a) $\nu = 0.25$ and (b) $\nu = 0.75$ for different values of θ.

Example 4.13 The power variance function frailty model for the udder quarter infection data

We fit the power variance function frailty model with Weibull baseline hazard to the udder quarter infection data in Example 1.4 including the binary covariate heifer (primiparous versus multiparous) in the model. We set the parameter μ equal to one. The loglikelihood can be obtained using (4.85). We make use of the profile loglikelihood for ν. We fix the value for ν, then maximise the loglikelihood for the other parameters, and obtain the loglikelihood at that particular value. Next, a grid search is done for the value of ν that maximises the profile loglikelihood. We use the profile loglikelihood idea for two reasons. First, ν is restricted to a narrow interval so that it is straightforward to use the profile loglikelihood. Second, for particular values of ν we obtain specific frailty distributions and it is useful to be able to compare this extended model to the different specific models (see Section 4.6). The profile loglikelihood is maximised for $\hat{\nu} = 0.65$ (Figure 4.30) with estimates for the other parameters given by $\hat{\lambda} = 0.894$ (s.e. $= 0.272$), $\hat{\rho} = 2.081$ (s.e. $= 0.113$), $\hat{\beta} = 0.483$ (s.e. $= 0.353$), and $\hat{\theta} = 3.956$ (s.e. $= 1.025$). ∎

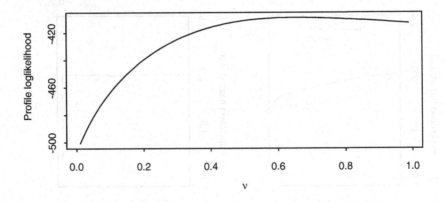

Fig. 4.30. Profile loglikelihood for ν with the power variance function frailty distribution for the udder quarter infection data.

4.5.3 Updating

The frailty density conditional on having survived up to a certain time t belongs to the power variance function family (closure property). As we did in the previous subsections on updating we assume, for simplicity, no covariate information. We investigate the closure property for the specific case of power variance function distributions with $\mu = 1$. Indeed,

$$f_U(u \mid T > t) = \frac{\exp\left(-uH_0(t)\right) f_U(u)}{\exp\left\{\dfrac{\nu}{\theta(1-\nu)}\left[1 - \left(1 + \dfrac{\theta H_0(t)}{\nu}\right)^{1-\nu}\right]\right\}}$$

$$= \exp\left(\frac{-\nu}{\theta A^{\nu-1}}\left(\frac{u}{A^{-\nu}} + \frac{1}{\nu-1}\right)\right)$$

$$\times \frac{1}{\pi u} \sum_{k=1}^{\infty} \frac{\left(\nu/\theta A^{\nu-1}\right)^{k\nu} \left(u/A^{-\nu}\right)^{k(\nu-1)} \Gamma\left(1 - k(\nu-1)\right) \sin\left(\pi k(\nu-1)\right)}{k! \left(\nu-1\right)^k}$$

with $A = 1 + \theta H_0(t)/\nu$ (we assume $\mu = 1$). Therefore, the frailty density of the survivors at time t is still a power variance function density with the same parameter ν but with the mean $E(U)$ equal to $A^{-\nu}$ and squared coefficient of variation equal to $\theta A^{\nu-1}$. Therefore, the mean and the squared coefficient of variation both decrease with time.

4.5.4 Copula form representation

The joint survival function can be rewritten as a copula. For bivariate survival data we obtain

$$S_f(t_1, t_2) = \exp\left[\frac{\nu}{\theta(1-\nu)}\left(1 - \left(b_1^{1/(1-\nu)} + b_2^{1/(1-\nu)} - 1\right)^{1-\nu}\right)\right]$$

with $b_j = 1 + \theta(1 - 1/\nu) \log S_{j,f}(t_j)$, $j = 1, 2$. The joint density function for bivariate data is given by

$$\frac{\partial^2}{\partial t_1 \partial t_2} S_f(t_1, t_2) = \frac{S_f(t_1, t_2)}{S_{1,f}(t_1) S_{2,f}(t_2)} f_{1,f}(t_1) f_{2,f}(t_2)$$

$$\times b_1^{\nu/(1-\nu)} b_2^{\nu/(1-\nu)} \left(b^{-2\nu} + \theta b^{-\nu-1}\right) \qquad (4.86)$$

with $b = \left(b_1^{1/(1-\nu)} + b_2^{1/(1-\nu)} - 1\right)$.

4.5.5 Dependence measures

The global dependence measure, Kendall's τ, is given by (see Hougaard (2000), p. 242: rewrite his (7.58) using our parameterisation)

$$\tau = \nu - \frac{2\nu}{\theta} + \frac{4\nu^2}{\theta^2 (1-\nu)} \exp\left(\frac{2\nu}{\theta(1-\nu)}\right) \int_1^\infty t^{-\nu/(1-\nu)} \exp\left(\frac{-2\nu t}{\theta(1-\nu)}\right) dt \tag{4.87}$$

The ratio of the joint survival function and the product of the population survival functions, $\psi(t_1, t_2)$, is presented in Figures 4.31a and 4.31b for $\nu = 0.35$ and in Figures 4.32a and 4.32b for $\nu = 0.65$ with Kendall's $\tau = 0.25$.

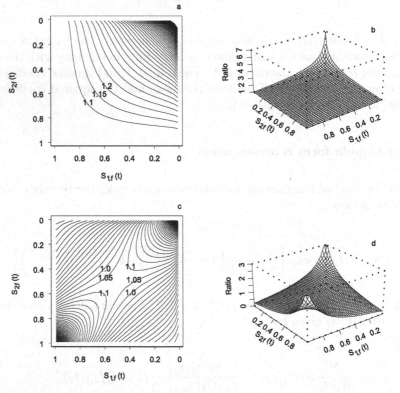

Fig. 4.31. The ratio of the joint survival function and the product of the population survival functions (a,b) and the ratio of the joint density function and the product of the population density functions (c,d) for the power variance function frailty distribution with $\nu = 0.35$ and $\tau = 0.25$.

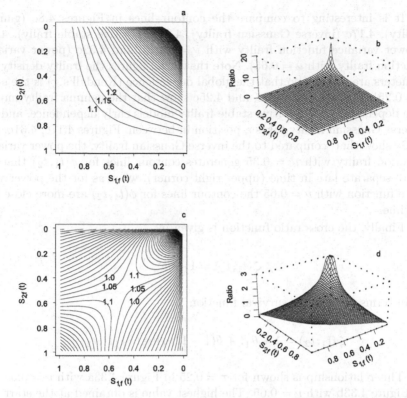

Fig. 4.32. The ratio of the joint survival function and the product of the population survival functions (a,b) and the ratio of the joint density function and the product of the population density functions (c,d) for the power variance function frailty distribution with $\nu = 0.65$ and $\tau = 0.25$.

These parameter values are chosen in order to compare the resulting distributions with the inverse Gaussian distribution function. Indeed, with $\nu = 0.50$ and $\theta = 1.282$, we obtain the inverse Gaussian distribution used in Section 4.3.5 with $\alpha = 1/\theta = 0.78$ resulting in $\tau = 0.25$.

The ratio of the joint density function and the product of the population density functions can be derived from (4.86) and equals

$$\phi(t_1, t_2) = \frac{S_f(t_1, t_2)}{S_{1,f}(t_1)S_{2,f}(t_2)} b_1^{\nu/(1-\nu)} b_2^{\nu/(1-\nu)} \left(b^{-2\nu} + \theta b^{-\nu-1} \right)$$

and a graphical representation of this relationship is given in Figures 4.31c and 4.31d for $\nu = 0.35$ and in Figures 4.32c and 4.32d for $\nu = 0.65$.

It is interesting to compare the contour lines in Figures 4.8c (gamma frailty), 4.17c (inverse Gaussian frailty), 4.25c (positive stable fraily), 4.31c (power variance function frailty with $\nu = 0.35$), and 4.32c (power variance function frailty with $\nu = 0.65$). Note that in all figures the frailty density parameters are selected so that the global dependence (Kendall's τ) is the same ($\tau=0.25$). Figures 4.8c, 4.17c, and 4.25c show that the gamma frailty models late dependence, the positive stable frailty models early dependence, and the inverse Gaussian frailty takes a position in between. Figures 4.17c, 4.31c, and 4.32c show that, compared to the inverse Gaussian frailty, the power variance function frailty with $\nu = 0.35$ generates contour lines for $\phi(t_1, t_2)$ that are more separate late in time (upper right corner), whereas for the power variance function with $\nu = 0.65$ the contour lines for $\phi(t_1, t_2)$ are more close late in time.

Finally, the cross ratio function is given by

$$\zeta(t_1, t_2) = 1 + \theta b^{\nu - 1}$$

or in terms of the joint survival function

$$\zeta(t_1, t_2) = 1 + \theta \left[1 + \theta(1 - 1/\nu) \log(S_f(t_1, t_2)) \right]^{-1}$$

This relationship is shown for $\tau = 0.25$ in Figure 4.33a with $\nu = 0.35$ and in Figure 4.33b with $\nu = 0.65$. The highest value is obtained at the start and goes to one (independence) as the survival goes to zero.

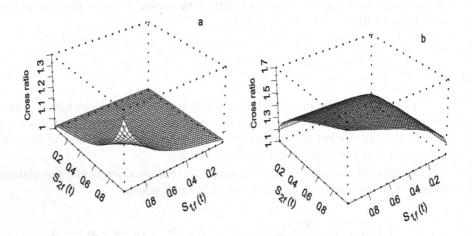

Fig. 4.33. Cross ratio function for the power variance function frailty distribution.

4.5.6 Diagnostics

We can make use of the estimate of $\gamma(r)$ which is asymptotically equivalent to the cross ratio function proposed in Section 4.2.6 and compare it to the estimate based on the frailty model with power variance function family distribution, as is demonstrated in Example 4.14.

Example 4.14 Diagnostics for the power variance function frailty distribution for time to diagnosis of being healed based on the cross ratio function

We first need to fit the frailty model for the time to diagnosis data (Example 1.2). The loglikelihood can be obtained using (4.85). We make use of the profile loglikelihood for ν. We fix the value for ν, then maximise the loglikelihood for the other parameters, and obtain the loglikelihood at that particular value. Next, a grid search is done for the value of ν that maximises the profile loglikelihood. The profile loglikelihood takes its maximum value for $\hat{\nu} = 0.52$. For $\hat{\nu} = 0.52$, the loglikelihood is maximised for $\hat{\lambda} = 0.394$ (s.e. = 0.163), $\hat{\rho} = 4.426$ (s.e. = 0.317), $\hat{\beta} = -0.836$ (s.e. = 0.165), and $\hat{\theta} = 10.73$ (s.e. = 6.283). Figure 4.34 shows the estimate of $\gamma(r)$, together with the estimate of the cross ratio function based on the power variance function frailty model with $\hat{\nu} = 0.52$ and $\hat{\theta} = 10.73$. This curve is very similar to the curve obtained from the inverse Gaussian frailty distribution (Figure 4.19) but requires one additional parameter. ∎

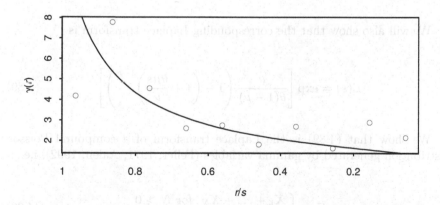

Fig. 4.34. The estimate of $\gamma(r)$ plotted against r/s for the time to diagnosis data. Adjacent r_a values are combined in groups 1–10, 11–20, ..., 91–100, and the average of the r_a values within each group, divided by s, is used as value to be plotted on the x-axis. The solid line is the cross ratio function estimated from the power variance function distribution frailty model.

4.6 The compound Poisson distribution

4.6.1 Definitions and basic properties

In some applications a proportion of the subjects is not susceptible for the event under consideration. To model this we use a frailty term U for which $P(U = 0)$ is positive. We therefore consider a distribution of the frailty term that has two parts: the positive probability at zero and a continuous subdensity on the positive real line. It will become clear from the further discussion that, with $\mu > 0$, $\theta > 0$, and $\nu > 1$, appropriate definitions are

$$P(U = 0) = \exp\left(\frac{-\nu}{\theta(\nu - 1)}\right)$$

and

$$f_U(u) = \exp\left(-\frac{\nu}{\theta}\left(\frac{u}{\mu} + \frac{1}{\nu - 1}\right)\right)$$

$$\times \frac{1}{\pi u} \sum_{k=1}^{\infty} \frac{(\nu/\theta)^{k\nu} (u/\mu)^{k(\nu-1)} \Gamma\left(1 - k(\nu - 1)\right) \sin\left(\pi k(\nu - 1)\right)}{k! \, (\nu - 1)^k} \quad (4.88)$$

We will also show that the corresponding Laplace transform is

$$\mathcal{L}(s) = \exp\left[\frac{\nu}{\theta(1 - \nu)}\left(1 - \left(1 + \frac{\theta \mu s}{\nu}\right)^{1-\nu}\right)\right] \quad (4.89)$$

We show that (4.89) is the Laplace transform of a compound Poisson distribution generated by gamma variables (Feller, 1971; Aalen, 1992), i.e.,

$$U = \begin{cases} X_1 + \ldots + X_N & \text{for } N > 0 \\ 0 & \text{for } N = 0 \end{cases} \quad (4.90)$$

where $X_1, X_2, \ldots$ are independent random variables with gamma distribution Gamma(η, ω) with $\eta > 0$, $\omega > 0$, and N is independent of $X_1, X_2, \ldots$ and Poisson distributed with intensity $\kappa > 0$.

The Laplace transform for U is

$$\mathcal{L}(s) = \mathrm{P}(N = 0) + \sum_{k=1}^{\infty} \mathrm{E}\left[\exp\left(-s\left(X_1 + \ldots + X_N\right)\right) \mid N = k\right] \mathrm{P}(N = k)$$

$$= \exp(-\kappa) + \sum_{k=1}^{\infty} \left(\prod_{j=1}^{k} \left(\frac{\omega}{\omega + s}\right)^{\eta}\right) \exp(-\kappa) \frac{\kappa^k}{k!}$$

$$= \sum_{k=0}^{\infty} \frac{\left(\kappa\left(\frac{\omega}{\omega + s}\right)^{\eta}\right)^k}{k!} \exp(-\kappa)$$

$$= \exp\left(-\kappa + \kappa\left(\frac{\omega}{\omega + s}\right)^{\eta}\right) \tag{4.91}$$

With

$$\kappa = \frac{\nu}{\theta(\nu - 1)}$$

$$\omega = \frac{\nu}{\theta\mu}$$

$$\eta = \nu - 1$$

the Laplace transform (4.91) takes the form (4.89). Note that $\eta = \nu - 1 > 0$ implies $\nu > 1$, hence the extension of the class of Laplace transforms defined in (4.80) for $0 < \nu \le 1$ ($\nu = 1$ is the limiting case that gives the gamma frailty distribution).

Due to the fact that the Laplace transforms of the power variance function and the compound Poisson are the same (except for the range of the parameter ν) all properties obtained from the Laplace transform of the power variance function family also hold for the compound Poisson distribution, e.g.,

$$\mathrm{E}(U) = \mu$$

and

$$\frac{\mathrm{Var}(U)}{(\mathrm{E}(U))^2} = \theta$$

with μ the mean and θ the squared coefficient of variation.

For the choice $\mu = 1$, θ is the heterogeneity parameter.

Using the explicit definition (4.90) of the frailty term it is easy to show the validity of (4.88). We indeed have

$$f_U(u) = \sum_{k=1}^{\infty} f_U(u \mid N = k) \mathrm{P}(N = k) \tag{4.92}$$

where $f_U(u \mid N = k)$ denotes the density of $X_1 + \ldots + X_k$. Since $X_1, \ldots, X_k$ are independent random variables with distribution $\mathrm{Gamma}(\eta, \omega)$ we have $X_1 + \ldots + X_k \sim \mathrm{Gamma}(k\eta, \omega)$. Therefore, (4.92) can be rewritten as

$$f_U(u) = \exp(-\kappa) \sum_{k=1}^{\infty} \frac{\omega^{k\eta} u^{k\eta-1} \exp(-\omega u)}{\Gamma(k\eta)} \frac{\kappa^k}{k!}$$

$$= \exp(-\kappa - \omega u) \frac{1}{u} \sum_{k=1}^{\infty} \frac{1}{k! \Gamma(k\eta)} \omega^{k\eta} u^{k\eta} \kappa^k$$

$$= \exp\left(-\frac{\nu}{\theta(\nu-1)} - \frac{\nu u}{\mu\theta}\right) \frac{1}{u}$$

$$\times \sum_{k=1}^{\infty} \frac{1}{k! \Gamma(k(\nu-1))} \left(\frac{\nu}{\mu\theta}\right)^{k(\nu-1)} u^{k(\nu-1)} \left(\frac{\nu}{\theta(\nu-1)}\right)^k$$

$$= \exp\left(-\frac{\nu}{\theta}\left(\frac{u}{\mu} + \frac{1}{\nu-1}\right)\right) \frac{1}{u}$$

$$\times \sum_{k=1}^{\infty} \frac{1}{k! \Gamma(k(\nu-1))} \left(\frac{\nu}{\theta}\right)^{k\nu} \frac{1}{(\nu-1)^k} \left(\frac{u}{\mu}\right)^{k(\nu-1)}$$

Since

$$\frac{1}{\Gamma(k(\nu-1))} = \frac{1}{\pi}\Gamma(1 - k(\nu-1)) \sin(\pi k(\nu-1))$$

we obtain the density function (4.88).

4.6.2 Joint and population survival functions

The joint survival function, the likelihood contributions, and the population survival and density functions are the same as in the case of the power variance function.

The population hazard function is therefore given by

$$h_{\mathbf{x},f}(t) = (1 + \theta H_{\mathbf{x},c}(t)/\nu)^{-\nu} h_{\mathbf{x},c}(t)$$

Now integrating the population hazard function from zero to ∞ we obtain

$$\int_0^\infty h_{\mathbf{x},f}(v)dv = \int_0^\infty (1 + \theta H_{\mathbf{x},c}(v)/\nu)^{-\nu} dH_{\mathbf{x},c}(v)$$

$$= \int_0^\infty (1 + \theta r/\nu)^{-\nu} dr$$

$$= \frac{\nu}{\theta} \int_1^\infty w^{-\nu} dw$$

$$= \frac{\nu}{\theta(\nu - 1)}$$

This shows (as expected) that the "survival function" obtained from the population hazard function is defective; for $t \to \infty$ it takes the value $\exp\left(\frac{-\nu}{\theta(\nu-1)}\right)$ rather than zero. For instance, for $\nu = 2.5$ and $\theta = 1$ the population survival function goes only up to 0.189, which is the fraction of subjects in the population not susceptible for the event.

Example 4.15 The compound Poisson frailty model for the udder quarter infection data

To fit a compound Poisson frailty model with Weibull baseline hazard to the udder quarter infection data in Example 1.4 we can make use again of the profile loglikelihood for ν using the marginal likelihood expressions (4.85), but now varying the value for ν from one upwards. The profile loglikelihood for the whole range of ν is shown in Figure 4.35. It is clear that with increasing values for ν starting from one, the loglikelihood decreases. Therefore, the data do not support a compound Poisson distribution. ∎

4.6.3 Updating

The frailty density of the survivors at time t is still compound Poisson. We demonstrate this for the case without covariates. For the probability of zero susceptibility, we have

$$P(U = 0 \mid T > t) = \frac{P(U = 0)}{P(T > t)}$$

as $U = 0$ implies $T > t$ for all t.

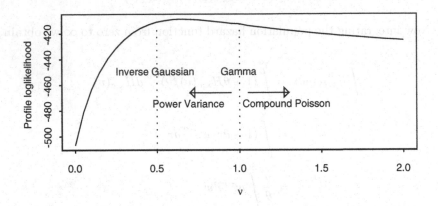

Fig. 4.35. Profile loglikelihood for ν including the compound Poisson and the power variance function frailty distribution for the udder quarter infection data.

Therefore, we have

$$P(U = 0 \mid T > t) = \frac{\exp\left(\dfrac{-\nu}{\theta(\nu - 1)}\right)}{\mathcal{L}\left(H_0(t)\right)}$$

$$= \exp\left(\frac{-\nu}{\theta(\nu - 1)}\right)$$

$$\times \exp\left[\frac{\nu}{\theta(\nu - 1)}\left(1 - \left(1 + \frac{\theta\mu H_0(t)}{\nu}\right)^{1-\nu}\right)\right]$$

$$= \exp\left[\frac{-\nu}{\theta(\nu - 1)}\left(1 + \frac{\theta\mu H_0(t)}{\nu}\right)^{1-\nu}\right]$$

For the continuous part, ν remains the same, the mean corresponds to $\mu\left(1 + \theta\mu H_0(t)/\nu\right)^{-\nu}$ and the squared coefficient of variation to $\theta\left(1 + \theta\mu H_0(t)/\nu\right)^{\nu-1}$ (see Aalen (1992), Section 4.2 for the details).

As can be expected, the probability of being equal to zero increases over time and will eventually become one.

The mean of the continuous density function decreases over time, but contrary to the power variance function, the squared coefficient of variation increases with time.

All the dependence measures are essentially the same as for the power variance function, so we do not discuss them separately here.

4.7 The lognormal distribution

McGilchrist (1993) developed methodology for fitting frailty models that parallels the classical mixed models theory. He therefore proposes the model $h_{ij}(t) = h_0(t)\exp\left(\mathbf{x}_{ij}^t\boldsymbol{\beta} + w_i\right)$, where w_i is the actual value of the random effect W_i which follows a zero-mean normal distribution with variance γ. The corresponding frailty has a lognormal distribution. It is easy to show that

$$f_U(u) = \frac{1}{u\sqrt{2\pi\gamma}}\exp\left(-\frac{(\log u)^2}{2\gamma}\right)$$

with $\gamma > 0$. The mean and variance of the frailty are given by

$$\mathrm{E}(U) = \exp\left(\gamma/2\right) \quad \text{and} \quad \mathrm{Var}(U) = \exp(2\gamma) - \exp(\gamma)$$

Lognormal density functions with zero mean for the random effect and different variances are depicted in Figure 4.36.

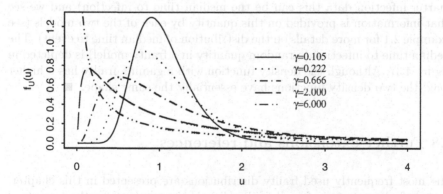

Fig. 4.36. Lognormal density functions.

For the frailty distributions studied so far we have chosen the parameterisation so that $\mathrm{E}(U)=1$. However, for the lognormal distribution, it is natural to assume a zero-mean normal distribution for the random effect W. As a consequence the mean of the frailty U is not one.

For a lognormal frailty distribution no explicit evaluation of the Laplace transform is possible. Analytic expressions for $\psi(t_1, t_2)$ and $\zeta(t_1, t_2)$ are therefore not available. Also for Kendall's τ no explicit formula exists.

Although the lognormal frailty distribution is, for reasons discussed above, less tractable, it has been used on a regular basis to fit frailty models (McGilchrist and Aisbett, 1991; Vaida and Xu, 2000; Ripatti and Palmgren, 2000). Also in the context of accelerated failure time models one often assumes normal random effects.

Example 4.16 The lognormal frailty model for the udder quarter infection data

No explicit form exists for the marginal likelihood for the lognormal frailty model. Instead of integrating out the frailties analytically, we therefore have to use other techniques. One such technique is numerical integration of the normal distributed random effects based on Gaussian quadrature. This technique is available in SAS (nlmixed procedure). Assuming a Weibull baseline hazard, the parameter estimates are $\hat{\lambda} = 0.317$ (s.e. $= 0.094$), $\hat{\rho} = 2.490$ (s.e. $= 0.135$), $\hat{\beta} = 0.460$ (s.e. $= 0.378$) and $\hat{\gamma} = 2.999$ (s.e. $= 0.610$). It is not straightforward to compare this model with the other frailty distributions, as the mean of the frailty is no longer one. In this particular case, the mean is estimated as $\exp(\hat{\gamma}/2) = 4.459$.

To compare the lognormal frailty model and the gamma frailty model we consider a quantity that is relevant for the actual study (for the udder quarter infection data this can be the median time to infection) and we see what information is provided on this quantity by each of the two models (see Example 2.1 for more details on the distribution of median time to event). The median time to infection (a random quantity in a frailty model) is depicted in Figure 4.37. Although the density function with a gamma frailty has a higher peak, the two density functions have essentially the same shape. ∎

4.8 Further extensions and references

The most frequently used frailty distributions are presented in this chapter. A typical characteristic for all frailty distributions except for the lognormal frailty distribution is that they have a simple Laplace transform representation from which the different properties follow easily.

Balakrishnan and Peng (2006) extended the often used gamma frailty distribution to the generalised gamma frailty distribution.

The compound Poisson distribution leads to a model with a cure rate fraction (Moger et al., 2004; Moger and Aalen, 2005). Other frailty models

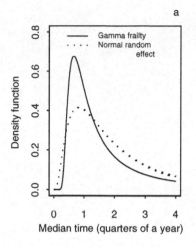
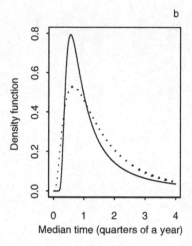

Fig. 4.37. Density of median time to infection for the gamma and the lognormal frailty distribution with (a) primiparous and (b) multiparous cows.

with a cure rate fraction have been proposed by Chen et al. (2002), Price and Manatunga (2001), and Longini and Halloran (1996).

Frailties are also modelled nonparametrically assuming a restricted number of values for the frailties with an associated probability for each of these values. McLachlan and McGiffin (1994) discuss such models, also called finite mixture models, and Ng et al. (2004) discuss the case of a two-component survival mixture model.

In the models discussed in this chapter it is assumed that the frailty is constant over time for a particular cluster. Time-varying frailties, however, have been proposed by a number of authors (Harkanen et al., 2003; Wintrebert et al., 2004; Manda and Meyer, 2005). Aalen and Hjort (2002) and Gjessing et al. (2003) used the Lévy process to model time-varying frailties. Time-varying frailties were introduced for recurrent events by Yau and McGilchrist (1998) and Fong et al. (2001).

We also discussed two diagnostic techniques to evaluate the frailty distribution assumption. There are only a few additional diagnostic techniques available for this problem (Glidden, 1999; Cui and Sun, 2004; Economou and Caroni, 2005; Gupta and Kirmani, 2006) and further research in this area is needed.

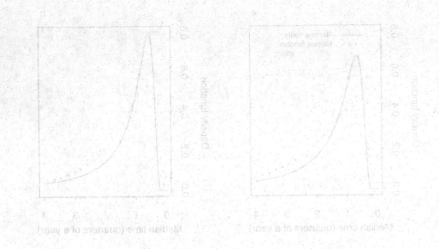

Fig. 4.27. Density of survival time or life function for the gamma, and the lognormal (right) distributions, with the prior/proper and the malignancies power ...

with a survivor function have been proposed by Chen et al. (2002), Price and Manatunga (2001) and Copput and Haberan (1999).

Features are also models that competing risks, assuming a restricted number of values for the failures, with an associated probability for each of these values. Mccall and MacMillan (1994) discuss such models, also called finite mixture models, and Ng et al. (2001) discuss the use of a two-component survival mixture model.

In the models discussed in this chapter it is assumed that the frailty is constant over time for an individual cluster. Time varying frailties, however, have been proposed by a number of authors (Manatunga et al., 2003; Wintrebert et al., 2004; Manda and Meyer, 2005; Aalen and Gjessing (2002) and Gjessing et al. (2003) used the stochastic process time varying frailties. Time-varying frailties were introduced for univariate events by Yau and McGilchrist (1998) and Paik et al. 2004.

We also discuss two diagnostic techniques to evaluate the frailty distributional assumption. There are only a few additional diagnostic techniques available for this model. Childs et al. (1999; Cui and Sun, 2004; Economou and Caroni, 2005; Glidden and Farewell, 2000) and further research in this area is needed.

5

The semiparametric frailty model

In Section 1.4.2 we briefly reviewed some ideas on parametric and semiparametric proportional hazards modelling in univariate survival analysis. The extension of the parametric proportional hazards model to the parametric proportional hazards model with a gamma frailty term, a model that can be used to fit multivariate survival data, is discussed at length in Chapter 2. In this chapter we study in detail the extension of the semiparametric proportional hazards model to the semiparametric frailty model. This model is a standard statistical tool to analyse multivariate or clustered survival data. A detailed discussion will be given on the different techniques that are available to fit these models. Section 5.1 deals with the EM algorithm approach for semiparametric gamma frailty models. In Section 5.2 an alternative approach to fit semiparametric gamma frailty models based on penalised partial likelihood maximisation is introduced. It is shown that this technique leads to the same estimates as the EM algorithm. This technique, however, can be extended to a semiparametric model with normal distributed random effects. In Section 5.3 we show how Bayesian techniques based on Gibbs sampling can be used to fit semiparametric frailty models.

5.1 The EM algorithm approach

5.1.1 Description of the EM algorithm

In Section 2.2 we demonstrated how gamma distributed frailties appearing in the conditional likelihood $\prod_{i=1}^{s} L_i(\xi, \beta \mid u_i)$ can be integrated out to obtain the marginal likelihood $\prod_{i=1}^{s} L_{marg,i}(\zeta)$ with $\zeta = (\xi, \theta, \beta)$. Maximisation of the marginal likelihood leads to estimation of ξ, the parameters related to the baseline hazard $h_0(t)$, β, and θ in a straightforward manner.

The approach taken in Chapter 2 is fully parametric. In survival analysis, however, the more classical approach is to assume that the hazard function is the product of an unspecified baseline hazard $h_0(t)$ and a parametric function of the covariates, i.e., we model the hazard function in a semiparametric way. In this chapter we will study model (2.2) with $h_0(t)$ unspecified: the semiparametric frailty model. For such a model direct maximisation of the marginal likelihood is no longer possible.

Semiparametric hazard models without frailty terms are fitted by maximisation of the partial likelihood (Cox, 1972). For semiparametric frailty models, however, we need to account for the contribution of the unobserved frailty terms. The solution will be that we rely on partial likelihood ideas in combination with the Expectation–Maximisation algorithm (the EM algorithm; an algorithm that is typically used in the presence of unobserved information).

The EM algorithm iterates between an expectation and maximisation step. In the expectation step, the expected values of the unobserved frailties conditional on the observed information and the current parameter estimates are obtained. In the maximisation step, these expected values are considered to be the true information, and new estimates of the parameters of interest are obtained by maximisation of the likelihood, given the expected values.

Note that the usefulness of the EM algorithm for a particular problem depends on two conditions. First, it should be easy to obtain expected values for the unobserved information. Second, the maximisation of the likelihood, conditional on the expected values of the unobserved information, should be straightforward as the EM algorithm is based on performing these two steps iteratively.

Those two conditions are satisfied for the semiparametric gamma frailty model. The collection of frailty terms is the unobserved information. As shown below, closed form expressions exist for the conditional expectation of the frailties (the expectation step). Using these expressions as fixed offset terms we can now perform a maximisation step using partial likelihood ideas. The details of the application of the iterative EM principle are given in Section 5.1.2.

5.1.2 Expectation and maximisation for the gamma frailty model

We first consider the complete or full data loglikelihood with the frailties assumed to be observed random variables. The full data loglikelihood follows from the joint density of $\mathbf{z}$ and $\mathbf{u}$, with $\mathbf{z}$ containing the observed times y_{ij} and the censoring indicators δ_{ij}.

With $h_0(.)$ the unspecified baseline hazard function we have, using ideas developed in Section 2.2,

$$l_{full}(h_0(.), \theta, \boldsymbol{\beta}) = \log f(\mathbf{z}, \mathbf{u} \mid h_0(.), \theta, \boldsymbol{\beta})$$

$$= \log f(\mathbf{z} \mid h_0(.), \boldsymbol{\beta}, \mathbf{u}) + \log f(\mathbf{u} \mid \theta)$$

$$= l_{full,1}(h_0(.), \boldsymbol{\beta}) + l_{full,2}(\theta) \tag{5.1}$$

with

$$
l_{full,1}(h_0(.), \beta) = \sum_{i=1}^{s} \sum_{j=1}^{n_i} \left[\delta_{ij} \log \left(h_0(y_{ij}) u_i \exp(\mathbf{x}_{ij}^t \beta) \right) \right.
$$

$$
\left. - H_0 (y_{ij}) u_i \exp \left(\mathbf{x}_{ij}^t \beta \right) \right] \tag{5.2}
$$

the loglikelihood of $\mathbf{z}$ conditional on the frailties, which is only a function of β and $h_0(.)$, and

$$
l_{full,2}(\theta) = \sum_{i=1}^{s} \log f_U (u_i) \tag{5.3}
$$

Note that (5.2) is the sum of the logarithm of likelihood contributions given by (2.4) over the different clusters, but for the further discussion it will be useful to have that $l_{full,1}(\beta, h_0(.))$ is a part of the full likelihood.

If the u_i's were actually observed, estimates for β could be obtained by first rewriting in $l_{full,1}(h_0(.), \beta)$ the $u_i \exp \left(\mathbf{x}_{ij}^t \beta \right)$ factors as $\exp \left(\mathbf{x}_{ij}^t \beta + \log u_i \right)$ and by then maximising with respect to β the partial likelihood corresponding to $l_{full,1}(h_0(.), \beta)$ with the $\log u_i$'s considered as fixed offset values.

That is the reason why we look in the expectation step for the expected values of the frailties, and then use these expected values as known entities to find, in the maximisation step, estimates for the other parameters.

Let us first consider the **maximisation step**.

We use $l_{full,1}(h_0(.), \beta)$ to estimate β, here $h_0(.)$ is a nuisance function, and $l_{full,2}(\theta)$ to estimate θ. Within the framework of the EM algorithm, the expected value of the full loglikelihood needs to be maximised.

The loglikelihood in (5.2) is first profiled to a partial loglikelihood by considering the frailties as fixed offset terms leading to

$$
l_{part,1}(\beta) = \sum_{i=1}^{s} \sum_{j=1}^{n_i} \delta_{ij} \left[\log u_i + \mathbf{x}_{ij}^t \beta \right.
$$

$$
\left. - \log \left(\sum_{qw \in R(y_{ij})} u_q \exp \left(\mathbf{x}_{qw}^t \beta \right) \right) \right]
$$

Next, the u_i's and $\log u_i$'s in this expression are replaced by the current expected values (at iteration step k) $E_{(k)}(U_i)$ and $E_{(k)}(\log U_i)$ (see (5.6), (5.8), and (5.9) for precise definitions) and these expected values are considered to be the true values leading to

$$
l_{part,1}(\boldsymbol{\beta}) = \sum_{i=1}^{s} \sum_{j=1}^{n_i} \delta_{ij} \left[E_{(k)}(\log U_i) + \mathbf{x}_{ij}^t \boldsymbol{\beta} \right.
$$
$$
\left. - \log \left(\sum_{qw \in R(y_{ij})} E_{(k)}(U_q) \exp\left(\mathbf{x}_{qw}^t \boldsymbol{\beta}\right) \right) \right]
$$

from which new estimates $\boldsymbol{\beta}^{(k)}$ can be obtained. A new estimate $\theta^{(k)}$ follows immediately by maximisation of $l_{full,2}(\theta)$ replacing also the u_i's and $\log u_i$'s in (5.3) by the current expected values at iteration step k.

Using the current estimate $\boldsymbol{\beta}^{(k)}$, we can derive the Nelson–Aalen estimator of the baseline hazard with the frailties considered to be known offset terms:

$$
H_0^{(k)}(t) = \sum_{y_{(l)} \leq t} h_{0l}^{(k)} \tag{5.4}
$$

and

$$
h_{0l}^{(k)} = \frac{N_{(l)}}{\sum_{qw \in R(y_{(l)})} E_{(k)}(U_q) \exp\left(\mathbf{x}_{qw}^t \boldsymbol{\beta}^{(k)}\right)} \tag{5.5}
$$

with $y_{(1)} < \ldots < y_{(r)}$ the ordered event times (r denotes the number of different event times) and $N_{(l)}$ the number of events at time $y_{(l)}$, $l = 1, \ldots, r$.

This expression for the baseline hazard is required in the **expectation step**. Assume that the current parameter estimates at iteration k of the EM algorithm are given by $\boldsymbol{\zeta}^{(k)} = \left(h_0^{(k)}(.), \theta^{(k)}, \boldsymbol{\beta}^{(k)} \right)$. In order to find the expectation

$$
E_{(k+1)}(U_i) = E_{\boldsymbol{\zeta}^{(k)}}(U_i \mid \mathbf{z}) \tag{5.6}
$$

we need the conditional distribution $f_U(u_i \mid \mathbf{z})$. Define $L_i(h_0(.), \boldsymbol{\beta} \mid u_i)$ as in (2.4) and $L_{marg,i}(h_0(.), \theta, \boldsymbol{\beta})$ as in (2.6) with now $h_0(.)$ unspecified (instead of parametrically specified as in Chapter 2).

From the Bayes theorem we have

$$f_U \left(u_i \mid \mathbf{z} \right) = \frac{L_i \left(h_0(.), \boldsymbol{\beta} \mid u_i \right) f_U \left(u_i \right)}{L_{marg,i} \left(h_0(.), \theta, \boldsymbol{\beta} \right)}$$

$$= \frac{u_i^{d_i+1/\theta-1} \exp \left(-u_i \left(1/\theta + H_{\mathbf{x}_i,c} \left(\mathbf{y}_i \right) \right) \right) \left(1/\theta + H_{\mathbf{x}_i,c} \left(\mathbf{y}_i \right) \right)^{d_i+1/\theta}}{\Gamma \left(d_i + 1/\theta \right)} \quad (5.7)$$

with $H_{\mathbf{x}_i,c} \left(\mathbf{y}_i \right) = \sum_{j=1}^{n_i} H_{\mathbf{x}_{ij},c} \left(y_{ij} \right)$. This expression corresponds to a gamma density with parameters $(d_i + 1/\theta)$ and $(1/\theta + H_{\mathbf{x}_i,c} \left(\mathbf{y}_i \right))$ and therefore the expected value is given by

$$\mathrm{E}_{(k+1)} \left(U_i \right) = \frac{\left(d_i + 1/\theta^{(k)} \right)}{1/\theta^{(k)} + H_{\mathbf{x}_i,c}^{(k)} \left(\mathbf{y}_i \right)} \quad (5.8)$$

where $H_{i.,c}^{(k)}$ is the version of $H_{i.,c}$ with $H_0 \left(y_{ij} \right)$ replaced by $H_0^{(k)} \left(y_{ij} \right)$ and $\boldsymbol{\beta}$ replaced by $\boldsymbol{\beta}^{(k)}$. Furthermore, as the conditional distribution of U_i is gamma distributed, the conditional distribution of $\log U_i$ has a loggamma distribution with expected value

$$\mathrm{E}_{(k+1)} \left(\log U_i \right) = \psi \left(d_i + 1/\theta^{(k)} \right) - \log \left(1/\theta^{(k)} + H_{\mathbf{x}_i,c}^{(k)} \left(\mathbf{y}_i \right) \right) \quad (5.9)$$

with $\psi(.)$ the digamma function, i.e., the first derivative of the logarithm of the gamma function.

The EM algorithm for the semiparametric gamma frailty model is presented in Figure 5.1.

In the initialisation step (iteration 0), θ is set to one and an ordinary Cox model is fitted leading to estimates $\hat{\boldsymbol{\beta}}_{IWM}$. We set $\boldsymbol{\beta}^{(0)} = \hat{\boldsymbol{\beta}}_{IWM}$. Next, we iterate between the expectation and maximisation step until convergence. To assess convergence of the algorithm, the marginal loglikelihood expression in (2.7) is used. At iteration level k, we insert $h_0^{(k)}(.)$, $\theta^{(k)}$, $\boldsymbol{\beta}^{(k)}$, and $H_0^{(k)}(.)$ into (2.7) to obtain the marginal loglikelihood value at iteration level k, $l_{marg} \left(h_0^{(k)}(.), \theta^{(k)}, \boldsymbol{\beta}^{(k)} \right)$. Convergence is reached if the absolute difference between $l_{marg} \left(h_0^{(k-1)}(.), \theta^{(k-1)} \boldsymbol{\beta}^{(k-1)} \right)$ and $l_{marg} \left(h_0^{(k)}(.), \theta^{(k)} \boldsymbol{\beta}^{(k)} \right)$ is smaller than a preset value ϵ. We note that in the above expressions for the full data loglikelihood, the terms $\mathrm{E}_{(k-1)}(\mathbf{U})$ and $\mathrm{E}_{(k)}(\mathbf{U})$ are also used to obtain $h_0^{(k)}(.)$ and $H_0^{(k)}(.)$, but since they are considered as fixed offset terms, we do not include this in our notation in an explicit way.

The rate of convergence of the EM algorithm can be improved by using a modified profile likelihood (Nielsen et al., 1992). We consider now two levels

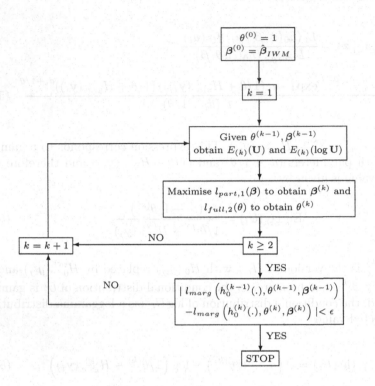

Fig. 5.1. The EM algorithm for the semiparametric gamma frailty model. $\hat{\beta}_{IWM}$ are the estimates for the regression coefficients in the classical Cox regression model (without frailties). For further explanation, see text.

of iteration, one at the level of θ, the parameter that is profiled out, and a lower level where estimates for β are obtained using the EM algorithm, but now conditional on a fixed value for θ. As demonstrated in Figure 5.2, the algorithm consists of an inner loop and an outer loop.

In the inner loop, the EM algorithm is used to obtain estimates for β and $\mathbf{u}$ for a particular value of θ, $\theta^{(l)}$. Therefore, two indices for β and $\mathbf{u}$ are required, a first index, l, for the outer loop referring to the fixed value of θ and a second index, k, for the inner loop. Assessing convergence for the inner loop is again based on the marginal likelihood, but now with fixed value for θ, $\theta^{(l)}$, and therefore we compare in the inner loop sequential values $l_{marg}\left(h_0^{(l,k)}(.), \theta^{(l)}, \beta^{(l,k)}\right)$, $k = 1, 2, \ldots$ with $\theta^{(l)}$ fixed.

Upon convergence of the EM algorithm for a fixed value of θ ($\theta = \theta^{(l)}$), we set $\hat{\beta}_{\theta^{(l)}} = \beta^{(l,k)}$, $\hat{\mathbf{u}}_{\theta^{(l)}} = \mathrm{E}_{(l,k)}(\mathbf{U})$ (modify (5.8) in the appropriate way).

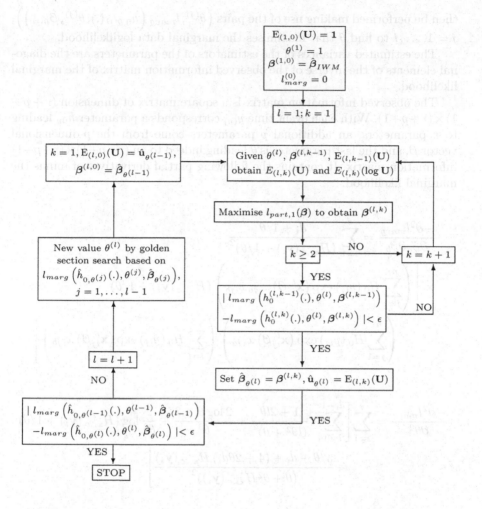

Fig. 5.2. The modified profile likelihood EM algorithm for the semiparametric gamma frailty model. $\hat{\beta}_{IWM}$ are the estimates for the regression coefficients in the classical Cox regression model (without frailties). For further explanation, see text.

Based on these values and using appropriate modifications of (5.4) and (5.5) we obtain, for the fixed value $\theta^{(l)}$, $\hat{h}_{0,\theta^{(l)}}(.)$ and $\hat{H}_{0,\theta^{(l)}}(.)$.

Furthermore, the marginal likelihood is then evaluated at $\theta^{(l)}$ plugging in the corresponding values $\hat{\beta}_{\theta^{(l)}}$, $\hat{u}_{\theta^{(l)}}$, $\hat{h}_{0,\theta^{(l)}}(.)$, and $\hat{H}_{0,\theta^{(l)}}(.)$ and is denoted by $l_{marg}\left(\hat{h}_{0,\theta^{(l)}}(.), \theta^{(l)}, \hat{\beta}_{\theta^{(l)}}\right)$. At the θ level, a golden section search can then be performed making use of the pairs $\left(\theta^{(j)}, l_{marg}\left(\hat{h}_{0,\theta^{(j)}}(.), \theta^{(j)}, \hat{\boldsymbol{\beta}}_{\theta^{(j)}}\right)\right)$, $j = 1, \ldots, l$ to find θ that maximises the marginal data loglikelihood.

The estimated variances of the estimators of the parameters are the diagonal elements of the inverse of the observed information matrix of the marginal likelihood.

The observed information matrix is a square matrix of dimension $(r+p+1) \times (r+p+1)$. With each event time $y_{(v)}$ corresponds a parameter h_{0v} leading to r parameters, an additional p parameters come from the p-dimensional vector $\boldsymbol{\beta}$, and the last parameter is θ leading indeed to an $(r+p+1) \times (r+p+1)$ information matrix. It contains the following partial derivatives of minus the marginal likelihood:

$$\frac{-\partial^2 l_{marg}}{\partial \beta_a \partial \beta_b} = \sum_{i=1}^{s} \frac{d_i + 1/\theta}{\left(H_{\mathbf{x}_i,c}(\mathbf{y}_i) + 1/\theta\right)^2}$$

$$\times \left[\left(\sum_{j=1}^{n_i} H_0(y_{ij}) \exp\left(\mathbf{x}_{ij}^t \boldsymbol{\beta}\right) x_{ija} x_{ijb} \right) \left(H_{\mathbf{x}_i,c}(\mathbf{y}_i) + 1/\theta \right) \right.$$

$$\left. - \left(\sum_{j=1}^{n_i} H_0(y_{ij}) \exp\left(\mathbf{x}_{ij}^t \boldsymbol{\beta}\right) x_{ija} \right) \left(\sum_{j=1}^{n_i} H_0(y_{ij}) \exp\left(\mathbf{x}_{ij}^t \boldsymbol{\beta}\right) x_{ijb} \right) \right]$$

$$\frac{-\partial^2 l_{marg}}{\partial \theta^2} = \sum_{i=1}^{s} \left[\sum_{l=0}^{d_i-1} -\frac{1 + 2l\theta}{(l\theta^2 + \theta)^2} + \frac{2\log\theta - 3}{\theta^3} + \frac{2}{\theta^3}\log\left(H_{\mathbf{x}_i,c}(\mathbf{y}_i) + 1/\theta\right) \right.$$

$$\left. + \frac{3/\theta + d_i + (4 + 2\theta d_i) H_{\mathbf{x}_i,c}(\mathbf{y}_i)}{\left(\theta + \theta^2 H_{\mathbf{x}_i,c}(\mathbf{y}_i)\right)^2} \right]$$

$$\frac{-\partial^2 l_{marg}}{\partial h_{0c} \partial h_{0d}} = \sum_{i=1}^{s} \frac{-(d_i + 1/\theta) \sum_{y_{ij} \geq y_{(c)}} \exp\left(\mathbf{x}_{ij}^t \boldsymbol{\beta}\right) \sum_{y_{ij} \geq y_{(d)}} \exp\left(\mathbf{x}_{ij}^t \boldsymbol{\beta}\right)}{\left(H_{\mathbf{x}_i,c}(\mathbf{y}_i) + 1/\theta\right)^2}$$

$$+ I(c = d) \frac{N_{(c)}}{(h_{0c})^2}$$

$$\frac{-\partial^2 l_{marg}}{\partial \beta_a \partial \theta} = \sum_{i=1}^{s} \frac{d_i - H_{\mathbf{x}_i,c}(\mathbf{y}_i) \sum_{j=1}^{n_i} H_0(y_{ij}) \exp\left(\mathbf{x}_{ij}^t \boldsymbol{\beta}\right) x_{ija}}{\left(1 + \theta H_{\mathbf{x}_i,c}(\mathbf{y}_i)\right)^2}$$

$$\frac{-\partial^2 l_{marg}}{\partial \beta_a \partial h_{0c}} = \sum_{i=1}^{s} \frac{d_i + 1/\theta}{\left(H_{\mathbf{x}_i,c}\left(\mathbf{y}_i\right) + 1/\theta\right)^2}$$

$$\times \left[\left(\sum_{y_{ij} \geq y_{(c)}} \exp\left(\mathbf{x}_{ij}^t \boldsymbol{\beta}\right) x_{ija} \right) \left(H_{\mathbf{x}_i,c}\left(\mathbf{y}_i\right) + 1/\theta\right) \right.$$

$$\left. - \left(\sum_{j=1}^{n_i} H_0\left(y_{ij}\right) \exp\left(\mathbf{x}_{ij}^t \boldsymbol{\beta}\right) x_{ija} \right) \left(\sum_{y_{ij} \geq y_{(c)}} \exp\left(\mathbf{x}_{ij}^t \boldsymbol{\beta}\right) \right) \right]$$

$$\frac{-\partial^2 l_{marg}}{\partial \theta \partial h_{0c}} = \sum_{i=1}^{s} \frac{\left(d_i - H_{\mathbf{x}_i,c}\left(\mathbf{y}_i\right)\right) \left(\sum\limits_{y_{ij} \geq y_{(c)}} \exp\left(\mathbf{x}_{ij}^t \boldsymbol{\beta}\right) \right)}{\left(1 + \theta H_{\mathbf{x}_i,c}\left(\mathbf{y}_i\right)\right)^2}$$

Example 5.1 Using the EM algorithm to fit the semiparametric gamma frailty model for the ductal carcinoma in situ trial

The semiparametric gamma frailty model is fitted to the ductal carcinoma in situ data described in Example 1.6 using the EM algorithm based on the SAS macro developed by Klein and Moeschberger (1997). Standard errors of the parameter estimates are obtained from the inverse of the observed information matrix. The radiotherapy effect estimate is -0.628 (s.e. $= 0.167$) corresponding to a hazard ratio of treated versus untreated of 0.53 with the 95% confidence interval $[0.38; 0.74]$. The actual value of the Wald test statistic is $(-0.628/0.167)^2 = 14.06$ leading to a p-value $P(\chi_1^2 \geq 14.06) = 0.0002$. So the local recurrence hazard is about half in the treated group compared to the untreated group. The estimate of the variance of the frailties, θ, is 0.086 (s.e. $= 0.080$). The survival functions for the treated and untreated group are obtained from the Nelson–Aalen estimator of the baseline hazard given in (5.5) and evaluated at the estimates for β and $\mathbf{u}$ at convergence. The two survival curves shown in Figure 5.3 refer to the treated and untreated group of patients in a centre with the frailty equal to one. ■

5.1.3 Why the EM algorithm works for the gamma frailty model

In applications of the EM algorithm, we typically have observed and unobserved information. In the particular case of the frailty model, the observed and unobserved information correspond to $\mathbf{z}$ and $\mathbf{u}$, respectively.

In Section 2.2 we obtained the marginal likelihood expression (2.7) by integrating out the unobserved frailties. We would like to base inference on an expression like (2.7) that no longer contains the unobserved information, but in the semiparametric model this expression still contains the unspecified

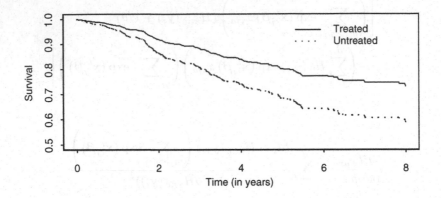

Fig. 5.3. The survival functions for the treated and untreated group of the ductal carcinoma in situ trial based on the Nelson–Aalen estimator in the semiparametric gamma frailty model in a centre with frailty equal to one.

baseline hazard. In such cases, the EM algorithm can solve the problem as described below.

We start from the joint density function of the observed and unobserved information (using again f as generic notation)

$$f(\mathbf{z}, \mathbf{u} \mid \zeta) = f(\mathbf{z} \mid \zeta) f(\mathbf{u} \mid \mathbf{z}, \zeta)$$

The loglikelihood function based on the observed and the unobserved information can therefore be written as

$$l(\zeta \mid \mathbf{z}, \mathbf{u}) = l(\zeta \mid \mathbf{z}) + \log f(\mathbf{u} \mid \mathbf{z}, \zeta)$$

from which follows that

$$l(\zeta \mid \mathbf{z}) = l(\zeta \mid \mathbf{z}, \mathbf{u}) - \log f(\mathbf{u} \mid \mathbf{z}, \zeta) \tag{5.10}$$

with the left-hand side now consisting of a loglikelihood expression that only depends on the observed information. The two terms on the right-hand side contain the unobserved information $\mathbf{U}$. We have, however, an expression for the density of $\mathbf{U}$ conditional on $\mathbf{z}$ and ζ, $f(\mathbf{u} \mid \mathbf{z}, \zeta)$. In order to make use of the conditional density $f(\mathbf{u} \mid \mathbf{z}, \zeta)$, however, we require a value for ζ. Denote by

$\zeta^{(k)}$ the estimate at iteration level k of the EM algorithm. We can then plug in this value so that the conditional density of the unobserved information is fully specified. This distribution can then be used to integrate out the unobservable information and obtain the expectation of these expressions

$$\int l(\zeta \mid \mathbf{z})f(\mathbf{u} \mid \mathbf{z}, \zeta^{(k)})du = \int l(\zeta \mid \mathbf{z}, \mathbf{u})f(\mathbf{u} \mid \mathbf{z}, \zeta^{(k)})du$$

$$- \int \log f(\mathbf{u} \mid \mathbf{z}, \zeta)f(\mathbf{u} \mid \mathbf{z}, \zeta^{(k)})du$$

Since obviously

$$\int l(\zeta \mid \mathbf{z})f(\mathbf{u} \mid \mathbf{z}, \zeta^{(k)})du = l(\zeta \mid \mathbf{z}) \int f(\mathbf{u} \mid \mathbf{z}, \zeta^{(k)})du$$

$$= l(\zeta \mid \mathbf{z})$$

we have

$$l(\zeta \mid \mathbf{z}) = \int l(\zeta \mid \mathbf{z}, \mathbf{u})f(\mathbf{u} \mid \mathbf{z}, \zeta^{(k)})du - \int \log f(\mathbf{u} \mid \mathbf{z}, \zeta)f(\mathbf{u} \mid \mathbf{z}, \zeta^{(k)})du$$

$$= Q\left(\zeta, \zeta^{(k)}\right) - H\left(\zeta, \zeta^{(k)}\right) \qquad (5.11)$$

The aim is to maximise the left-hand side of (5.11) but equivalently the right-hand side can be maximised. We first concentrate on the term $Q\left(\zeta, \zeta^{(k)}\right)$. This term actually corresponds to the full likelihood expression $l_{full}(h_0(.), \theta, \beta)$ given in (5.1) of the previous section. The expected value can be obtained by replacing $\mathbf{u}$ and functions of $\mathbf{u}$ with their expected values conditional on $\mathbf{z}$ and $\zeta^{(k)}$. This is actually the E-step described in the previous section. Next, $Q\left(\zeta, \zeta^{(k)}\right)$ is maximised for ζ. This is the maximisation step of the previous section. In this way a new estimate $\zeta^{(k+1)}$ is obtained.

A central property in the derivation of the EM algorithm by Dempster et al. (1977) is that, due to Jensen's inequality,

$$H\left(\zeta^{(k+1)}, \zeta^{(k)}\right) - H\left(\zeta^{(k)}, \zeta^{(k)}\right) \leq 0$$

Using this expression it follows easily that

$$l(\zeta^{(k+1)} \mid \mathbf{z}) - l(\zeta^{(k)} \mid \mathbf{z}) = Q\left(\zeta^{(k+1)}, \zeta^{(k)}\right) - Q\left(\zeta^{(k)}, \zeta^{(k)}\right)$$
$$+ H\left(\zeta^{(k)}, \zeta^{(k)}\right) - H\left(\zeta^{(k+1)}, \zeta^{(k)}\right) > 0$$

Therefore, the EM algorithm converges to the parameter estimates that maximise the likelihood of the observed information. An interesting reference for further reading is Section 8.6 in Gill (2002).

5.2 The penalised partial likelihood approach

The penalised partial likelihood approach leads to the same estimates as the EM algorithm in the case of the semiparametric gamma frailty model. The penalised partial likelihood approach, however, can also be used to fit a semiparametric model with normal distributed random effects, which is the topic of the next section.

5.2.1 The penalised partial likelihood for the normal random effects density

The full data loglikelihood (5.1) consists of two parts. The first part is the conditional likelihood of the data given the frailties, whereas the second part corresponds to the distribution of the frailties. McGilchrist and Aisbett (1991) used this expression to derive the penalised partial likelihood approach but starting from the alternative representation of the frailty model

$$h_{ij}(t) = h_0(t) \exp\left(\mathbf{x}_{ij}^t \boldsymbol{\beta} + w_i\right)$$

where $w_i = \log u_i$. We will call u_i the frailty and w_i the random effect to distinguish between the two. We will use γ to denote the variance of the random effects w_i to distinguish between the variance of the frailties given by θ.

In this approach the second part of the likelihood is considered to be a penalty term: if the actual value of the random effect is far away from its (zero) mean, the absolute value of the logarithm of the density function evaluated at this value will typically be large and the penalty term typically has a large negative contribution to the full data loglikelihood. Additionally, taking the random effects as another set of parameters in the first part of the likelihood, this likelihood part can be transformed into a partial likelihood expression resulting in

$$l_{ppl}\left(\gamma, \boldsymbol{\beta}, \mathbf{w}\right) = l_{part}\left(\boldsymbol{\beta}, \mathbf{w}\right) - l_{pen}\left(\gamma, \mathbf{w}\right) \tag{5.12}$$

where, with $\eta_{ij} = \mathbf{x}_{ij}^t \boldsymbol{\beta} + w_i$ and $\boldsymbol{\eta} = (\eta_{11}, \ldots, \eta_{sn_s})$,

$$l_{part}(\boldsymbol{\beta}, \mathbf{w}) = \sum_{i=1}^{s} \sum_{j=1}^{n_i} \delta_{ij} \left[\eta_{ij} - \log \left(\sum_{qw \in R(y_{ij})} \exp\left(\eta_{qw}\right) \right) \right] \tag{5.13}$$

and

$$l_{pen}(\gamma, \mathbf{w}) = - \sum_{i=1}^{s} \log f_W\left(w_i\right)$$

For random effects $w_i, i = 1, \ldots, s$, having a zero-mean normal density with variance γ, we then have

$$l_{pen}(\gamma, \mathbf{w}) = \frac{1}{2} \sum_{i=1}^{s} \left(\frac{w_i^2}{\gamma} + \log\left(2\pi\gamma\right) \right)$$

The maximisation of the penalised partial (log)likelihood consists of an inner and an outer loop. In the inner loop the Newton–Raphson procedure is used to maximise, for a provisional value of γ, $l_{ppl}(\gamma, \boldsymbol{\beta}, \mathbf{w})$ for $\boldsymbol{\beta}$ and $\mathbf{w}$ (best linear unbiased predictors, BLUPs). In the outer loop, the restricted maximum likelihood estimator for γ is obtained using the BLUPs. The process is iterated until convergence.

The details are as follows. Let l denote the outer loop index and k the inner loop index. Let $\gamma^{(l)}$ be the estimate for γ at the lth iteration in the outer loop. Given $\gamma^{(l)}$, $\boldsymbol{\beta}^{(l,k)}$ and $\mathbf{w}^{(l,k)}$ are the estimates and predictions for $\boldsymbol{\beta}$ and $\mathbf{w}$ at the kth iterative step in the inner loop.

Starting from initial values $\boldsymbol{\beta}^{(1,0)}$, $\mathbf{w}^{(1,0)}$, $\gamma^{(0)}$, and $\gamma^{(1)}$, the kth iterative step for Newton–Raphson, given $\gamma^{(l)}$, is given by

$$\begin{bmatrix} \boldsymbol{\beta}^{(l,k)} \\ \mathbf{w}^{(l,k)} \end{bmatrix} = \begin{bmatrix} \boldsymbol{\beta}^{(l,k-1)} \\ \mathbf{w}^{(l,k-1)} \end{bmatrix} - \mathbf{V} \begin{bmatrix} \mathbf{0} \\ (\gamma^{(l)})^{-1}\mathbf{w}^{(l,k-1)} \end{bmatrix}$$

$$+ \mathbf{V} \begin{bmatrix} \mathbf{X} & \mathbf{Z} \end{bmatrix} \frac{dl_{part}(\boldsymbol{\beta}, \mathbf{w})}{d\boldsymbol{\eta}}$$

where

$$\mathbf{V} = \begin{bmatrix} \mathbf{V}_{11} & \mathbf{V}_{12} \\ \mathbf{V}_{21} & \mathbf{V}_{22} \end{bmatrix}$$

is the inverse of the square $(p+s)$-dimensional matrix $\mathbf{A}$ with $\mathbf{A}$ given by

$$\mathbf{A} = \begin{bmatrix} \mathbf{A}_{11} & \mathbf{A}_{12} \\ \mathbf{A}_{21} & \mathbf{A}_{22} \end{bmatrix} = \begin{bmatrix} \mathbf{X}^t \\ \mathbf{Z}^t \end{bmatrix} \left(\frac{-d^2 l_{part}(\boldsymbol{\beta}, \mathbf{w})}{d\boldsymbol{\eta}\, d\boldsymbol{\eta}^t} \right) \begin{bmatrix} \mathbf{X} & \mathbf{Z} \end{bmatrix}$$

$$+ \begin{bmatrix} \mathbf{0} & \mathbf{0} \\ \mathbf{0} & (\gamma^{(l)})^{-1} \mathbf{I}_G \end{bmatrix}$$

Once the Newton–Raphson procedure has converged for the current value of $\gamma^{(l)}$, a REML estimate for γ is given by

$$\gamma^{(l+1)} = \frac{\sum\limits_{i=1}^{s} \left(w_i^{(l,k)} \right)^2}{s-r}$$

where $r = \mathrm{trace}\,(\mathbf{V}_{22})\,/\gamma^{(l)}$.

This outer loop is iterated until the absolute difference between two sequential values for γ, $|\gamma^{(l)} - \gamma^{(l-1)}|$, is sufficiently small (see Figure 5.4).

The asymptotic variance for $\hat{\beta}$ is given by $\mathbf{V}_{11}$ (Henderson, 1975; Schall, 1991; McGilchrist and Aisbett, 1991).

Additionally, the asymptotic variance for $\hat{\gamma}$ (McGilchrist, 1993) is generally given by

$$\frac{2\gamma^2}{s - 2r + \gamma^{-2}\mathrm{trace}\,(\mathbf{V}_{22}^2)}$$

Example 5.2 Using penalised partial likelihood to fit the semiparametric normal random effects model for the ductal carcinoma in situ trial

The semiparametric normal random effects model is fitted to the ductal carcinoma in situ data described in Example 1.6 through the penalised partial likelihood approach. The parameter estimates are almost the same as in Example 5.1. The radiotherapy effect estimate equals -0.627 (s.e. $= 0.167$) corresponding to the hazard ratio of treated versus untreated equal to 0.53 with the 95% confidence interval $[0.38; 0.74]$; also the p-value for the Wald statistic is the same as in Example 5.1. The estimate of the variance of the random effects, γ, is given by 0.087 (s.e. = 0.080). In Section 5.2.4 it will be shown that the variance of gamma distributed frailties and normal distributed random effects is virtually the same as long as the variance is reasonably small, which is the case here. ■

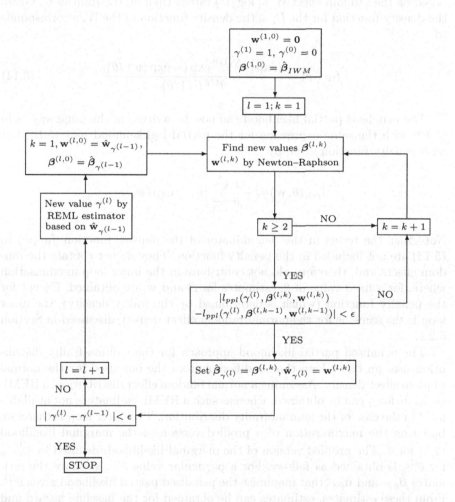

Fig. 5.4. The penalised partial likelihood maximisation algorithm for the semiparametric normal random effects model. For further explanation, see text.

5.2.2 The penalised partial likelihood for the gamma frailty distribution

The semiparametric gamma frailty model can also be fitted by the penalised partial likelihood approach. We will demonstrate in this section that the EM algorithm and the penalised partial likelihood approach lead to the same estimates. We assume again a one-parameter gamma frailty distribution with mean one and variance θ. As in the previous section, however, the modelling is based on the random effect $W = \log(U)$ rather than on the frailties U. Given the density function for the U_i's, the density function of the W_i's corresponds to

$$f_W(w) = \frac{(\exp(w))^{1/\theta} \exp(-\exp(w)/\theta)}{\theta^{1/\theta} \Gamma(1/\theta)} \tag{5.14}$$

The penalised partial likelihood can now be written in the same way as in (5.12) with the same expression for the partial loglikelihood part (5.13) but with penalty function given by

$$l_{pen}(\theta, \mathbf{w}) = -\frac{1}{\theta} \sum_{i=1}^{s} (w_i - \exp(w_i))$$

Note that the terms in the denominator of the density function $f_W(w)$ in (5.14) are not included in the penalty function. They do not contain the random effects and, therefore, do not contribute in the inner loop maximisation where, for a fixed value of θ, estimates for β and $\mathbf{w}$ are obtained. Except for the penalty function (which is determined by the frailty density), the inner loop is the same as for the normal random effect density discussed in Section 5.2.1.

The penalised partial likelihood approach for the gamma frailty distribution uses an outer loop that is different from the one used for the normal random effect density. Assuming a normal random effect distribution, a REML estimate for γ can be obtained, whereas such a REML estimate is not available for θ in the case of the gamma frailty distribution. The outer loop is therefore based on the maximisation of a profiled version of the marginal likelihood (2.7) for θ. The profiled version of the marginal likelihood, denoted by $l_{marg}^{(l)}$ for $\theta^{(l)}$, is obtained as follows. For a particular value $\theta^{(l)}$, we have the estimates $\hat{\beta}_{\theta^{(l)}}$ and $\hat{\mathbf{u}}_{\theta^{(l)}}$ that maximise the penalised partial likelihood given $\theta^{(l)}$. From these estimates, estimates can be obtained for the baseline hazard and cumulative baseline hazard function based on the Nelson–Aalen estimates as given in (5.4) and (5.5), replacing the expected values of the frailties in (5.5) by the estimates $\hat{\mathbf{u}}_{\theta^{(l)}}$ and replacing $\beta^{(k)}$ by $\hat{\beta}_{\theta^{(l)}}$.

As in the modified EM algorithm, this profile marginal likelihood for θ is used to find an estimate for θ. The algorithm stops if the absolute difference between two sequential values for θ is sufficiently small. The algorithm is given in Figure 5.5 and is very similar to the one for the penalised partial likelihood approach for the normal random effects model; the main difference is the use of the golden section search based on $l_{marg}^{(l)}$ to obtain a new value for θ.

Example 5.3 Using penalised partial likelihood to fit the semiparametric gamma frailty model for the ductal carcinoma in situ trial

The semiparametric normal random effects model is fitted to the ductal carcinoma in situ data described in Example 1.6 through the penalised partial likelihood approach. The parameter estimates are almost the same as in Example 5.1 where the EM algorithm was used to fit the semiparametric gamma frailty model. The radiotherapy effect estimate equals -0.627 (s.e. $= 0.167$) corresponding to the hazard ratio of treated versus untreated equal to 0.53 with the 95% confidence interval $[0.38; 0.74]$ and we obtain the same p-value equal to 0.0002 for the Wald statistic. The estimate of the variance of the random effects, θ, is given as 0.087.

We now study the behaviour of the two terms of the penalised partial likelihood separately as a function of θ. We vary θ between 0 and 0.5 and obtain estimates $\hat{\boldsymbol{\beta}}_{\theta^{(l)}}$ and $\hat{\mathbf{u}}_{\theta^{(l)}}$ for values $\theta^{(l)}$ in the considered range. From these estimates, the penalised partial likelihood and its two parts, the partial likelihood alone and the penalty term, can be determined (see Figure 5.6). Obviously, the partial likelihood part alone increases and the penalty term increases with increasing values of θ. The penalised partial likelihood as a whole also increases with increasing values of θ. It is therefore obvious that the penalised partial likelihood can only be used to obtain estimates for $\boldsymbol{\beta}$ and the baseline hazard, not for θ. ■

We now prove that the penalised partial likelihood approach and the modified EM algorithm lead to the same estimates. The outer loop is the same implying that there is equivalence at the level of θ.

We therefore only need to prove that for given $\theta^{(l)}$, the two approaches lead to the same solutions for $\boldsymbol{\beta}$ and $\mathbf{w}$.

For $\boldsymbol{\beta}$ both approaches maximise the same partial likelihood for $\boldsymbol{\beta}$ with fixed offset terms $\hat{\mathbf{w}}$ and $\hat{\mathbf{u}}$ for the penalised partial likelihood approach and the modified EM algorithm, respectively. So in case that $\exp(\hat{\mathbf{w}})$, with $\hat{\mathbf{w}}$ the estimate from the penalised partial likelihood approach, equals the estimate $\hat{\mathbf{u}}$ from the EM algorithm, the same estimate for $\boldsymbol{\beta}$ will be obtained.

We now consider the score equations for w_a in the penalised partial likelihood approach

$$\frac{\partial l_{ppl}}{\partial w_a} = \frac{\partial l_{part}}{\partial w_a} - \frac{\partial l_{pen}}{\partial w_a} \tag{5.15}$$

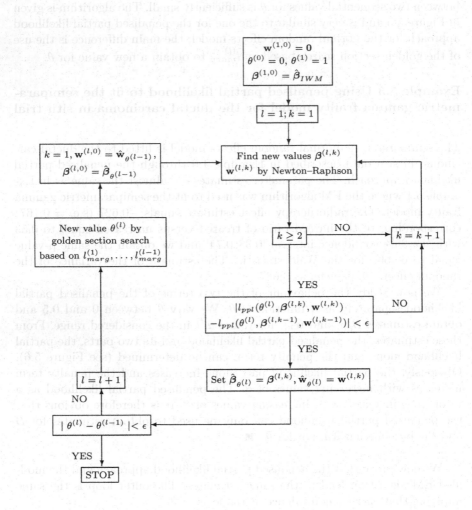

Fig. 5.5. The penalised partial likelihood maximisation algorithm for the semiparametric gamma frailty model. For further explanation, see text.

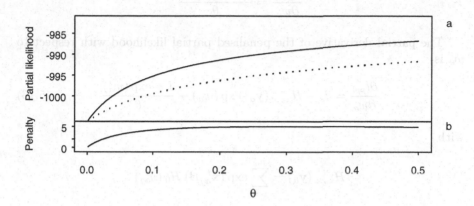

Fig. 5.6. Profile penalised partial likelihood for θ: in (a) the penalised partial likelihood (dashed line) and the partial likelihood part (solid line); in (b) the penalty term.

The first term on the right-hand side of (5.15), the partial derivative of the partial loglikelihood with fixed offset term as in (5.13), can be written as

$$
\frac{\partial l_{part}}{\partial w_a} = \sum_{i=1}^{s} \sum_{j=1}^{n_i} \delta_{ij} \left(Z_{ij,a} - \frac{\sum\limits_{qw \in R(y_{ij})} Z_{qw,a} \exp\left(\mathbf{x}_{qw}^t \boldsymbol{\beta} + w_q\right)}{\sum\limits_{qw \in R(y_{ij})} \exp\left(\mathbf{x}_{qw}^t \boldsymbol{\beta} + w_q\right)} \right)
$$

with $Z_{ij,a} = 1$ if $i = a$, i.e., the subject belongs to cluster a.

This can be rewritten as

$$
\frac{\partial l_{part}}{\partial w_a} = \sum_{j=1}^{n_a} \delta_{aj} - \sum_{j=1}^{n_a} \exp\left(\mathbf{x}_{aj}^t \boldsymbol{\beta} + w_a\right) H_0\left(y_{aj}\right)
$$

with

$$
H_0\left(y_{aj}\right) = \sum_{y(l) \leq y_{aj}} \frac{N_{(l)}}{\sum\limits_{qw \in R(y(l))} \exp\left(\mathbf{x}_{qw}^t \boldsymbol{\beta} + w_q\right)}
$$

On the other hand,

$$\frac{\partial l_{pen}}{\partial w_a} = \frac{1 - \exp(w_a)}{\theta}$$

The partial derivative of the penalised partial likelihood with respect to w_a is

$$\frac{\partial l_{ppl}}{\partial w_a} = d_a - H_{\mathbf{x}_a,c}(\mathbf{y}_a)\exp(w_a) - \frac{1 - \exp(w_a)}{\theta} \qquad (5.16)$$

with

$$H_{\mathbf{x}_a,c}(\mathbf{y}_a) = \sum_{j=1}^{n_a} \exp\left(\mathbf{x}_{aj}^t \boldsymbol{\beta}\right) H_0(y_{aj})$$

Now consider the solution for u_a from the modified EM algorithm for a particular value $\theta^{(l)}$. When the algorithm has converged at step $k+1$ within outer loop iteration l, the estimate for u_a, $\hat{u}_{a,\theta^{(l)}}$, can be taken as the expected value in (5.8), but with $\theta^{(k)}$ replaced by the fixed value for θ, $\theta^{(l)}$, as only the inner loop of the modified EM algorithm is currently considered. Similarly, we consider $H_{\mathbf{x}_a,c}^{(k)}(\mathbf{y}_a)$ to be, upon convergence, the estimate $\hat{H}_{\mathbf{x}_a,c,\theta^{(l)}}(\mathbf{y}_a)$. We need to convert the estimated frailty $\hat{u}_{a,\theta^{(l)}}$ to the random effect $\hat{w}_{a,\theta^{(l)}}$ to evaluate it in the context of the penalised partial likelihood approach, so denote by $\hat{w}_{a,\theta^{(l)}}$ the logarithm of the estimate $\hat{u}_{a,\theta^{(l)}}$.

We then have, by transforming (5.8), that

$$\hat{H}_{\mathbf{x}_a,c,\theta^{(l)}}(\mathbf{y}_a) = \exp\left(-\hat{w}_{a,\theta^{(l)}}\right)\left(d_a + 1/\theta^{(l)}\right) - 1/\theta^{(l)} \qquad (5.17)$$

If we substitute this expression in the score equation (5.16) and evaluate it at the estimates $\boldsymbol{\beta}$ and $\mathbf{w}$ derived from the EM algorithm, we obtain

$$\frac{\partial l_{part}}{\partial w_a} = d_a - \left(\exp\left(-\hat{w}_{a,\theta^{(l)}}\right)\left(d_a + 1/\theta^{(l)}\right) - 1/\theta^{(l)}\right)\exp\left(\hat{w}_{a,\theta^{(l)}}\right)$$

$$-\frac{1 - \exp\left(\hat{w}_{a,\theta^{(l)}}\right)}{\theta^{(l)}} \qquad (5.18)$$

and this equals zero. Therefore, the two approaches lead to the same estimates.

Finally, the following relationship exists between the marginal likelihood obtained by plugging in estimates for $\boldsymbol{\beta}$, $h_0(.)$, and $H_0(.)$ from the inner loop of the penalised partial likelihood approach for a fixed value of θ and the penalised partial likelihood:

$$l_{marg}^{(l)} = l_{ppl} + \sum_{i=s}^{s} 1/\theta^{(l)} - \left(1/\theta^{(l)} + d_i\right) \log\left(1/\theta^{(l)} + d_i\right) + \log(1/\theta^{(l)})/\theta^{(l)}$$

$$+ \log\left(\frac{\Gamma(1/\theta^{(l)} + d_i)}{\Gamma(1/\theta^{(l)})}\right) \tag{5.19}$$

This relation is of interest since the value of l_{ppl} is already available from the inner loop. It is therefore computationally efficient to calculate the marginal likelihood from the penalised partial likelihood.

This relationship can be proven as follows. We start from the marginal likelihood expression (2.7), and now evaluate this function at $\theta^{(l)}$ and the corresponding estimates $\hat{\boldsymbol{\beta}}_{\theta^{(l)}}$, $\hat{h}_{0,\theta^{(l)}}(.)$, and $\hat{H}_{0,\theta^{(l)}}(.)$. We will drop the subscript $\theta^{(l)}$ from the estimates $\hat{\boldsymbol{\beta}}_{\theta^{(l)}}$, $\hat{h}_{0,\theta^{(l)}}(.)$ and $\hat{w}_{a,\theta^{(l)}}$ in the expressions below.

This leads to the expression

$$l_{marg}^{(l)} = \sum_{i=1}^{s}\sum_{j=1}^{n_i} \delta_{ij}\left(\mathbf{x}_{ij}^t\hat{\boldsymbol{\beta}} + \log\hat{h}_0(y_{ij})\right)$$

$$+ \sum_{i=1}^{s}\left[d_i\log\theta^{(l)} + \log\left(\frac{\Gamma(1/\theta^{(l)} + d_i)}{\Gamma(1/\theta^{(l)})}\right)\right.$$

$$\left. -(1/\theta^{(l)} + d_i)\log\left(1 + \theta^{(l)}\hat{H}_{i\cdot,c}\right)\right]$$

Now use (5.17) to rewrite $l_{marg}^{(l)}$ as

$$l_{marg}^{(l)} = \sum_{i=1}^{s}\sum_{j=1}^{n_i} \delta_{ij}\left(\mathbf{x}_{ij}^t\hat{\boldsymbol{\beta}} + \log\hat{h}_0(y_{ij})\right)$$

$$+ \sum_{i=1}^{s}\left[\log\left(\frac{\Gamma(1/\theta^{(l)} + d_i)}{\Gamma(1/\theta^{(l)})}\right) + \log\left(\exp\left(\hat{w}_i/\theta^{(l)}\right)\right)/\theta^{(l)}\right.$$

$$\left. + d_i\log\left(\exp\left(\hat{w}_i\right)\right) - \left(d_i + 1/\theta^{(l)}\right)\log\left(d_i + 1/\theta^{(l)}\right)\right]$$

We can include the term $d_i\log\left(\exp\left(\hat{w}_i\right)\right)$ in the double sum term

This gives

$$l_{marg}^{(l)} = \sum_{i=1}^{s} \sum_{j=1}^{n_i} \delta_{ij} \left(\mathbf{x}_{ij}^t \hat{\boldsymbol{\beta}} + \hat{w}_i + \log \hat{h}_0(y_{ij}) \right)$$

$$+ \sum_{i=1}^{s} \left[\log \left(\frac{\Gamma(1/\theta^{(l)} + d_i)}{\Gamma(1/\theta^{(l)})} \right) + \log \left(\exp \left(\hat{w}_i/\theta^{(l)} \right) \right) / \theta^{(l)} \right.$$

$$\left. - \left(d_i + 1/\theta^{(l)} \right) \log \left(d_i + 1/\theta^{(l)} \right) \right]$$

Now we subtract and add the penalty term

$$l_{pen}(\theta, \hat{\mathbf{w}}) = - \sum_{i=1}^{s} \left(\hat{w}_i/\theta^{(l)} - \exp(\hat{w}_i)/\theta^{(l)} \right)$$

which leads to

$$l_{marg}^{(l)} = \sum_{i=1}^{s} \sum_{j=1}^{n_i} \delta_{ij} \left(\mathbf{x}_{ij}^t \hat{\boldsymbol{\beta}} + \hat{w}_i + \log \hat{h}_0(y_{ij}) \right) - l_{pen}(\theta, \hat{\mathbf{w}})$$

$$+ \sum_{i=1}^{s} \left[-\hat{w}_i/\theta^{(l)} + \exp \left(\hat{w}_i \right) / \theta^{(l)} + \log \left(\frac{\Gamma(1/\theta^{(l)} + d_i)}{\Gamma(1/\theta^{(l)})} \right) \right.$$

$$\left. + \log \left(\exp \left(\hat{w}_i/\theta^{(l)} \right) \right) / \theta^{(l)} - \left(d_i + 1/\theta^{(l)} \right) \log \left(d_i + 1/\theta^{(l)} \right) \right] \quad (5.20)$$

The first line on the right-hand side of (5.20) corresponds to the penalised partial likelihood. This can be seen by plugging in (5.5) for the baseline hazard estimate $\hat{h}_0(y_{ij})$ where we have shown in (5.18) that $\mathrm{E}_{(k)}(U_q)$ can be replaced by the $\exp(\hat{w}_q)$ with $\hat{w}_q$ the estimate obtained from the penalised partial likelihood maximisation.

The second part can be simplified by using the fact that $\sum_{i=1}^{s} \exp(\hat{w}_i) = s$. This restriction indeed minimises the penalised partial likelihood. The restriction has no influence on the partial likelihood part. Adding or subtracting a constant value to the frailties does not change the partial likelihood value as the constant term appears in both the numerator and denominator and can be cancelled out. The penalty term, however, is minimised when using this restriction. Applying this restriction to the equation above leads to (5.19).

5.2.3 Performance of the penalised partial likelihood estimates

Asymptotic properties for the estimated heterogeneity parameter are only available for a limited number of semiparametric models (Murphy, 1995; Parner, 1998). Therefore, the properties of the variance parameter estimate in the semiparametric model with normal distributed random effects or gamma distributed frailties are studied in this section through simulations. The simulations are based on the perioperative cancer clinical trial described in Example 1.5. We therefore first analyse this data set in the following example before embarking on the simulation study.

Example 5.4 Semiparametric frailty models for the perioperative breast cancer clinical trial

We consider Example 1.5, the perioperative breast cancer clinical trial. Fitting the semiparametric model to the disease-free survival endpoint without taking the clustering of patients in centres into account leads to an estimated treatment effect of 0.157 (s.e. = 0.063), corresponding to a hazard ratio of untreated versus treated of 1.17 with the 95% confidence interval [1.03; 1.32]. The hazard ratio differs significantly from 1 (the p-value is 0.013).

Now add gamma distributed frailty terms for the centres to the model. The hazard ratio for an untreated versus a treated patient in a centre is now estimated as 1.17 with the 95% confidence interval [1.03; 1.33], so it is virtually the same except that the confidence interval is slightly larger. This similarity is expected as the treatment assignment is balanced within an institute (see Table 5.1) due to the fact that institute was one of the stratification factors in the central randomisation.

The variance of the frailties is estimated as 0.087. To test the null hypothesis $H_0 : \theta = 0$ versus the alternative hypothesis $H_0 : \theta > 0$, Andersen et al. (1993) proposed a likelihood ratio test comparing the model with and without frailties. The likelihood ratio test statistic is compared with a χ_1^2 distribution. The likelihood ratio test statistic for this example equals 46.86 (the p-value is < 0.0001). Note, however, that the use of the χ_1^2 distribution is questionable since the value for θ in the null hypothesis is at the boundary of the parameter space. We come back to the boundary problem in this section and study the distribution of the likelihood ratio test by simulation.

Furthermore, the profile marginal likelihood can be used to determine confidence intervals. For instance, when approximating the profile marginal likelihood by χ_1^2, we need to take those two values of θ for which the marginal profile likelihood lies 1.92 units below the maximum profile likelihood value for the 95% confidence interval (Morgan, 1992). For our data example, the maximum value for the marginal profile likelihood at $\theta = 0.087$ equals -7621.82. For $\theta = 0.0255$ and $\theta = 0.1842$ the profile marginal likelihood corresponds to -7623.74, and thus differs 1.92 from the maximal value. The 95% confidence interval for θ is therefore given by [0.026; 0.184] and is depicted in Figure 5.7.

A similar comparison for the effect of the prognostic factor nodal status leads to a hazard of nodal involvement versus no nodal involvement of 1.80 with the 95% confidence interval $[1.59; 2.04]$ in the model without frailties which changes to 1.82 with the 95% confidence interval $[1.60; 2.07]$ for the model including gamma distributed frailties. The difference is again small although larger than for the treatment effect, which is due to the fact that there is more imbalance for this prognostic factor over the different institutes (see Table 5.1).

The same analysis can be done but now assuming a normal distribution for the random effects. The hazard ratio for the treatment effect of untreated versus treated is now estimated as 1.17 with 95% confidence interval $[1.03; 1.33]$, which is exactly the same as for the gamma frailty model. The variance of the random effects is estimated as 0.069. The variance estimate is similar to the one obtained from the gamma frailty model, although it relates now to the random effects rather than the frailties. The relationship between normal distributed random effects and gamma distributed frailties will be discussed in detail in the next subsection. ∎

Table 5.1. Distribution of patients with respect to treatment and nodal status over the different institutes.

Institute	Nodal status			Treatment	
	0	1	Missing	0	1
11	31	22	0	26	27
12	18	7	0	12	13
13	99	81	4	92	92
21	16	23	1	19	21
22	24	54	0	40	38
31	140	169	2	154	157
32	346	276	0	310	312
33	108	76	1	91	94
34	515	378	9	455	447
41	18	36	0	28	26
42	25	35	0	31	29
43	13	12	0	14	11
44	13	33	2	24	24
51	101	101	4	102	104

In the simulation study we investigate how the bias and the spread of estimates of θ around its true value depend on

(i)   the size of the multicentre trial (which is determined by the number of clusters (s) and the number of patients per cluster $(n_i = n)$);

(ii)   the event rate $h_0(t)$ (assumed to be constant over time: $h_0(t) = h_0$);

(iii)   the size of the true heterogeneity parameter θ and γ;

(iv)   the size of the true treatment effect β (expressed in terms of the hazard ratio $HR = \exp(\beta)$).

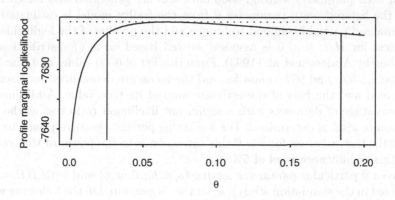

Fig. 5.7. Profile marginal loglikelihood for θ with the 95% confidence interval based on the profile marginal likelihood.

The simulations will also provide information on size and power for the likelihood ratio test for heterogeneity. The choice of the parameter settings $(s, n, h_0, \theta$ or $\gamma, \beta)$ used in the simulations is based on the parameter estimates obtained in the perioperative cancer clinical trial.

The number of centres in breast cancer clinical trials typically varies from 15 to 30 centres; for the number of patients per centre we take 20, 40, and 60. We study two different types of breast cancer trials: the early breast cancer clinical trials, with a typically low hazard rate, set here at $h_0 = 0.07$ yearly constant hazard rate (median time to event equals 9.9 years); and metastatic breast cancer clinical trials, with a typically high hazard rate, set here at $h_0 = 0.22$ yearly constant hazard rate (median time to event equals 3.15 years). We assume an accrual period of 5 years (with constant accrual rate) and a further follow-up period of 3 years. Time at risk for a particular patient thus consists of the time at risk before the end of the accrual period (ranging from 0 to 5 years) plus the follow-up time. This results in approximately 30% and 70% of the patients having the event in the early breast cancer and metastatic breast cancer clinical trial, respectively, at the end of the study with the remaining patients censored. As true values for the heterogeneity parameter, 0, 0.1, and 0.2 are used as this is the most likely range of values to be observed in breast cancer clinical trials.

Finally, for the treatment effect, we only use a hazard ratio of 1.3, as this is a typical effect expected for a new promising treatment compared to the standard treatment. Simulation results obtained for this setting were basically the same as for no treatment effect, so that we do not vary the value for the treatment effect β.

For each parameter setting, 6500 data sets are generated and for each of them the heterogeneity parameter θ from the frailty model is estimated by the penalised partial likelihood technique and the p-value of the loglikelihood ratio test for $H_0 : \theta = 0$ is assessed as well based on a χ_1^2 distribution as described by Andersen et al. (1993). From this list of 6500 values of θ, the 5%, 25%, 50%, 75%, and 95% quantiles and the mean are determined to describe the spread and the bias of the estimate around its true value. Additionally, the percentage of data sets with a significant likelihood ratio test at the 5% significance level is determined. For $\theta = 0$ this percentage corresponds to the size of the test, whereas for $\theta > 0$ this corresponds to the power of the test at a nominal significance level of 5%.

Given a particular parameter setting $(s, n, h_0, \theta$ or $\gamma)$ and with $HR = 1.3$ (β is fixed in the simulation study), a data set is generated in the following way. First, s random centre effects $w_1, \ldots, w_s$ are generated from the appropriate normal density or s frailties $u_1, \ldots, u_s$ from the appropriate gamma density. The time to event outcome for each patient is randomly generated from an exponential distribution with parameter h_{ij} for patient j from centre i given by

$$h_{ij} = \begin{cases} h_0 \exp\left(\beta x_{ij} + w_i\right) & \text{for normal distributed random effects} \\ h_0 u_i \exp\left(\beta x_{ij}\right) & \text{for gamma distributed random effects} \end{cases}$$

A patient for which the time to event is longer than the time at risk is censored with censoring time equal to time at risk. The results of the simulation studies are summarised below. First we discuss the bias using the mean and the interquantile range, for both the gamma and the normal distribution, and also compare the results for the two distributions. Next we report on the size and power for the gamma distribution.

Mean and 90% interquantile range

In all cases studied for $\theta = 0.1$ and $\theta = 0.2$ (or $\gamma = 0.1$ and $\gamma = 0.2$), the estimate of θ (or γ) is biased downward as the mean of the estimates of the heterogeneity parameter from the simulated data sets is smaller than the true parameter value. The patterns in the results are basically the same for the gamma and normal distribution. The normal distribution seems to do slightly better with respect to bias and interquantile range for $\gamma = 0.1$ and $\theta = 0.1$, whereas for $\gamma = 0.2$ and $\theta = 0.2$, the least biased and least variable results are sometimes obtained for the gamma distribution, sometimes for the normal distribution. For the further discussion, we do not make a distinction anymore between the gamma and the normal distribution.

For a fixed number of centres, either 15 or 30, there is little effect on bias when increasing the patient numbers (see Table 5.2). Increasing the number of centres from 15 to 30 reduces the bias, especially when $\theta = 0.2$ and less so for $\theta = 0.1$. The 90% interquantile range is decreasing substantially with increasing number of patients per centre and with increasing number of centres whatever the parameter setting. A pronounced effect is observed when increasing the number of patients per centre up to 40. When increasing the number of patients per centre further, the gain in terms of a smaller interquantile range is only marginal in most cases. The interquantile range shrinks considerably when increasing the number of centres from 15 to 30.

For fixed total sample size of 600 patients but distributed either over 15 centres or over 30 centres, the results are dependent on the event rate and the true heterogeneity parameter θ. With low event rate and $\theta = 0.1$, it is preferable to have only 15 centres with 40 patients each instead of 30 centres with 20 patients each. In all other cases studied, the interquantile range is smaller for 30 centres with 20 patients each. A higher event rate, however, reduces the interquantile range substantially, especially for $\theta = 0.1$ and for the smaller trials with fewer patients.

Size and power

In all cases, the size of the likelihood ratio test stays well below 5% and comes closer to 5% with larger trials (see Table 5.3). With respect to power based on the likelihood ratio test, it is obvious that a trial with 15 centres and only 20 patients per centre is inadequate when the event rate is low, or when $\theta = 0.1$ with a high event rate as in these cases the power stays well below 0.8. When increasing the sample size to 40 patients per centre, the trial has only a power of 0.568 when $\theta = 0.1$ and $h_0 = 0.07$. The power stays also well below 80% with only 20 patients per centre and 30 centres if the event rate is low and $\theta = 0.1$. In all other cases the power is above 0.8.

The power can also be derived based on the simulated results alone by determining the percentage of data sets for which the estimate of the heterogeneity parameter is above the 95% quantile for $\theta = 0$. For instance, 42.5% of the data sets with 15 centres and 20 patients per centre generated with parameters $h_0 = 0.07$, $\theta = 0.1$, and $HR = 1.3$ have an estimated heterogeneity parameter θ above 0.086, the 95% quantile for the same setting but with $\theta = 0$. Using this simulation-derived power leads to the same conclusions as when using the likelihood ratio test-based power. The simulation-derived power, however, is in most instances much higher. Thus, the likelihood ratio test is often too conservative. This is due to the fact that the value for θ in the null hypothesis is at the boundary of the parameter space, a fact well known in mixed models (Stram and Lee, 1994; Self and Liang, 1987). Therefore, the approximation of the loglikelihood ratio statistic by a χ_1^2 distribution is inadequate (see Figure 5.8). Rather, a mixture of a chi-square distribution with one and zero degrees of freedom should be used. This would result in a decrease of the critical value of the loglikelihood ratio statistic. Theoretical support for these findings is given in Maller and Zhou (2003) and Claeskens et al. (2007).

Table 5.2. Simulation study with $\theta = 0.1, 0.2$ and $\gamma = 0.1, 0.2$.

θ/γ	Statistic	20/15	40/15	60/15	20/30	40/30	60/30
Gamma distributed frailties — Hazard rate 0.07
0.1	5%	0.000	0.000	0.015	0.000	0.027	0.038
	50%	0.070	0.078	0.082	0.086	0.089	0.091
	95%	0.245	0.200	0.188	0.207	0.175	0.162
	Mean	0.088	0.087	0.090	0.093	0.093	0.095
	PowerLR	0.254	0.568	0.802	0.478	0.881	0.983
	PowerSim	0.425	0.751	0.904	0.654	0.941	0.991
0.2	5%	0.000	0.041	0.056	0.054	0.087	0.098
	50%	0.156	0.169	0.172	0.180	0.186	0.186
	95%	0.424	0.360	0.344	0.352	0.317	0.303
	Mean	0.179	0.181	0.183	0.188	0.192	0.191
	PowerLR	0.556	0.870	0.969	0.879	0.995	1.000
	PowerSim	0.737	0.945	0.986	0.937	0.999	1.000
Gamma distributed frailties — Hazard rate 0.22
0.1	5%	0.002	0.023	0.030	0.029	0.045	0.050
	50%	0.080	0.084	0.086	0.090	0.093	0.093
	95%	0.203	0.180	0.171	0.176	0.157	0.151
	Mean	0.089	0.091	0.092	0.095	0.095	0.096
	PowerLR	0.614	0.893	0.975	0.892	0.999	1.000
	PowerSim	0.770	0.961	0.990	0.953	0.999	1.000
0.2	5%	0.048	0.072	0.075	0.089	0.107	0.110
	50%	0.171	0.176	0.176	0.186	0.188	0.190
	95%	0.361	0.333	0.333	0.317	0.298	0.295
	Mean	0.184	0.186	0.186	0.192	0.193	0.194
	PowerLR	0.899	0.992	0.998	0.995	1.000	1.000
	PowerSim	0.959	0.998	1.000	0.998	1.000	1.000
Normal distribution — Hazard rate 0.07
0.1	5%	0.001	0.008	0.019	0.005	0.032	0.040
	50%	0.079	0.084	0.086	0.089	0.092	0.092
	95%	0.252	0.200	0.190	0.204	0.172	0.163
	Mean	0.095	0.092	0.093	0.095	0.095	0.096
0.2	5%	0.013	0.049	0.060	0.058	0.086	0.096
	50%	0.164	0.171	0.173	0.178	0.183	0.181
	95%	0.406	0.364	0.351	0.338	0.311	0.300
	Mean	0.183	0.184	0.184	0.185	0.188	0.188
Normal distribution — Hazard rate 0.22
0.1	5%	0.008	0.027	0.032	0.031	0.044	0.050
	50%	0.088	0.087	0.088	0.092	0.093	0.093
	95%	0.211	0.181	0.174	0.176	0.157	0.151
	Mean	0.096	0.093	0.093	0.096	0.096	0.096
0.2	5%	0.052	0.068	0.074	0.088	0.102	0.109
	50%	0.171	0.174	0.175	0.184	0.187	0.186
	95%	0.368	0.342	0.329	0.313	0.300	0.292
	Mean	0.186	0.186	0.185	0.191	0.192	0.192

Table 5.3. Simulation study with $\theta = 0$, $\gamma = 0$.

Statistic	20/15	40/15	60/15	20/30	40/30	60/30
Hazard rate 0.07						
5%	0.000	0.000	0.000	0.000	0.000	0.000
50%	0.000	0.000	0.000	0.000	0.000	0.000
95%	0.086	0.042	0.027	0.061	0.030	0.020
Mean	0.016	0.008	0.005	0.012	0.006	0.004
Size	0.012	0.016	0.017	0.014	0.022	0.021
Hazard rate 0.22						
5%	0.000	0.000	0.000	0.000	0.000	0.000
50%	0.000	0.000	0.000	0.000	0.000	0.000
95%	0.041	0.020	0.014	0.029	0.015	0.009
Mean	0.007	0.004	0.003	0.006	0.003	0.002
Size	0.011	0.013	0.014	0.018	0.022	0.022

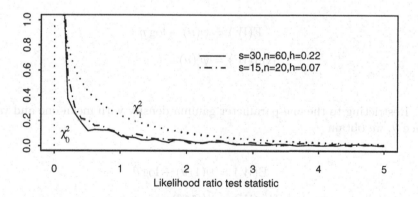

Fig. 5.8. The estimated density function of the likelihood ratio test statistic from the simulated data of two different settings ($s=30$, $n=60$, $h_0=0.22$ and $s=15$, $n=20$, $h_0=0.07$). The other two lines correspond to the density functions for χ_0^2 and χ_1^2.

5.2.4 Robustness of the frailty distribution assumption

In this subsection we consider the robustness of the gamma frailty distribution assumption. We generate frailties from a lognormal density with mean one and a particular variance and investigate by simulations whether the semiparametric gamma frailty model is capable of retrieving this variance.

Note that there is a difference between generating frailties from a lognormal density with mean one and generating random effects from a normal density with mean zero. If the distributional assumption is stated in terms of the random effect with $E(W) = 0$, then generally $E(U) \neq 1$, and vice versa, if the distributional assumption is stated in terms of the frailty with $E(U) = 1$, then generally $E(W) \neq 0$.

We first consider the particular situation of gamma distributed frailties, and start from the two-parameter gamma density

$$f_U(u) = \frac{\eta^\nu u^{\nu-1} \exp(-\eta u)}{\Gamma(\nu)} \quad 0 \leq u < \infty$$

This leads to the distribution for the random effects W

$$f_W(w) = \frac{\eta^\nu \exp(\nu w - \eta \exp(w))}{\Gamma(\nu)} \quad -\infty < w < \infty$$

with (see A.3 in Hougaard (2000))

$$E(W) = \psi(\nu) - \log \eta$$

$$\text{Var}(W) = \psi'(\nu)$$

Restricting to the one-parameter gamma density with mean one and variance θ, we obtain

$$E(W) = \psi(1/\theta) + \log \theta$$

$$\text{Var}(W) = \psi'(1/\theta)$$

with $\psi(.)$ the digamma function, i.e., the first derivative of the logarithm of the gamma function, and with $\psi'(.)$ the trigamma function, i.e., the second derivative of the logarithm of the gamma function. The relationship between $E(W)$ and the variance θ is shown in Figure 5.9. The expected value of W is always below zero, and deviates more and more from zero with increasing θ. On the other hand, the variance of W is always larger than θ and deviates more and more with larger values for θ, as shown in Figure 5.10. For relatively small values of θ, the two variances are virtually the same.

On the other hand, consider the situation of a normal distributed random effect with mean μ and variance γ. We obtain for the frailties the lognormal distribution

$$f_U(u) = \frac{1}{\sqrt{2\pi\gamma}} \frac{1}{u} \exp\left(\frac{-1}{2\gamma}(\log u - \mu)^2\right)$$

with

$$E(U) = \exp(\mu + \gamma/2) \tag{5.21}$$

$$\mathrm{Var}(U) = \exp(2\mu + \gamma)(\exp(\gamma) - 1) \tag{5.22}$$

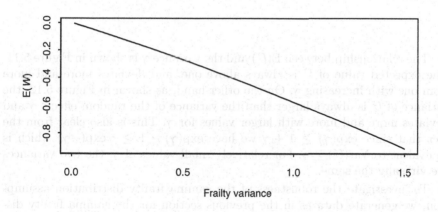

Fig. 5.9. Relationship between the variance of the frailties from the gamma frailty density with mean one and the expected value of the random effects $E(W)$.

Restricting to the normal density function with mean zero, we obtain

$$E(U) = \exp(\gamma/2) \tag{5.23}$$

$$\mathrm{Var}(U) = \exp(\gamma)(\exp(\gamma) - 1) \tag{5.24}$$

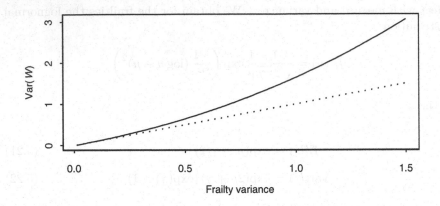

Fig. 5.10. Relationship between the variance of the frailties from the gamma frailty density θ with mean one and the variance of the random effects $\mathrm{Var}(W) = \gamma$. The dotted line represents equality between the frailty variance and $\mathrm{Var}(W)$.

The relationship between $E(U)$ and the variance γ is shown in Figure 5.11. The expected value of U is always above one, and deviates more and more from one with increasing γ. On the other hand, as shown in Figure 5.12, the variance of U is always larger than the variance of the random effects γ and deviates more and more with larger values for γ. This is also clear from the fact that since $\exp(\gamma) \geq 1 + \gamma$ we have $\exp(\gamma) - 1 \geq \gamma \exp(-\gamma)$ which is equivalent to $\mathrm{Var}(U) \geq \gamma$. For relatively small values of γ, the two variances are virtually the same.

To investigate the robustness of the gamma frailty distribution assumption, we generate data as in the previous section for the gamma frailty distribution, but now replacing the gamma frailty distribution by the lognormal distribution with mean equal to one. From (5.21) and (5.22) it follows that, in order to obtain a lognormal distribution with mean one and variance θ, we require

$$\mu = -\log(\theta + 1)/2 \tag{5.25}$$

$$\gamma = \log(\theta + 1) \tag{5.26}$$

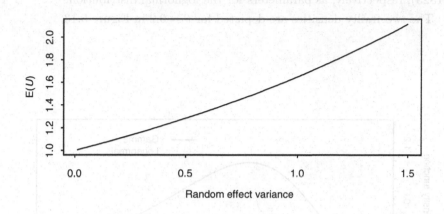

Fig. 5.11. Relationship between the variance of the random effects from a normal density with mean zero, γ , and the expected value of the frailties $E(U)$.

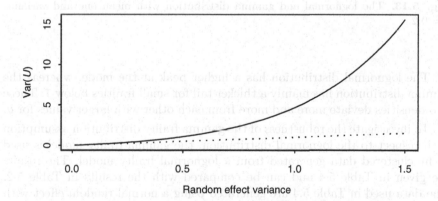

Fig. 5.12. Relationship between the variance of the random effects from a normal density with mean zero, γ, and the variance of the frailties $\text{Var}(U) = \theta$. The dotted line represents equality between the random effect variance and $\text{Var}(U)$.

In the simulations we use frailty variances $\theta = 0.1$ and $\theta = 0.2$ and these choices correspond to parameters $(\mu, \gamma) = (-0.0477, 0.0953)$ and $(-0.0917, 0.1823)$, respectively, as parameters for the lognormal distribution.

The two frailty densities are depicted for $\theta = 0.2$ in Figure 5.13.

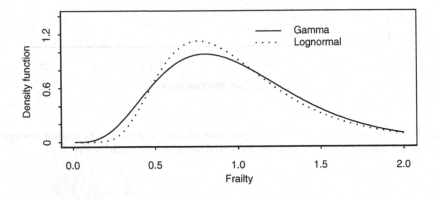

Fig. 5.13. The lognormal and gamma distribution with mean one and variance $\theta = 0.2$.

The lognormal distribution has a higher peak at the mode, whereas the gamma distribution has mainly a thicker tail for small frailties below 1. These two densities deviate more and more from each other with larger values for θ.

To investigate the robustness of the gamma frailty distribution assumption with respect to the lognormal distribution, the gamma frailty model is used to fit clustered data generated from a lognormal frailty model. The results are given in Table 5.4 and can be compared with the results in Table 5.2. The data used in Table 5.4 are generated using a normal random effect with mean and variance as in (5.25) and (5.26). The model we use to fit the data is the gamma frailty model (model misspecification). The comparison of the two tables reveals that the downward bias of the variance estimator is more pronounced in the misspecified model, for both the mean and the median of the variance estimates. Increasing $\theta = 0.1$ to $\theta = 0.2$ leads to further discrepancy. We can conclude that for small values of θ working with a misspecified model still leads to acceptable estimates for the heterogeneity parameter. On the other hand, robustness is an issue for larger values of the heterogeneity parameter.

Table 5.4. Robustness: the gamma frailty model is used to fit clustered data generated from a lognormal frailty model with $\theta = 0.1, 0.2$.

θ	Statistic	20/15	40/15	60/15	20/30	40/30	60/30
Hazard rate 0.07							
0.1	5%	0.000	0.000	0.011	0.000	0.025	0.035
	50%	0.065	0.075	0.077	0.081	0.084	0.086
	95%	0.243	0.194	0.178	0.202	0.166	0.155
	Mean	0.083	0.083	0.083	0.088	0.088	0.090
	PowerLR	0.225	0.552	0.755	0.452	0.849	0.969
	PowerSim	0.370	0.692	0.848	0.585	0.921	0.988
0.2	5%	0.000	0.033	0.049	0.038	0.073	0.082
	50%	0.140	0.149	0.153	0.160	0.166	0.166
	95%	0.379	0.327	0.315	0.323	0.287	0.275
	Mean	0.157	0.161	0.164	0.168	0.171	0.170
	PowerLR	0.499	0.852	0.952	0.807	0.988	0.999
	PowerSim	0.656	0.920	0.973	0.887	0.996	1.000
Hazard rate 0.22							
0.1	5%	0.000	0.020	0.027	0.025	0.040	0.045
	50%	0.075	0.078	0.079	0.083	0.086	0.087
	95%	0.185	0.166	0.158	0.163	0.147	0.142
	Mean	0.082	0.084	0.084	0.087	0.089	0.089
	PowerLR	0.554	0.887	0.969	0.856	0.994	1.000
	PowerSim	0.714	0.953	0.985	0.931	0.997	1.000
0.2	5%	0.033	0.056	0.063	0.073	0.090	0.094
	50%	0.147	0.150	0.155	0.162	0.165	0.164
	95%	0.322	0.298	0.288	0.279	0.263	0.257
	Mean	0.158	0.160	0.163	0.167	0.169	0.168
	PowerLR	0.849	0.986	0.998	0.989	1.000	1.000
	PowerSim	0.922	0.997	1.000	0.997	1.000	1.000

5.3 Bayesian analysis for the semiparametric gamma frailty model through Gibbs sampling

Also Bayesian techniques can be used to fit gamma frailty models with non-parametric baseline hazard. Kalbfleisch (1978) introduced a Bayesian analysis of the semiparametric Cox model. The Bayesian analysis for frailty models is discussed in Clayton (1991). A good overview of Bayesian survival analysis in general and frailty models in particular is given in the book by Ibrahim et al. (2001).

In Section 2.4 we demonstrated how the Metropolis algorithm can be applied for the parametric gamma frailty model. The Metropolis algorithm is based on sampling from the joint (multivariate) posterior density of the parameters of interest. For the semiparametric model this approach is problematic due to the fact that, for this model, the hazard rate at each event time is considered as a parameter. This results in a high-dimensional sampling problem for which the Metropolis algorithm is no longer efficient. The more efficient approach is to use Gibbs sampling, which is based on the posterior density of each parameter, conditional on all the other parameters. Gibbs sampling is also called alternating conditional sampling. The parameter vector is divided into a number of subvectors (in our case a subvector consists of just one parameter). In each iteration, sampling cycles through the different subvectors and draws a random sample for the subvector using the posterior density of the subvector conditional on the current values of the other subvectors. The main advantage is that a high-dimensional problem can be reduced to a number of unidimensional or lower-dimensional problems. Furthermore, the conditional posterior densities are often easy to obtain and to draw a sample from.

We will demonstrate in this section how Gibbs sampling can be applied to obtain posterior densities for the parameters of interest of the semiparametric gamma frailty model. To arrive at the conditional likelihood (5.34) used in a Bayesian analysis of semiparametric frailty models, it is useful to first derive, in Section 5.3.1, the conditional likelihood for a semiparametric frailty model in case of grouped (within disjoint intervals) multivariate survival data subject to right censoring. To construct the likelihood we assume that the increments over an interval of the cumulative baseline hazard are independent and we further assume a gamma process prior for the cumulative baseline hazard. See Kalbfleisch (1978) for a precise definition of the independent increments gamma process. We will explain in general terms how (expressions proportional to) conditional posterior densities can be obtained on which Gibbs sampling is based. In Section 5.3.2, we consider Gibbs sampling for the semiparametric gamma frailty model with the independent increments gamma process for the cumulative baseline hazard but now for right-censored multivariate survival data. Based on ideas from Section 5.3.1 we obtain an approximate conditional likelihood of Poisson form that is a key expression for the Bayesian analysis. In Section 5.3.3, we consider Gibbs sampling for the semiparametric frailty model with normal random effects. The sampling technique used to generate samples from a conditional density depends on the properties of that density . Different sampling techniques used for the semiparametric frailty models are discussed in Section 5.3.4. Finally, in Section 5.3.5, the basic theory behind Gibbs sampling is given and it is explained why the Gibbs sampling approach works.

5.3.1 The frailty model with a gamma process prior for the cumulative baseline hazard for grouped data

We consider the frailty model

$$h_{ij}(t) = h_0(t) u_i \exp\left(\mathbf{x}_{ij}^t \boldsymbol{\beta}\right)$$

with u_i the actual value of $U_i \sim \text{Gamma}(1/\theta, 1/\theta)$. Using the Gibbs sampler, we need to sample iteratively from the conditional posterior density of each parameter (conditional on all the other parameters) in order to obtain samples from the posterior densities of the parameters of interest. To derive these conditional posterior densities, we need the data likelihood as well as the prior densities of the parameters. As explained above, we first discuss the data likelihood assuming an independent increments gamma process for the cumulative baseline hazard and assuming grouped data. Next, we introduce the prior distributions and continue with a general discussion and a scheme for the derivation of the conditional posterior densities from which samples can be drawn.

Data likelihood specification

In this section, we consider the case of grouped data, which is the most appropriate data structure when the cumulative baseline hazard is specified in terms of increments over particular intervals with no information on the hazard function itself. With grouped data, the time axis is partitioned in z disjoint intervals $(L_{(0)}, L_{(1)}], \ldots, (L_{(z-1)}, L_{(z)}]$ with $(L_{(0)}, L_{(1)}] \equiv (0, L_{(1)}]$. For a particular interval $(L_{(k-1)}, L_{(k)}]$ and a particular subject three situations are possible: (i) the subject experienced the event in $(L_{(k-1)}, L_{(k)}]$; (ii) the subject did not experience the event in $(L_{(k-1)}, L_{(k)}]$ and is still at risk at $L_{(k)}$, the end of the interval; (iii) the subject is no longer in the study at time $L_{(k)}$ and is lost to follow-up in the interval $(L_{(k-1)}, L_{(k)}]$.

To fix the idea, we give a discussion for a simple but explicit data example for which we show how information on actual event and censoring times is reduced when looking at grouped data. Consider the time to first insemination data (see Example 1.8) for six cows from two different farms a and b, with their actual event or censoring times observed (Figure 5.14a), with first insemination and removal of the cow from the farm recorded individually on a daily basis. Assume, however, that insemination or removal of the cow is recorded only on a monthly basis when the farm is visited by the investigator. Therefore, information on insemination or censoring is only available at the end of each monthly interval (Figure 5.14b), which then reduces the time to event information to the grouped data structure.

The increase of the cumulative baseline hazard in interval $(L_{(k-1)}, L_{(k)}]$ is denoted by

$$h_{(k)} = H_0(L_{(k)}) - H_0(L_{(k-1)})$$

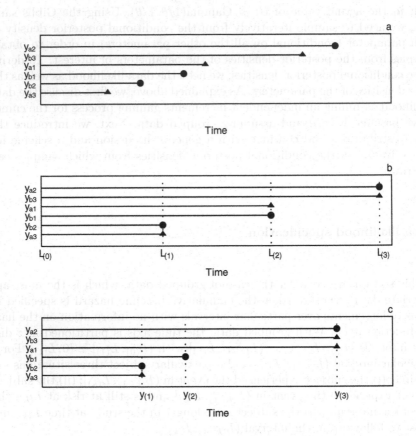

Fig. 5.14. Survival data for two clusters with three subjects with: (a) information on the actual times to event/censoring; (b) grouped data information given prespecified intervals; (c) grouped data information with event times as interval boundaries. Information on event/censoring times is denoted as ●/▲, respectively.

The conditional likelihood contributions of the six subjects are given by

$$L(y_{a3}) = 1$$

$$L(y_{b2}) = 1 - \exp\left(-u_b \exp(\mathbf{x}_{b2}^t\boldsymbol{\beta})h_{(1)}\right)$$

$$L(y_{b1}) = \exp\left(-u_b \exp(\mathbf{x}_{b1}^t\boldsymbol{\beta})h_{(1)}\right)\left[1 - \exp\left(-u_b \exp(\mathbf{x}_{b1}^t\boldsymbol{\beta})h_{(2)}\right)\right]$$

$$L(y_{a1}) = \exp\left(-u_a \exp(\mathbf{x}_{a1}^t\boldsymbol{\beta})h_{(1)}\right)$$

$$L(y_{b3}) = \exp\left(-u_b \exp(\mathbf{x}_{b3}^t\boldsymbol{\beta})\left(h_{(1)} + h_{(2)}\right)\right)$$

$$L(y_{a2}) = \exp\left(-u_a \exp(\mathbf{x}_{a2}^t\boldsymbol{\beta})\left(h_{(1)} + h_{(2)}\right)\right)\left[1 - \exp\left(-u_a \exp(\mathbf{x}_{a2}^t\boldsymbol{\beta})h_{(3)}\right)\right]$$

$$(5.27)$$

In general we can write the conditional likelihood either in terms of the contributions of the subjects

$$\prod_{i=1}^{s}\prod_{j=1}^{n_i}\exp\left(-u_i\exp(\mathbf{x}_{ij}^t\boldsymbol{\beta})\sum_{k:L_{(k)}<y_{ij}}h_{(k)}\right)\left[1-\exp\left(-u_i\exp(\mathbf{x}_{ij}^t\boldsymbol{\beta})h_{(m,ij)}\right)\right]^{\delta_{ij}}$$

with $m, ij = \min\{k : L_{(k)} \geq y_{ij}\}$, or in terms of the intervals

$$\prod_{k=1}^{z}\left\{\exp\left(-h_{(k)}\sum_{qw:y_{qw}>L_{(k)}}u_q\exp(\mathbf{x}_{qw}^t\boldsymbol{\beta})\right)\right.$$

$$\left.\times\prod_{qw:L_{(k-1)}<y_{qw}\leq L_{(k)}}\left[1-\exp\left(-h_{(k)}u_q\exp(\mathbf{x}_{qw}^t\boldsymbol{\beta})\right)\right]^{\delta_{ij}}\right\}\qquad(5.28)$$

The fact that this likelihood is different from previous survival likelihood expressions follows from the fact that only the cumulative hazard increments are specified, not the hazard function itself. This likelihood therefore resembles the likelihood used for interval-censored data.

Specification of the prior distributions

We assume an independent increments gamma process prior for the cumulative baseline hazard. For a particular increment we have

$$h_{(k)} \sim \text{Gamma}\left[c\left(H_0^*\left(L_{(k)}\right) - H_0^*\left(L_{(k-1)}\right)\right), c\right]\qquad(5.29)$$

with H_0^* an increasing continuous function such that $H_0^*(0) = 0$ and independence between the different increments contained in the vector $\mathbf{h} = \left(h_{(1)}, \ldots, h_{(z)}\right)^t$. For the cumulative baseline hazard we have

$$H_0\left(L_{(l)}\right) = \sum_{k=1}^{l}h_{(l)} \sim \text{Gamma}\left(cH_0^*\left(L_{(l)}\right), c\right)\qquad(5.30)$$

and $\text{E}\left(H_0\left(L_{(l)}\right)\right) = H_0^*\left(L_{(l)}\right)$ and $\text{Var}\left(H_0\left(L_{(l)}\right)\right) = H_0^*\left(L_{(l)}\right)/c$. In (5.29) we need to specify both H_0^* and c. The parametric function H_0^* is often taken to be based on a time-constant hazard h_0^*, and thus $H_0^*\left(L_{(l)}\right) = h_0^*L_{(l)}$. On the other hand, the parameter c reflects the belief that is put in this prior. For c large, the increments have small variances and therefore the prior belief in h_0^* is strong.

Note that other processes have been proposed as prior for the cumulative baseline hazard, e.g., Hjort (1990) considered beta processes.

For each β_j, $j = 1, \ldots, p$, we assume the improper uniform prior $f(\beta_j) \propto 1$. We will further assume independence between all the parameters, also between the β_j's, so that $f(\beta) = \prod_{j=1}^{p} f(\beta_j) \propto 1$. This prior is improper because it does not correspond to a density function; the integral of the assumed f is infinite. For the frailties, the one-parameter gamma distribution with mean one and variance θ, $U \sim \text{Gamma}(1/\theta, 1/\theta)$, is taken as prior distribution. For θ, which is also a (hyper)parameter of interest, Clayton (1991) proposed the gamma distribution with parameters η and μ as prior distribution, i.e., $\theta \sim \text{Gamma}(\eta, \mu)$. For the usual vague improper prior for a variance, we take $\mu = \eta = 0$ as proposed by Clayton (1991). Alternatively, a uniform prior for $\sqrt{\theta}$ can be used. Gelman (2003) advocates the use of this prior for variance parameters in hierarchical models (for further motivation, see Gelman (2003)). The posterior density for θ will be derived for the gamma prior on θ (see 5.41) as well as for the uniform prior on $\sqrt{\theta}$ (see 5.42).

Derivation of the posterior distributions

As explained in Section 2.4, the Bayes theorem leads to the following joint posterior density function of the parameter vector

$$f(\omega \mid \mathbf{y}) = \frac{f(\mathbf{y} \mid \omega) f(\omega)}{f(\mathbf{y})}$$

with $\omega = (\mathbf{h}^t, \theta, \beta^t, \mathbf{u}^t)^t$, a $(z+p+s+1) \times 1$ vector with $\mathbf{h} = (h_{(1)}, \ldots, h_{(z)})^t$, $\beta = (\beta_1, \ldots, \beta_p)^t$ and $\mathbf{u} = (u_1, \ldots, u_s)^t$.

The Bayes theorem can also be applied to one of the parameters ω_i while conditioning on the other parameters. We will denote the parameter vector without the ith component, ω_i, by $\omega_{(-i)}$.

We generally have for the ith component of ω the following conditional posterior density

$$f(\omega_i \mid \mathbf{y}, \omega_{(-i)}) = \frac{f(\mathbf{y} \mid \omega) f(\omega_i \mid \omega_{(-i)})}{f(\mathbf{y} \mid \omega_{(-i)})} \tag{5.31}$$

Furthermore, since the conditioning of the prior density of ω_i on the other parameters is not instrumental (we assume independence of prior densities) we drop here and everywhere in the further discussion this type of conditioning. In the right-hand side of the conditional posterior density (5.31) the denominator does not depend on ω_i. Therefore, the numerator on the right-hand side of (5.31) and the conditional posterior density of ω_i are proportional:

$$f(\omega_i \mid \mathbf{y}, \omega_{(-i)}) \propto f(\mathbf{y} \mid \omega) f(\omega_i) \tag{5.32}$$

Using the likelihood function (5.28), we will make use of the unnormalised conditional posterior densities of form (5.32) for all the parameters since the normalising factor (i.e., the denominator on the right-hand side of 5.31) is, in most cases, difficult to obtain. A further reason is that, in case of grouped data, including the normalisation does, in general, not result in a particular form for the conditional posterior density from which sampling is easy.

In the next section, however, it will be demonstrated that an alternative, approximate likelihood expression will lead to more simple conditional posterior densities from which sampling is easy. We will further concentrate on that likelihood formulation since it is the one that is used in WinBUGS.

5.3.2 The frailty model with a gamma process prior for the cumulative baseline hazard for observed event times

In this section, we still use the grouped data idea of the previous section, but the interval boundaries now correspond to the observed event times. Furthermore, we will obtain an approximation of Poisson form for the likelihood in (5.28). We first derive this approximation. We then specify prior densities for the parameters and finally obtain the conditional posterior densities. We will find that some of the conditional posterior densities are well known density functions. Sampling will therefore be easy.

Approximated likelihood of Poisson form

We still use an independent increments gamma process for the cumulative baseline hazard but we take as intervals $(0, y_{(1)}], \ldots, (y_{(r-1)}, y_{(r)}]$ with $y_{(1)}, \ldots, y_{(r)}$ the ordered event times and thus $\mathbf{h} = (h_{(1)}, \ldots, h_{(r)})^t$ (Figure 5.14c) with $h_{(l)} = H_0(y_{(l)}) - H_0(y_{(l-1)})$. We now give approximations for the likelihood contributions (5.27).

First consider a subject for which an event time is observed. For instance, the likelihood contribution for y_{b1} is given by

$$L(y_{b1}) = \exp\left(-u_b \exp(\mathbf{x}_{b1}^t \boldsymbol{\beta}) h_{(1)}\right) - \exp\left[-u_b \exp(\mathbf{x}_{b1}^t \boldsymbol{\beta})(h_{(1)} + h_{(2)}))\right]$$

$$= \phi(h_{(1)}) - \phi(h_{(1)} + h_{(2)}) \qquad (5.33)$$

This expression can be approximated by rewriting the second term as a first-order Taylor series approximation around $h_{(1)}$

$$L(y_{b1}) \approx \left(h_{(1)} - (h_{(1)} + h_{(2)})\right)\phi'(h_{(1)} + h_{(2)})$$

$$= -h_{(2)}\left[-u_b \exp(\mathbf{x}_{b1}^t \boldsymbol{\beta})\exp\left(-u_b \exp(\mathbf{x}_{b1}^t \boldsymbol{\beta})(h_{(1)} + h_{(2)}))\right)\right]$$

$$= u_b h_{(2)} \exp(\mathbf{x}_{b1}^t \boldsymbol{\beta})\exp\left(-u_b \exp(\mathbf{x}_{b1}^t \boldsymbol{\beta})(h_{(1)} + h_{(2)}))\right)$$

The contribution of censored subjects, on the other hand, is based on the cumulative hazard corresponding to the sum of the cumulative hazard increments of all event times before or at the actual censoring time. This leads to the following likelihood expression

$$\prod_{i=1}^{s}\prod_{j=1}^{n_i} \exp\left(-u_i \exp(\mathbf{x}_{ij}^t\boldsymbol{\beta}) \sum_{k:y_{(k)}\leq y_{ij}} h_{(k)}\right) \left(u_i \exp(\mathbf{x}_{ij}^t\boldsymbol{\beta})h_{(m,ij)}\right)^{\delta_{ij}}$$

with $m, ij = \min\{k : y_{(k)} \geq y_{ij}\}$, or to the alternative expression

$$\prod_{i=1}^{s}\prod_{j=1}^{n_i} \prod_{k:y_{(k)}\leq y_{ij}} \left(u_i h_{(k)} \exp(\mathbf{x}_{ij}^t\boldsymbol{\beta})\right)^{\delta_{ij}(y_{(k)})} \exp\left(-u_i h_{(k)} \exp(\mathbf{x}_{ij}^t\boldsymbol{\beta})\right) \quad (5.34)$$

with $\delta_{ij}(y_{(k)}) = 1$ if $\delta_{ij} = 1$ and $y_{ij} = y_{(k)}$.

This likelihood function thus resembles the likelihood of Poisson distributed data, a fact that is used to fit semiparametric survival models in Win-BUGS (Spiegelhalter et al., 2003). Consider the likelihood contribution of subject j from cluster i at time $y_{(k)}$, then this term is indeed similar to the likelihood contribution of a Poisson distributed random variable with expected value $u_i h_{(k)} \exp(\mathbf{x}_{ij}^t\boldsymbol{\beta})$ when it takes values zero or one.

Specification of the prior distributions

The prior distributions are the same as in the the previous section.

Derivation of the posterior densities

The conditional posterior densities for all the parameters of interest are derived in this section with results for the regression parameters given in (5.35), for the discretised hazard in (5.39), for the frailties in (5.40), and finally for θ in (5.41) and (5.42).

We first consider the conditional posterior density of one component of $\boldsymbol{\beta}$, say β_a. Using the conditional version of the Bayes theorem (5.31) and due to the fact that β_a has a uniform prior, we can write

$$f\left(\beta_a \mid \mathbf{y}, \mathbf{h}, \theta, \boldsymbol{\beta}_{(-a)}, \mathbf{u}\right) \propto f\left(\mathbf{y} \mid \mathbf{h}, \theta, \boldsymbol{\beta}, \mathbf{u}\right)$$

$$= \prod_{i=1}^{s}\prod_{j=1}^{n_i} \prod_{k:y_{(k)}\leq y_{ij}} \left(h_{(k)}u_i \exp(\mathbf{x}_{ij}^t\boldsymbol{\beta})\right)^{\delta_{ij}(y_{(k)})} \exp\left(-h_{(k)}u_i \exp(\mathbf{x}_{ij}^t\boldsymbol{\beta})\right) \quad (5.35)$$

with $\beta_{(-a)}$ the β-vector without the ath component β_a and $\mathbf{h}=(h_{(1)},\ldots,h_{(r)})$. The vector β on the right-hand side of (5.35) is considered as a vector of fixed constants except for β_a which is the argument of the conditional posterior density. An important property of this conditional posterior density is its logconcavity. It allows us to make use of the adaptive rejection sampling algorithm (Gilks and Wild, 1992) to generate a sample. A detailed discussion on the adaptive rejection sampling algorithm is given in Section 5.3.4. In order to demonstrate logconcavity of this conditional posterior density, we need to prove that its second derivative is nonpositive. Now, with $\mathbf{x}_{ij} = (x_{ij1},\ldots,x_{ijp})$,

$$\frac{\partial^2}{\partial \beta_a^2} \log f\left(\beta_a \mid \mathbf{y}, \mathbf{h}, \theta, \beta_{(-a)}, \mathbf{u}\right)$$

$$= \frac{\partial^2}{\partial \beta_a^2} \sum_{i=1}^{s} \sum_{j=1}^{n_i} \sum_{k:y_{(k)} \leq y_{ij}} \left[\delta_{ij}(y_{(k)}) \log\left(h_{(k)} u_i \exp\left(\mathbf{x}_{ij}^t \beta\right)\right) - h_{(k)} u_i \exp\left(\mathbf{x}_{ij}^t \beta\right)\right]$$

$$= -\sum_{i=1}^{s} \sum_{j=1}^{n_i} \sum_{k:y_{(k)} \leq y_{ij}} h_{(k)} u_i \exp\left(\mathbf{x}_{ij}^t \beta\right) x_{ija}^2$$

and this last expression is always less than or equal zero.

We now apply (5.31), the conditional version of the Bayes theorem, to obtain the conditional posterior density of $h_{(k)}$, $k = 1,\ldots,r$

$$f\left(h_{(k)} \mid \mathbf{y}_{(k)}, \mathbf{h}_{(-k)}, \theta, \beta, \mathbf{u}\right) = \frac{f\left(\mathbf{y}_{(k)} \mid \mathbf{h}, \theta, \beta, \mathbf{u}\right) f\left(h_{(k)} \mid \mathbf{h}_{(-k)}, \theta, \beta, \mathbf{u}\right)}{f\left(\mathbf{y}_{(k)} \mid \mathbf{h}_{(-k)}, \theta, \beta, \mathbf{u}\right)}$$

(5.36)

with $\mathbf{y}_{(k)}$ referring to all the subjects having an event at time $y_{(k)}$. We can simplify the general expression (5.36) by noting that the assumed independence between all the parameters implies that $f\left(h_{(k)} \mid \mathbf{h}_{(-k)}, \theta, \beta, \mathbf{u}\right) = f\left(h_{(k)}\right)$, and that $\mathbf{h}_{(-k)}$ is not required in the conditioning leading to

$$f\left(h_{(k)} \mid \mathbf{y}_{(k)}, \theta, \beta, \mathbf{u}\right) = \frac{f\left(\mathbf{y}_{(k)} \mid h_{(k)}, \theta, \beta, \mathbf{u}\right) f\left(h_{(k)}\right)}{f\left(\mathbf{y}_{(k)} \mid \theta, \beta, \mathbf{u}\right)}$$

(5.37)

The conditional likelihood expression of $\mathbf{y}_{(k)}$ in the numerator of (5.37) is given by

$$f\left(\mathbf{y}_{(k)} \mid h_{(k)}, \theta, \beta, \mathbf{u}\right) = \prod_{i=1}^{s} \prod_{j=1}^{n_i} \left(h_{(k)} u_i \exp\left(\mathbf{x}_{ij}^t \beta\right)\right)^{\delta_{ij}\left(y_{(k)}\right)} \exp\left(-h_{(k)} B_{(k)}\right)$$

with

$$B_{(k)} = \sum_{qw \in R(y_{(k)})} u_q \exp\left(\mathbf{x}_{qw}^t \boldsymbol{\beta}\right)$$

where $R\left(y_{(k)}\right)$ is the risk set at time $y_{(k)}$ as in (1.11). This simplifies to

$$f\left(\mathbf{y}_{(k)} \mid h_{(k)}, \theta, \boldsymbol{\beta}, \mathbf{u}\right) = \prod_{i=1}^{s} \prod_{j=1}^{n_i} \left[\left(u_i \exp\left(\mathbf{x}_{ij}^t \boldsymbol{\beta}\right)\right)^{\delta_{ij}\left(y_{(k)}\right)}\right]$$

$$\times h_{(k)}^{N_{(k)}} \exp\left(-N_{(k)} h_{(k)} B_{(k)}\right) \tag{5.38}$$

with $N_{(k)}$ the number of events at event time $y_{(k)}$. We can obtain the denominator of the right-hand side of (5.37) by integrating out in (5.38) the cumulative baseline hazard increment $h_{(k)}$ with respect to its prior distribution given in (5.29):

$$\prod_{i=1}^{s} \prod_{j=1}^{n_i} \left[\left(u_i \exp\left(\mathbf{x}_{ij}^t \boldsymbol{\beta}\right)\right)^{\delta_{ij}\left(y_{(k)}\right)}\right.$$

$$\left. \times \int_{0}^{\infty} h_{(k)}^{N_{(k)}} \exp\left(-N_{(k)} h_{(k)} B_{(k)}\right) f\left(h_{(k)}\right) dh_{(k)}\right]$$

This equals

$$\prod_{i=1}^{s} \prod_{j=1}^{n_i} \left[\left(u_i \exp\left(\mathbf{x}_{ij}^t \boldsymbol{\beta}\right)\right)^{\delta_{ij}\left(y_{(k)}\right)}\right.$$

$$\left. \times \frac{c^{ch_{(k)}^*}}{\Gamma\left(ch_{(k)}^*\right)} \left(c + N_{(k)} B_{(k)}\right)^{-ch_{(k)}^* - N_{(k)}} \Gamma\left(ch_{(k)}^* + N_{(k)}\right)\right]$$

with $h_{(k)}^* = H_0^*(y_{(k)}) - H_0^*(y_{(k-1)})$.

Therefore, we now have

$$f\left(h_{(k)} \mid \mathbf{y}_{(k)}, \theta, \boldsymbol{\beta}, \mathbf{u}\right) = \frac{f\left(\mathbf{y}_{(k)} \mid h_{(k)}, \theta, \boldsymbol{\beta}, \mathbf{u}\right) f\left(h_{(k)}\right)}{f\left(\mathbf{y}_{(k)} \mid \theta, \boldsymbol{\beta}, \mathbf{u}\right)}$$

$$= \left(c + N_{(k)} B_{(k)}\right)^{ch_{(k)}^* + N_{(k)}} h_{(k)}^{ch_{(k)}^* + N_{(k)} - 1}$$

$$\times \exp\left(-h_{(k)} \left(c + N_{(k)} B_{(k)}\right)\right) \left(\Gamma\left(ch_{(k)}^* + N_{(k)}\right)\right)^{-1}$$

This corresponds to a gamma density

$$f\left(h_{(k)} \mid \mathbf{y}_{(k)}, \theta, \boldsymbol{\beta}, \mathbf{u}\right) = \text{Gamma}\left(ch_{(k)}^* + N_{(k)}, c + N_{(k)} B_{(k)}\right) \qquad (5.39)$$

Hence, we can immediately sample from the gamma density.

In this specific case, the conditional posterior density for the baseline hazard increments is also an independent increments gamma process. Therefore, the independent increments gamma process prior is the conjugate prior for the cumulative baseline hazard in the case of censored survival data. Generally, conjugacy means that the prior and posterior density belong to the same family of densities. For a more formal discussion on conjugacy, we refer to Gelman et al. (2004), p. 41. The independent increments gamma process prior for the cumulative baseline hazard is therefore often the preferred choice.

For the frailties, we already have shown in (5.7) of Section 5.1.2 that their conditional posterior distribution corresponds to a gamma density

$$f\left(u_i \mid \mathbf{y}, \boldsymbol{\beta}, \mathbf{h}, \theta\right) = \text{Gamma}\left(d_i + 1/\theta, H_{\mathbf{x}_i, c}\left(\mathbf{y}_i\right) + 1/\theta\right) \qquad (5.40)$$

and therefore samples can be drawn immediately from this gamma density.

Finally, we need the conditional posterior density of θ. The conditional posterior density of θ depends only on the frailties $\mathbf{u}$. The following relationship holds

$$f\left(\theta \mid \mathbf{u}\right) \propto f\left(\mathbf{u} \mid \theta\right) f(\theta)$$

With the prior distribution for the u_i's equal to the two-parameter gamma with parameters $1/\theta$ and $1/\theta$ and for θ also gamma with parameters η and μ, we have

$$f\left(\theta \mid \mathbf{u}\right) \propto \frac{\mu^\eta}{\Gamma(\eta)} \frac{\theta^{\eta - 1 - s/\theta} \exp\left(-\mu\theta - \sum_{i=1}^{s} u_i/\theta + (1/\theta - 1) \sum_{i=1}^{s} \log u_i\right)}{\left(\Gamma(1/\theta)\right)^s}$$

$$(5.41)$$

This is a more difficult conditional distribution to sample from, and therefore slice sampling, proposed by Neal (2003), will be used to generate a sample from this density. A detailed discussion on the slice sampling algorithm is given in Section 5.3.4.

Alternatively, a uniform prior distribution can be assumed for the standard deviation of the frailties

$$\sqrt{\theta} \sim \text{Uniform}(0, A)$$

from which it follows that

$$\theta \sim \frac{1}{2A}\theta^{-1/2}I\left(\theta \in (0, A^2)\right)$$

Therefore, the posterior distribution for θ is

$$f(\theta \mid \mathbf{u}) \propto \frac{\theta^{-1/2-s/\theta}\exp\left(-\sum_{i=1}^{s}u_i/\theta + (1/\theta - 1)\sum_{i=1}^{s}\log u_i\right)}{2A\left(\Gamma(1/\theta)\right)^s}I\left(\theta \in (0, A^2)\right) \tag{5.42}$$

5.3.3 The normal frailty model based on Poisson likelihood

We consider the same model as in the previous section, except that the heterogeneity is now modelled by normal distributed random effects. Therefore, the prior distribution for the random effects is now normal with mean zero and variance γ with independent random effects. The conditional posterior distributions for β_a and $h_{(k)}$, $k = 1, \ldots, r$ are the same as before as in (5.35) and (5.39), respectively, but with now

$$h_{ij}(t) = h_0(t)\exp\left(\mathbf{x}_{ij}^t\boldsymbol{\beta} + w_i\right)$$

$$B_{(k)} = \sum_{qw \in R\left(y_{(k)}\right)}\exp\left(\mathbf{x}_{qw}^t\boldsymbol{\beta} + w_q\right)$$

For the random effect w_i, $i = 1, \ldots, s$, the conditional posterior density is proportional to

$$f(w_i \mid \mathbf{y}, \mathbf{h}, \gamma, \boldsymbol{\beta}) \propto f(\mathbf{y} \mid \mathbf{h}, \gamma, \boldsymbol{\beta}, w_i)f(w_i)$$

$$= \prod_{j=1}^{n_i}\prod_{k:y_{(k)} \leq y_{ij}}\left(h_{(k)}\exp(\mathbf{x}_{ij}^t\boldsymbol{\beta} + w_i)\right)^{\delta_{ij}(y_{(k)})}\exp\left(-h_{(k)}\exp(\mathbf{x}_{ij}^t\boldsymbol{\beta} + w_i)\right)$$

$$\times \frac{1}{\sqrt{2\pi\gamma}}\exp\left(\frac{-w_i^2}{2\gamma}\right) \tag{5.43}$$

To demonstrate logconcavity of the conditional posterior density of the random effect w_i, observe that the first part of the conditional posterior density given by (5.43) is (5.35) with u_i replaced by $\exp(w_i)$. In this expression w_i occurs at the same position as the β_j's, i.e., in the exponential. Therefore, since the conditional posterior density of β_j is logconcave (same proof as logconcavity of conditional posterior density of β_a in the semiparametric gamma frailty model) it also follows that the first part of the conditional posterior density of w_i is logconcave. The second derivative of the second part of the conditional posterior density given by (5.43) is

$$\frac{\partial^2}{\partial w_i^2} \log\left(\frac{1}{2\pi\gamma}\exp\left(\frac{-w_i^2}{2\gamma}\right)\right) = \frac{-1}{\gamma} \tag{5.44}$$

and therefore, with $\gamma > 0$, this contribution is also negative which proves the logconcavity. Finally, the preferred option for the prior distribution of γ is the uniform (Gelman, 2003), $f(\gamma) \propto 1$ for γ in $[0, +\infty)$.

Example 5.5 Bayesian semiparametric frailty model for ductal carcinoma in situ

We revisit the DCIS example and fit the semiparametric frailty model with gamma distribution assumption for the frailties and normal distribution assumption for the random effects. The Gibbs sampling scheme based on the conditional posterior densities described in Sections 5.3.2 and 5.3.3 is actually what is applied in WinBUGS (Spiegelhalter et al., 2003). We set up four independent chains using 1000 iterations as burn-in period and another 5000 iterations are then used as sample to construct the posterior density. In all cases the $\hat{R}$ statistic given by (2.37) is very close to one.

The summary statistics of the univariate posterior densities of the parameters of interest for the model with gamma distributed frailties are given in Table 5.5.

Table 5.5. Summary statistics of posterior density functions based on the semiparametric frailty model with gamma distributed frailties for ductal carcinoma in situ data set.

Parameter	Mean	s.e.	2.5%	25%	Quantiles 50%	75%	97.5%
β	−0.628	0.167	−0.962	−0.740	−0.626	−0.514	−0.303
θ	0.216	0.895	0.005	0.054	0.109	0.187	0.451

The univariate posterior density functions can be estimated from the sample and visualised by using spline techniques. Recall that θ, the heterogeneity parameter, takes values in $[0, +\infty)$. For such cases Silverman (1986) first estimates the density g of $\log \theta$ and then proposes an estimate for f using the relation

$$f(\theta) = \frac{1}{\theta} g(\log \theta) \quad \text{for } \theta \geq 0$$

Spline techniques are applied to obtain $\hat{g}$, an estimate for the posterior density function of $\log \theta$. We then divide $\hat{g}(\log \theta)$ by θ to obtain an estimated density function $\hat{f}$ on the original scale θ. The univariate posterior density function for θ is obtained in this way, and depicted in Figure 5.15 together with the estimated univariate posterior density function of β. Both the mean and the standard error for β are very close to the estimates obtained from the EM algorithm in Example 5.1. The mean and the median of the variance, equal to 0.216 and 0.109, respectively, are higher than the variance of 0.086 obtained from the EM algorithm. However, as the EM algorithm is based on maximisation, the mode of the posterior density should be more equivalent to the solution from the EM algorithm. It can be seen from Figure 5.15 that the univariate posterior density function is not unimodal, and it is unclear how to compare the Bayesian and the EM approach. Furthermore, it is questionable whether the Gibbs sampler has actually converged to a stable distribution for θ. Consider the sequence of generated values of the four chains in Figure 5.16. There seems to be no problem for β; but for θ we see that at some places in the trace there are brief periods with sampled values of θ close to zero. Also high sampled values of θ occur. These findings correspond with the mode close to zero and with the heavy right tail of the density in Figure 5.15.

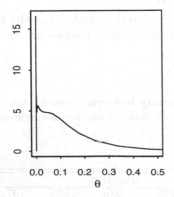 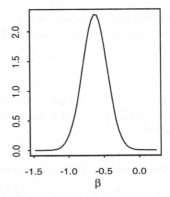

Fig. 5.15. The estimated univariate posterior densities of θ and β based on the semiparametric frailty model with gamma distributed frailties for the ductal carcinoma in situ data set.

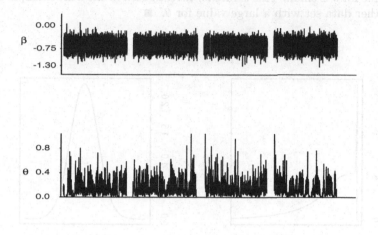

Fig. 5.16. The trace of θ and β based on the semiparametric frailty model with gamma distributed frailties for the ductal carcinoma in situ data set.

The summary statistics for the parameter β in the semiparametric frailty model with normal distributed random effects are very similar to the semiparametric gamma frailty model (Table 5.6), and the same is true for the univariate posterior density function (Figure 5.17). Furthermore, the same convergence problems occur as before (Figure 5.18).

Table 5.6. Summary statistics of marginal posterior density functions based on semiparametric frailty model with normal distributed random effects for ductal carcinoma in situ data set.

Parameter	Mean	s.e.	Quantiles				
			2.5%	25%	50%	75%	97.5%
β	−0.628	0.170	−0.960	−0.742	−0.627	−0.513	−0.294
γ	0.120	0.104	0.003	0.044	0.094	0.168	0.388

Although the results for the semiparametric gamma frailty model obtained by Gibbs sampling are similar to those obtained through the EM algorithm when taking the median of the estimated posterior density, it is clear from the example that it is important to look at convergence diagnostics such as the trace plots. The fact that the plots demonstrate some dependency from one generated value to the next makes the use of these techniques in this setting questionable. The convergence problems might be related to the fact that the true value for θ is small. This is further investigated in the next example based on another data set with a large value for θ. ∎

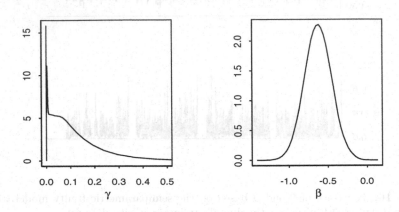

Fig. 5.17. The estimated univariate posterior densities of γ and β based on the semiparametric frailty model with normal distributed random effects for the ductal carcinoma in situ data set.

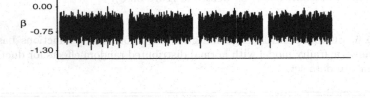

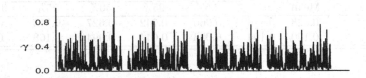

Fig. 5.18. The trace of γ and β based on the semiparametric frailty model with normal distributed random effects for the ductal carcinoma in situ data set.

Example 5.6 Bayesian semiparametric frailty model for the udder quarter infection data set

We revisit the udder infection example (Example 1.4) and fit the semiparametric frailty model with normal distribution assumption for the random effects to verify whether a stable solution is obtained for this application with typically a large variance of the random effects. Again we set up four independent chains using 1000 iterations as burn-in period and another 5000 iterations are then used as sample to construct the posterior density.

The summary statistics and a visual representation of the posterior distributions of the parameters of interest are given in Table 5.7 and Figure 5.19, respectively. It is clear from the trace plots for β and γ (Figure 5.20) that for this setting there is no problem with convergence. ■

Table 5.7. Summary statistics of posterior density functions based on the semiparametric frailty model with normal distributed random effects for the udder quarter infection data set.

Parameter	Mean	s.e.	Quantiles				
			2.5%	25%	50%	75%	97.5%
β	0.411	0.362	−0.301	0.165	0.411	0.654	1.111
γ	2.676	0.577	1.724	2.266	2.612	3.022	3.969

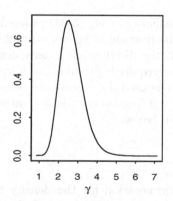 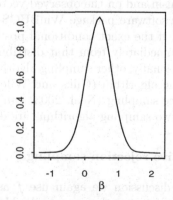

Fig. 5.19. The estimated univariate posterior densities of γ and β based on the semiparametric frailty model with normal distributed random effects for the udder infection data set.

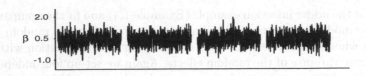

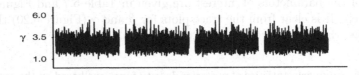

Fig. 5.20. The trace of γ and β based on the semiparametric frailty model with normal distributed random effects for the udder infection data set.

5.3.4 Sampling techniques used for semiparametric frailty models

In Gibbs sampling, values must be drawn at random from the conditional posterior distribution of each individual parameter, conditional on the values of the other parameters obtained in the previous step of the iterative sampling mechanism and on the observed vector **z**.

The software package WinBUGS (Spiegelhalter et al., 2003) proceeds as follows. If the exact conditional posterior distribution is known, sampling is done immediately from that distribution. If the distribution is only defined proportionally, other sampling algorithms are required: the adaptive rejection sampling algorithm (Gilks and Wild, 1992) is used for logconcave densities and slice sampling (Neal, 2003) can be used if logconcavity is not satisfied. These two sampling algorithms are described below.

Adaptive rejection sampling

In the discussion we again use f as generic notation for the density from which we want to draw a sample. Moreover, we assume that we only know g, a function that is proportional to f, i.e., $g(x) = cf(x)$. The precise meaning of the words "adaptive" and "rejection" will become clear from the discussion below. The logconcavity condition says that the first derivative of $\log g$ is a monotone decreasing function.

As an example, think $f\left(\beta_a \mid \mathbf{y}, \mathbf{h}, \theta, \boldsymbol{\beta}_{(-a)}, \mathbf{u}\right)$ as in (5.35) in the role of g. Then logconcavity means that the shape of the log of the conditional posterior density for β_a is as in Figure 5.21. Figure 5.21 depicts the conditional posterior density for β_a where we have taken as values for the parameters on which we condition the median of a sequence of values (of length 5000) generated by Gibbs sampling.

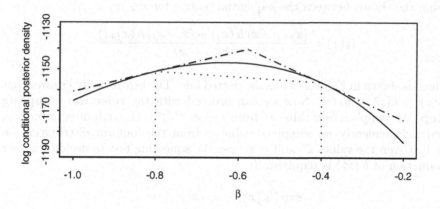

Fig. 5.21. Illustration of the initialisation step of the adaptive rejection sampling algorithm. For two points, $\beta = -0.8, -0.4$, the value of the logarithm of the conditional posterior distribution is obtained, together with their first derivatives. Based on this information, the linear hull for the logarithm of the conditional posterior distribution is constructed.

We start with the **initialisation step**. We first have to choose a set of points $T_k = \{x_1, \ldots, x_k\}$ with ordering $x_1 \leq \ldots \leq x_k$. For each of these points we determine $h(x_1) = \log g(x_1), \ldots, h(x_k) = \log g(x_k)$. Based on these points we define the rejection envelope on T_k as $\exp u_k(x)$ where $u_k(x)$ is the piecewise linear upper hull formed by the tangents to $h(x)$ at the points in T_k as shown in Figure 5.21 by the upper dashed lines. Often, only two starting points are taken, as depicted in Figure 5.21 where $T_2 = \{-0.8, -0.4\}$. The tangent lines intersect at a point with abcis z_j between x_j and x_{j+1}:

$$z_j = \frac{h\left(x_{j+1}\right) - h\left(x_j\right) - x_{j+1}h'\left(x_{j+1}\right) + x_jh'\left(x_j\right)}{h'\left(x_j\right) - h'\left(x_{j+1}\right)}$$

Thus, for $x \in [z_{j-1}, z_j]$ $(j = 1, \ldots, k)$, the convex upper hull is given by

$$u_k(x) = h(x_j) + (x - x_j) h'(x_j)$$

The density function corresponding to this convex hull is given by

$$f_k(x) = \frac{\exp u_k(x)}{\int_D \exp u_k(v) dv} \tag{5.45}$$

with D the domain of f. We further define a piecewise linear lower hull on T_k using the chords between the sequential points: for $x \in [x_j, x_{j+1}]$

$$l_k(x) = \frac{(x_{j+1} - x) h(x_j) + (x - x_j) h(x_{j+1})}{x_{j+1} - x_j}$$

which is shown in Figure 5.21 as the dotted line. The logconcavity ensures that $l_k(x) \leq h(x) \leq u_k(x)$. Now we can proceed with the **rejection sampling step**. We sample a new value x^* from f_k (see (5.45)) through direct sampling and independently we sample a value w from the uniform distribution on $[0, 1]$. Given the values x^* and w we use the squeezing test to decide whether evaluation of $h(x^*)$ is required: if

$$\exp(l_k(x^*) - u_k(x^*)) \geq w$$

the point x^* is accepted without deriving $h(x^*)$. It means that the function which is squeezed between the lower and upper hull is known with sufficient accuracy. Further justification for the squeezing test is given below. Otherwise, we need to determine $h(x^*)$. We accept the value x^* if $\exp(h(x^*) - u_k(x^*)) \geq w$, otherwise we do not consider this value as a sampled value and we go to the next iteration to obtain a sampled value.

We demonstrate such a situation in Figure 5.22. Assume that the random draw from f_k gives $x^* = -0.6$. According to the squeezing test, the value could not be accepted right away. Therefore, we derived the value $h(x^*)$ and based on the test $\exp(h(x^*) - u_k(x^*)) \geq w$, x^* was accepted. When an evaluation $h(x^*)$ is done, we proceed to the **adaptation step**. We include x^* in T_k leading to T_{k+1} and calculate $h'(x^*)$. Next, we reorder T_{k+1} so that $x_1 \leq \ldots \leq x_{k+1}$ and also obtain the lower and upper hull l_{k+1}, u_{k+1}, and the density f_{k+1}. The new lower and upper hull for our example are shown in Figure 5.22. It is clear that these hulls are more close to f than the previous hulls which were only based on two points. We can then go back to the start of the sampling step and sample a new value.

We now prove that this sampling algorithm leads to a random sample from f. Denote by $x^{(k)}$ the actual value of $X^{(k)}$, a random variable with density f_k and let H_k be the information about the lower and upper hull at

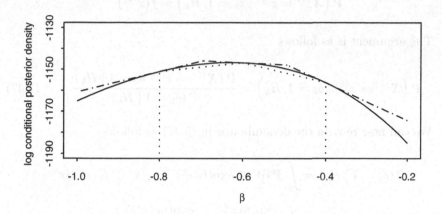

Fig. 5.22. Illustration of the sampling and adaptation step of the adaptive rejection sampling algorithm. The value $x^* = -0.6$ is drawn randomly from f_k via direct sampling. As this value did not pass the squeezing test, $h(x^*)$ was obtained and based on the fact that $\exp(h(x^*) - u_k(x^*)) \geq w$, the value x^* is accepted. Adding x^* to the set T_k, new linear hulls are obtained that are more close to f compared to the previous hulls.

iteration k. Let δ_k be a binary indicator taking value one, respectively zero, if $x^{(k)}$ is accepted, respectively not accepted. Given the information H_k, we need the "joint probability" that the continuous random variable $X^{(k)}$ takes value $x^{(k)}$ and that the binary random variable δ_k takes value one, i.e.,

$$P\left(X^{(k)} = x^{(k)}, \delta_k = 1 \mid H_k\right) = P\left(\delta_k = 1 \mid X^{(k)} = x^{(k)}, H_k\right) f_k(x^{(k)})$$

$$= \left\{ P\left[W \leq \exp(l_k(x^{(k)}) - u_k(x^{(k)}))\right] \right.$$

$$\left. + P\left[W > \exp(l_k(x^{(k)}) - u_k(x^{(k)})) \text{ and } W \leq \exp(h(x^{(k)}) - u_k(x^{(k)}))\right] \right\}$$

$$\times \frac{\exp(u_k(x^{(k)}))}{\int_D \exp(u_k(v))dv}$$

$$= P\left[W \leq \exp(h(x^{(k)}) - u_k(x^{(k)}))\right] \frac{\exp(u_k(x^{(k)}))}{\int_D \exp(u_k(v))dv}$$

$$= \frac{\exp(h(x^{(k)}))}{\int_D \exp(u_k(v))dv} \tag{5.46}$$

Using (5.46) we now show that

$$P\left(X^{(k)} = x^{(k)} \mid \delta_k = 1, H_k\right) = f(x^{(k)})$$

The argument is as follows

$$P\left(X^{(k)} = x^{(k)} \mid \delta_k = 1, H_k\right) = \frac{P\left(X^{(k)} = x^{(k)}, \delta_k = 1 \mid H_k\right)}{P\left(\delta_k = 1 \mid H_k\right)} \qquad (5.47)$$

We can now rewrite the denominator in (5.47) as follows

$$P\left(\delta_k = 1 \mid H_k\right) = \int_D P\left[W \le \exp(h(x^*) - u_k(x^*))\right] f_k(x^*) dx^*$$

$$= \int_D \frac{\exp(h(x^*))}{\exp(u_k(x^*))} \frac{\exp(u_k(x^*))}{\int_D \exp(u_k(v)) dv} dx^*$$

$$= \frac{\int_D \exp(h(x^*)) dx^*}{\int_D \exp(u_k(v)) dv} \qquad (5.48)$$

Now replacing the numerator and denominator in (5.47) by (5.46) and (5.48), respectively, we obtain

$$P\left(X^{(k)} = x^{(k)} \mid \delta_k = 1, H_k\right) = \frac{\exp(h(x^{(k)}))}{\int_D \exp(h(x^*)) dx^*} = f(x^{(k)}) \qquad (5.49)$$

and therefore the accepted values $x^{(k)}$ have underlying density f.

Note that Gibbs sampling consists of two levels of iteration (see Section 5.3.5 below). Within each outer loop, samples are drawn from the different components of the parameter vector sequentially, using the respective conditional posterior densities. Therefore, within each such outer loop, only one random draw from the conditional posterior density is required, after which the next component of the parameter vector is sampled. In the next iteration of the outer loop, we have to start with a new initialisation step to obtain the next value from the conditional posterior density, as the values of the other parameters upon which it is conditioned are different. We can, however, make a good initial choice for T_k based on the previous step in the Gibbs iteration process. One possibility is to take the 15th and 85th percentiles of f_k.

Slice sampling

An important assumption in the adaptive rejection sampling algorithm is the logconcavity of the density from which is sampled. For densities that do not satisfy the logconcavity assumption a more general procedure such as slice sampling is required. The main idea behind slice sampling is that one can sample from a univariate distribution by sampling points uniformly from the region under the curve of the density function, with the horizontal coordinate then corresponding to the sample value.

Slice sampling can be done in a multidimensional way, but we will restrict the discussion to the univariate case; this is what is required in our applications. Let x denote the parameter of interest, which is, in a Bayesian context, assumed to have a particular distribution. Further assume that the density function f is known up to a constant, i.e., the known function is $g(x) = cf(x)$.

We now need to sample uniformly from a two-dimensional region that lies under g, which is defined more formally as $R = \{(x, y) : x \in D, 0 < y < g(x)\}$ with D the domain of f.

The uniform bivariate density from which we have to sample is

$$f(x, y) = \begin{cases} 1/\int_D g(t)dt & (x, y) \in R \\ 0 & \text{otherwise} \end{cases}$$

The marginal density for x from this joint density is

$$\int_0^{g(x)} \frac{1}{\int_D g(t)dt} dy = \frac{g(x)}{\int_D g(t)dt} = f(x)$$

Therefore, to sample from f, we could sample from the joint density of (X, Y) and then ignore y.

However, it is not always easy to sample from R. So generally, a Markov Chain is set up which alternates between drawing a random sample from the conditional distribution of y given the current value for x and from the conditional distribution of x given the current value of y. Drawing a random sample from the conditional distribution of y given the current value for x corresponds to drawing uniformly a random sample from the vertical slice given by $(0, g(x))$. Similarly, drawing a random sample from the conditional distribution of x given the current value for y corresponds to drawing uniformly a random sample from the horizontal slice given by $S = \{x : y < g(x)\}$. Consider the function g given in Figure 5.23. Conditional on $Y = y$, S is the set of intervals depicted by the bold lines. Different methods have been developed to draw a sample from the horizontal slice. We will just discuss one such method; other methods are given by Neal (2003). Instead of defining the whole slice S, we start with an interval of size w which is put randomly around a randomly chosen initial point $x^{(0)}$. Next, this interval is expanded to the left and the right with steps of size w until both the lower and upper level of the resulting interval $I = (L, U)$ fall outside the slice S (see Figure 5.23). Now a new point is drawn through uniform sampling from the interval I. If the point is within the slice S, it is accepted and $x^{(1)}$ is set equal to this value. If it is not accepted, the interval I is shrunk with the sampled point x' as new upper or lower level. A new value is then drawn through uniform sampling from the newly defined interval. We proceed this way until a value is drawn that falls in the slice S, and then we set $x^{(1)}$ equal to that value. If more random draws are required, we draw a new value for y given $x^{(1)}$ and so on.

The proof that this algorithm generates a sample from the desired conditional distribution is somewhat harder and is given by Neal (2003).

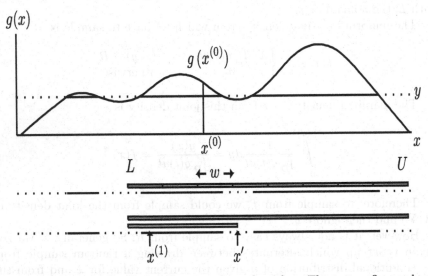

Fig. 5.23. Illustration of the slice sampling algorithm. The upper figure shows $g(x) = cf(x)$ with f the density of x. First a value $x^{(0)}$ is chosen at random. Next, a value for Y, say y, is sampled uniformly from the slice defined by $(0, g(x^{(0)}))$. Next, in the middle picture, an interval of width w is placed at random around $x^{(0)}$, and is further extended to left and right in steps of size w until the lower and upper limit of the extended interval are outside the horizontal slice depicted by the set of bold lines; i.e., we chose L (U) as the first value for which $g(L) < y$ $(g(U) < y)$. In the lower picture, a new point, say x', is drawn through uniform sampling from this extended interval that falls to the right of $x^{(0)}$ (see arrow) and is therefore outside the slice. This value is not accepted, but is used as the new upper limit of the extended interval. The next random draw from this interval falls in the slice and is therefore set as $x^{(1)}$.

5.3.5 Gibbs sampling, a special case of the Metropolis–Hastings algorithm

The Gibbs sampler is actually a special case of the Metropolis–Hastings algorithm presented in Section 2.4.2 with a specific transition kernel and an acceptance ratio equal to one. In Gibbs sampling, two levels of iterations are present. In the outer loop, indexed by n, a whole new parameter vector ζ is obtained. Within each outer loop, samples are drawn from the conditional posterior densities of the different components ζ_j, $j = 1, \ldots, q$, of the parameter vector ζ. So we have to define a transition kernel at each step j within step n. Consider the following transition kernel at step n for parameter ζ_j

$$J_{n,j}\left(\zeta^*, \zeta^{(n-1)}\right) = \begin{cases} f\left(\zeta_j^* \mid \zeta_{(-j)}^{(n-1)}, \mathbf{y}\right) & \text{if } \zeta_{(-j)}^* = \zeta_{(-j)}^{(n-1)} \\ 0 & \text{otherwise} \end{cases} \quad (5.50)$$

where $\zeta_{(-j)}^{(n-1)}$ is a vector containing the last values obtained for all the components except for parameter ζ_j. This means that, if the order of sampling is from ζ_1 to ζ_q, $\zeta_{(-j)}^{(n-1)} = \left(\zeta_1^{(n)}, \ldots, \zeta_{j-1}^{(n)}, \zeta_{j+1}^{(n-1)}, \ldots, \zeta_q^{(n-1)}\right)$. The only possible transitions at step j of the inner loop are therefore to parameter vectors ζ^* that match $\zeta^{(n-1)}$ on all components except for component ζ_j.

The acceptance ratio of the Metropolis–Hastings algorithm (see Section 2.4.2) is given by

$$r_{n,j} = \frac{f\left(\zeta^* \mid \mathbf{y}\right) / J_{n,j}\left(\zeta^*, \zeta^{(n-1)}\right)}{f\left(\zeta^{(n-1)} \mid \mathbf{y}\right) / J_{n,j}\left(\zeta^{(n-1)}, \zeta^*\right)}$$

As ζ^* only differs from $\zeta^{(n-1)}$ in the jth component, we can rewrite the transition kernel in the denominator of the expression above as follows:

$$J_{n,j}\left(\zeta^{(n-1)}, \zeta^*\right) = f\left(\zeta_j^{(n-1)} \mid \zeta_{(-j)}^{(n-1)}, \mathbf{y}\right)$$

Plugging in this expression in the acceptance ratio formula, we obtain

$$r_{n,j} = \frac{f\left(\zeta^* \mid \mathbf{y}\right) / f\left(\zeta_j^* \mid \zeta_{(-j)}^{(n-1)}, \mathbf{y}\right)}{f\left(\zeta^{(n-1)} \mid \mathbf{y}\right) / f\left(\zeta_j^{(n-1)} \mid \zeta_{(-j)}^{(n-1)}, \mathbf{y}\right)}$$

Using the fact that

$$f\left(\zeta^* \mid \mathbf{y}\right) = f\left(\zeta_j^* \mid \zeta_{(-j)}^{(n-1)}, \mathbf{y}\right) f\left(\zeta_{(-j)}^{(n-1)} \mid \mathbf{y}\right)$$

$$f\left(\zeta^{(n-1)} \mid \mathbf{y}\right) = f\left(\zeta_j^{(n-1)} \mid \zeta_{(-j)}^{(n-1)}, \mathbf{y}\right) f\left(\zeta_{(-j)}^{(n-1)} \mid \mathbf{y}\right)$$

and noting that $\zeta^*_{(-j)} = \zeta^{(n-1)}_{(-j)}$ we have

$$r_{n,j} = \frac{f\left(\zeta^{(n-1)}_j \mid \mathbf{y}\right)}{f\left(\zeta^{(n-1)}_j \mid \mathbf{y}\right)} = 1$$

Therefore, Gibbs sampling is a special case of the Metropolis–Hastings algorithm with transition kernel given in (5.50) and acceptance ratio equal to one. The Gibbs sampling algorithm has the same properties as the Metropolis–Hastings algorithm described in Section 2.4.2. We refer to Gelman et al. (2004), Section 11.3, for a more detailed account of these properties.

5.4 Further extensions and references

In this chapter, we only discussed the semiparametric frailty model with either gamma distributed frailties or normal distributed random effects. Other frailty distributions have been considered for the semiparametric model, although often the software is not available to fit these models. The positive stable shared frailty model was considered by Martinussen and Pipper (2005) and by Fine et al. (2003). Moger et al. (2004) developed techniques to fit the compound Poisson shared frailty model, which allows a nonsusceptible group. Fong et al. (2001) discuss time-varying random effects for recurrent event data in the framework of the semiparametric model.

6

Multifrailty and multilevel models

In previous chapters, we discussed models with one frailty term. In this chapter, frailty models with more than one frailty term will be studied. We distinguish two different cases. In the first case, the different frailty terms occur within the same cluster, whereas in the second case, the frailty terms are nested (hierarchical or multilevel models).

In Section 6.1 we consider models with only one cluster level but with two frailty terms within a cluster. A typical example of such a model is a multicentre clinical trial with a frailty term describing the heterogeneity between centres and a second frailty term modelling the centre by treatment interaction. The latter frailty term describes the treatment heterogeneity between centres. We call such models multifrailty models. If more than one frailty term occurs, the frailty terms can no longer be integrated out analytically to obtain a closed form expression for the marginal likelihood as was for instance the case for the gamma frailty model discussed in Chapter 2. Therefore, specific techniques have been developed to fit multifrailty models. In Section 6.1.1 we discuss a Bayesian technique making use of Laplacian integration to obtain posterior densities. The proposed technique is an extension of the method proposed by Ducrocq and Sölkner (1994) and Ducrocq and Casella (1996) for frailty models with one frailty term (Legrand et al., 2007). An advantage of the Laplacian integration is that it is computationally much faster than for instance the Gibbs sampling method discussed in Section 5.3.4. A second method to fit multifrailty models is discussed in Ripatti and Palmgren (2000). Their approach, which is discussed in Section 6.1.2, is frequentist and also uses Laplacian integration.

In Section 6.2 we discuss hierarchical models with two nested frailty terms. Again, two different techniques are considered. A first technique is based on numerical integration of the frailties at the higher level; the frailties at the lower level are assumed to be gamma distributed and are integrated out analytically (Rondeau et al., 2006). The second technique is Bayesian and uses Gibbs sampling.

6.1 Multifrailty models with one clustering level

In this section we consider models of clustered data with two frailty terms within the same cluster

$$h_{ij}(t) = h_0(t) \exp\left(w_{0i} + (\beta_1 + w_{1i})x_{ij1} + \mathbf{x}_{ij(-1)}^t \boldsymbol{\beta}_{(-1)}\right) \tag{6.1}$$

with $h_0(t)$ the baseline hazard and w_{0i} the random effect for cluster i ($j = 1, \ldots, n_i$, $i = 1, \ldots, s$). For the first covariate with covariate information x_{ij1} and fixed effect β_1, we also incorporate the random covariate by cluster interaction w_{1i}. The impact of the other covariates $\mathbf{x}_{ij(-1)}^t = (x_{ij2}, \ldots, x_{ijp})$ on the hazard function is given through the vector $\boldsymbol{\beta}_{(-1)}^t = (\beta_2, \ldots, \beta_p)$. We have $\boldsymbol{\beta}^t = \left(\beta_1, \boldsymbol{\beta}_{(-1)}^t\right)$. Different distributional assumptions will be made for the random effects in the two following subsections.

6.1.1 Bayesian analysis based on Laplacian integration

Ducrocq and Casella (1996) developed a Bayesian approach to fit frailty models with one frailty term. They use Laplacian integration to obtain the posterior distributions for the parameters of interest. Laplacian integration is computationally much faster than the Gibbs sampling techniques that are most often used in a Bayesian context. Laplacian integration provided the right technique to cope with the very large data sets typical in animal breeding.

Legrand et al. (2005, 2007) extended these techniques to model multivariate survival data with two frailty terms within a cluster and demonstrated that this technique works well for multicentre cancer clinical trials.

Within the Bayesian context, statistical inference is based on the univariate posterior distributions of the parameters of interest, obtained by integrating out the other parameters. The integral cannot be solved analytically, therefore an approximation based on Laplacian integration is proposed. Tierney and Kadane (1986) provide good insight in the accuracy of the Laplace approximation method.

Our discussion will be focused on the variance components. This technique was developed by animal breeders and therefore the parameters of interest are the variance components (which are related to heritability), the fixed effects being rather covariates to adjust for (e.g., season, parity, ...). Therefore, fixed effects estimates come only as a by-product and no posterior distributions are given. We start from the joint posterior density which is proportional to

$$f(\boldsymbol{\beta}, \mathbf{w}, \boldsymbol{\gamma} \mid \mathbf{y}) \propto L(\boldsymbol{\beta}, \mathbf{w} \mid \mathbf{y}) \times f(\mathbf{w} \mid \boldsymbol{\gamma}) \times f(\boldsymbol{\beta}) \times f(\boldsymbol{\gamma}) \tag{6.2}$$

where $\mathbf{w}^t = (\mathbf{w}_0^t, \mathbf{w}_1^t) = (w_{01}, \ldots, w_{0s}, w_{11}, \ldots, w_{1s})$, $\boldsymbol{\gamma}^t = (\gamma_0, \gamma_1)$. The parameters γ_0 and γ_1 are the variance of the random centre effect and the variance of the random covariate by cluster interaction effect, respectively. The first factor on the right-hand side of (6.2) is the likelihood of the observations. We will leave the baseline hazard unspecified, and therefore, based on the justification provided by Sinha et al. (2003), we use for $L(\boldsymbol{\beta}, \mathbf{w} \mid \mathbf{y})$ the following partial likelihood-based expression:

$$L_{part}(\boldsymbol{\beta}, \mathbf{w} \mid \mathbf{y}) =$$

$$\prod_{i=1}^{s} \prod_{j=1}^{n_i} \left[\frac{\exp\left(w_{0i} + (\beta_1 + w_{1i}) x_{ij1} + \mathbf{x}_{ij(-1)}^t \boldsymbol{\beta}_{(-1)}\right)}{\sum\limits_{qw \in R(y_{ij})} \exp\left(w_{0q} + (\beta_1 + w_{1q}) x_{qw1} + \mathbf{x}_{qw(-1)}^t \boldsymbol{\beta}_{(-1)}\right)} \right]^{\delta_{ij}}$$

The second factor on the right-hand side of (6.2) corresponds to the joint prior density of the random effects. The random effects w_{0i} and w_{1i}, $i = 1, \ldots, s$, are assumed to be independent and normal distributed with mean zero and variances γ_0 and γ_1 and therefore

$$f(\mathbf{w} \mid \boldsymbol{\gamma}) = \prod_{i=1}^{s} \frac{1}{2\pi \sqrt{\gamma_0 \gamma_1}} \exp\left(-\frac{1}{2}\left(\frac{w_{0i}^2}{\gamma_0} + \frac{w_{1i}^2}{\gamma_1}\right)\right)$$

The third and fourth factor of (6.2) represent the prior distributions for $\boldsymbol{\beta}$ and $\boldsymbol{\gamma}$. We take flat priors for these priors over their respective parameter space, i.e., $\gamma_0 \in [0, +\infty)$, $\gamma_1 \in [0, +\infty)$, and $\beta_i \subset I\!R$

$$f(\boldsymbol{\beta}) \propto 1 \text{ and } f(\boldsymbol{\gamma}) \propto 1$$

The logarithm of the joint posterior density can then be written as

$$\log f(\boldsymbol{\beta}, \mathbf{w}, \boldsymbol{\gamma} \mid \mathbf{y}) \propto \sum_{i=1}^{s} \sum_{j=1}^{n_i} \delta_{ij} \left\{ w_{0i} + (\beta_1 + w_{1i}) x_{ij1} + \mathbf{x}_{ij(-1)}^t \boldsymbol{\beta}_{(-1)} \right.$$

$$\left. - \log\left[\sum_{qw \in R(y_{ij})} \exp\left(w_{0q} + (\beta_1 + w_{1q}) x_{qw1} + \mathbf{x}_{qw(-1)}^t \boldsymbol{\beta}_{(-1)}\right)\right] \right\}$$

$$-s \log\left(2\pi \sqrt{\gamma_0 \gamma_1}\right) - \frac{1}{2} \sum_{i=1}^{s} \left(\frac{w_{0i}^2}{\gamma_0} + \frac{w_{1i}^2}{\gamma_1}\right) \tag{6.3}$$

Note that the expression above is only proportional to the posterior density since we ignore the normalising constant. In a Bayesian context, statistical inference on a particular subset of parameters of interest is based on the posterior density of the particular subset of parameters, which is obtained by integrating out the other parameters.

We first obtain the bivariate posterior density for γ which is obtained by integrating out both β and $\mathbf{w}$ from the joint posterior density

$$f(\gamma \mid \mathbf{y}) = \int \cdots \int f(\beta, \mathbf{w}, \gamma \mid \mathbf{y}) \, d\beta d\mathbf{w} \qquad (6.4)$$

where the integration is over $I\!R^{2s}$ for $\mathbf{w}$ and $I\!R^p$ for β. This integral cannot be solved analytically, but Laplacian integration can be used to approximate the integral for a particular value γ^* of γ. For a fixed value γ^* we use $f(\beta, \mathbf{w} \mid \mathbf{y}, \gamma^*)$ as notation for $f(\beta, \mathbf{w}, \gamma^* \mid \mathbf{y})$ and we write

$$\int \cdots \int f(\beta, \mathbf{w} \mid \mathbf{y}, \gamma^*) \, d\beta d\mathbf{w} = \int \cdots \int \exp\left(\log f(\beta, \mathbf{w} \mid \mathbf{y}, \gamma^*)\right) d\beta d\mathbf{w}$$

We now replace $\log f(\beta, \mathbf{w} \mid \mathbf{y}, \gamma^*)$ by the first terms of its Taylor expansion around the mode of the joint posterior density function $f(\beta, \mathbf{w} \mid \mathbf{y}, \gamma^*)$ given by

$$\hat{\mathbf{\Psi}}_{\gamma^*} = \left(\hat{\beta}^t_{\gamma^*}, \hat{\mathbf{w}}^t_{\gamma^*}\right)^t = \operatorname*{Arg\,max}_{\mathbf{\Psi}} f(\mathbf{\Psi} \mid \mathbf{y}, \gamma^*)$$

where $\mathbf{\Psi} = (\beta^t, \mathbf{w}^t)^t$. The mode $\hat{\mathbf{\Psi}}_{\gamma^*}$ can be found by maximising the logarithm of the joint posterior density (6.3) with respect to β and $\mathbf{w}$ taking $\gamma = \gamma^*$. Ducrocq and Sölkner (1994) use a limited memory quasi-Newton method for this maximisation which only requires the computation of the vector of first derivatives (Liu and Nocedal, 1989).

At the mode, the gradient vector equals zero:

$$\left.\frac{\partial \log f(\mathbf{\Psi} \mid \mathbf{y}, \gamma^*)}{\partial \mathbf{\Psi}}\right|_{\mathbf{\Psi}=\hat{\mathbf{\Psi}}_{\gamma^*}} = \mathbf{0}$$

and the second term in the Taylor series expansion therefore cancels. For the third term of the expansion we need the negative Hessian at $\hat{\mathbf{\Psi}}_{\gamma^*}$:

$$\mathbf{H}_{\gamma^*} = -\left.\frac{\partial^2 \log f(\mathbf{\Psi} \mid \mathbf{y}, \gamma^*)}{\partial \mathbf{\Psi} \partial \mathbf{\Psi}^t}\right|_{\mathbf{\Psi}=\hat{\mathbf{\Psi}}_{\gamma^*}}$$

The integral is then approximately given by

$$f\left(\gamma^{*} \mid \mathbf{y}\right) \approx \int \cdots \int \exp \left(\log f\left(\hat{\boldsymbol{\Psi}}_{\gamma^{*}} \mid \mathbf{y}, \gamma^{*}\right)\right.$$

$$\left.-\frac{1}{2}\left(\boldsymbol{\Psi}-\hat{\boldsymbol{\Psi}}_{\gamma^{*}}\right)^{t} \mathbf{H}_{\gamma^{*}}\left(\boldsymbol{\Psi}-\hat{\boldsymbol{\Psi}}_{\gamma^{*}}\right)\right) d\boldsymbol{\Psi}$$

Furthermore, we can write

$$\int \cdots \int (2\pi)^{-(2s+p)/2} \mid \mathbf{H}_{\gamma^{*}}^{-1} \mid^{-1/2}$$

$$\times \exp \left(-\frac{1}{2}\left(\boldsymbol{\Psi}-\hat{\boldsymbol{\Psi}}_{\gamma^{*}}\right)^{t} \mathbf{H}_{\gamma^{*}}\left(\boldsymbol{\Psi}-\hat{\boldsymbol{\Psi}}_{\gamma^{*}}\right)\right) d\boldsymbol{\Psi} = 1$$

as the expression is a multivariate normal density with mean $\hat{\boldsymbol{\Psi}}_{\gamma^{*}}$ and variance–covariance matrix $\mathbf{H}_{\gamma^{*}}^{-1}$. Thus, the approximation of the integral can be rewritten as

$$f\left(\gamma^{*} \mid \mathbf{y}\right) \approx (2\pi)^{(2s+p)/2} \mid \mathbf{H}_{\gamma^{*}}^{-1} \mid^{1/2} f\left(\hat{\boldsymbol{\Psi}}_{\gamma^{*}} \mid \mathbf{y}, \gamma^{*}\right) \tag{6.5}$$

Taking the logarithm on both sides we obtain the following approximation of the logarithm of the bivariate posterior density

$$\log f\left(\gamma^{*} \mid \mathbf{y}\right) \approx \text{constant} + \log f\left(\hat{\boldsymbol{\Psi}}_{\gamma^{*}} \mid \mathbf{y}, \gamma^{*}\right) - \frac{1}{2} \log \mid \mathbf{H}_{\gamma^{*}} \mid$$

The mode of the approximated density given by the right-hand side of (6.5) is used as an estimate for the variance components γ_0 and γ_1. It is denoted as $\hat{\gamma}$. Besides the mode $\hat{\gamma}$, other interesting measures such as the mean, variance, and skewness can be obtained from the bivariate posterior density. First, we can depict the bivariate posterior density by evaluating the right-hand side of (6.5) on a grid of equidistant points $\gamma_{ab} = (\gamma_{0a}, \gamma_{1b})$, $a = 1, \ldots, n_a$, $b = 1, \ldots, n_b$. These values can then be standardised by computing

$$p\left(\gamma_{ab} \mid \mathbf{y}\right) = \frac{f\left(\gamma_{ab} \mid \mathbf{y}\right)}{\sum\limits_{l=1}^{n_a} \sum\limits_{k=1}^{n_b} f\left(\gamma_{lk} \mid \mathbf{y}\right) \epsilon^2} \tag{6.6}$$

where ϵ is the distance between two adjacent points. With a sufficient number of pairs γ_{ab} evaluated in the relevant region, this procedure provides a good picture of the two-dimensional posterior density of γ. We can further obtain a figure of the univariate posterior density for each variance component separately. For instance, for $\gamma_0 = \gamma_{0a}$, an approximated value for the density is given by

$$p\left(\gamma_{0a} \mid \mathbf{y}\right) \approx \frac{\sum_{k=1}^{n_b} f\left(\gamma_{ak} \mid \mathbf{y}\right)}{\sum_{l=1}^{n_a} \sum_{k=1}^{n_b} f\left(\gamma_{lk} \mid \mathbf{y}\right) \epsilon} \tag{6.7}$$

We will demonstrate the use of (6.6) and (6.7) in Example 6.1.

Based on this discretised version of the univariate posterior density, we can also obtain good approximations of the first moments of γ_0 and γ_1. For instance, for γ_0 we have for the first moment

$$\mu_{1,\gamma_0} = \sum_{l=1}^{n_a} \gamma_{0l} p\left(\gamma_{0l} \mid \mathbf{y}\right) \epsilon$$

$$= \frac{\sum_{l=1}^{n_a} \sum_{k=1}^{n_b} \gamma_{0l} f\left(\gamma_{lk} \mid \mathbf{y}\right)}{\sum_{l=1}^{n_a} \sum_{k=1}^{n_b} f\left(\gamma_{lk} \mid \mathbf{y}\right)}$$

and in general for the cth moment

$$\mu_{c,\gamma_0} = \sum_{l=1}^{n_a} \gamma_{0l}^c p\left(\gamma_{0l} \mid \mathbf{y}\right) \epsilon$$

From these non-central moments, the mean, the variance, and the skewness can be obtained as

$$\mathrm{E}\left(\gamma_0\right) = \mu_{1,\gamma_0} \tag{6.8}$$

$$\mathrm{Var}\left(\gamma_0\right) = \mu_{2,\gamma_0} - \mu_{1,\gamma_0}^2 \tag{6.9}$$

$$\mathrm{Skewness}\left(\gamma_0\right) = \frac{\mu_{3,\gamma_0} - 3\mu_{1,\gamma_0}\mu_{2,\gamma_0} + 2\mu_{1,\gamma_0}^3}{\left(\mathrm{Var}\left(\gamma_0\right)\right)^{3/2}} \tag{6.10}$$

Example 6.1 Prognostic index heterogeneity for a bladder cancer multicentre trial: a Bayesian analysis

To investigate the relationship between the prognostic index and disease-free survival for the bladder cancer data (Example 1.10), we fit the frailty model (6.1) with the prognostic index as fixed effect and independent and normal distributed centre and centre by prognostic index interaction effects.

The parameter estimate for β_1 is 0.737, which can be interpreted as follows. For $x_{ij} = 0$ (good prognosis group) we have $h_{ij}(t) = h_0(t) \exp(w_{0i})$ and for $x_{ij} = 1$ (poor prognosis group) we have $h_{ij}(t) = h_0(t) \exp(w_{0i}) \exp(\beta_1 + w_{1i})$. Hence, the hazard ratio for cluster i is now the random variable $HR_i = \exp(\beta + w_{1i})$. Therefore, the hazard ratio for a cluster with $w_{1i} = 0$ (the mean of the random effect distribution) is estimated as $\exp(0.737) = 2.09$; the 95% confidence interval is $[1.73; 2.52]$. While the estimated hazard ratio and the corresponding confidence interval provide information on the overall effect and the precision of the estimated prognostic index effect, it does not provide information on the heterogeneity in the prognostic index effect over centres.

Results obtained when fitting model (6.1) assuming a normal distribution for the centre effect and for the prognostic index by centre interaction effect lead to estimates for the variance components of $\hat{\gamma}_0 = 0.095$ and $\hat{\gamma}_1 = 0.016$ corresponding to the mode of the approximated posterior density of γ given in (6.5). The bivariate posterior density can be approximated by (6.6) and is depicted in Figure 6.1. The univariate posterior densities for γ_0 and γ_1 can be approximated by (6.7) and are depicted in Figure 6.2.

Furthermore, the mean, standard deviation, and skewness of the univariate posterior densities for γ_0, respectively γ_1, can be obtained from (6.8)–(6.10) and are 0.087, 0.042, and 0.291, respectivey 0.052, 0.039, and 0.944. Note that the estimate for γ_0 is substantially larger than the estimate for γ_1. Therefore the variability of the conditional hazard due to the centre effect will be much bigger than the variability of the prognostic index effect over centres. To visualise the variability of the conditional hazard due to the centre effect, we plot $\exp(w_{0i})$ (Figure 6.3a); to see the variability of the prognostic index over centres, we plot the hazard ratio for cluster i: $HR_i = \exp(\beta + w_{1i})$ (Figure 6.3b).

A nice way to interpret the variance components is to consider their impact on clinically relevant quantities. This has already been mentioned in Example 2.1, where the median event time was considered. Considering the median event time in this particular clinical trial, however, is rather meaningless. At the time of analysis, less than 50% of the patients had already experienced the event in the good prognosis group. Therefore, the median event time can only be obtained from a parametric model by extrapolation.

We therefore rather rely on the five-year disease-free percentage. The five-year disease-free percentage can be obtained as follows. With time expressed

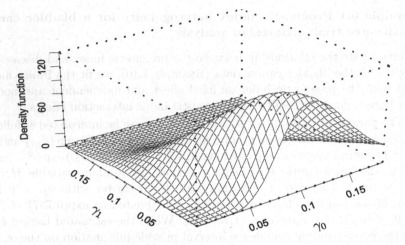

Fig. 6.1. The bivariate posterior density of γ_0 and γ_1.

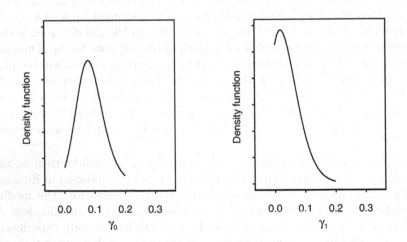

Fig. 6.2. The univariate posterior densities of γ_0 and γ_1.

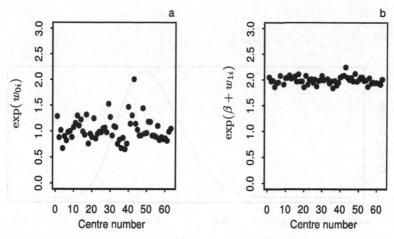

Fig. 6.3. Predicted frailties $\exp(w_{0i})$ (a) and $\exp(\beta + w_{1i})$ (b) of the different centres.

in number of years, fitting a frailty model with Weibull baseline hazard to the data, parameter estimates equal to $\hat{\lambda} = 0.7182$ and $\hat{\rho} = 0.1548$ are obtained. The five-year disease-free percentage in the good prognosis group for cluster i is then estimated by $\hat{S}_i(5)$ where

$$\hat{S}_i(t) = \exp\left(-\hat{\lambda} t^{\hat{\rho}} \exp(w_{0i})\right) \tag{6.11}$$

Due to the random centre effect w_{0i} in (6.11), the five-year disease-free percentage varies from centre to centre. The density of the five-year disease-free percentage can be obtained as follows:

$$P\left(S_i(5) \le a\right) \approx P\left(-\hat{\lambda} 5^{\hat{\rho}} \exp(w_{0i}) \le \log a\right)$$

$$= P\left(w_{0i} \le \log\left(-\frac{\log a}{\hat{\lambda} 5^{\hat{\rho}}}\right)\right)$$

$$\approx F_N\left(\frac{1}{\sqrt{\hat{\gamma}_0}} \log\left(-\frac{\log a}{\hat{\lambda} 5^{\hat{\rho}}}\right)\right) \tag{6.12}$$

where $0 \le a \le 1$ and with F_N the standard normal distribution function. The spread of the five-year disease-free percentage over the different clusters is shown in Figure 6.4.

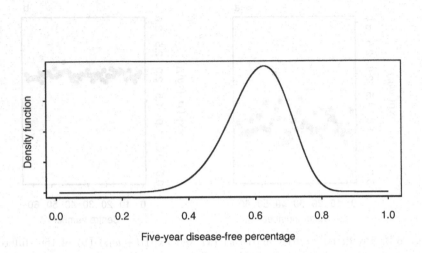

Fig. 6.4. Density of five-year disease-free percentage over centres in the good prognosis group.

To understand the impact of γ_1 we consider in Figure 6.5 the density of the $HR_i = \exp(\beta + w_{1i})$; we call this the density of the prognostic index effect over centres. This density function can be derived in an analogous way as (6.12). Considering the 5th and 95th quantiles of this density, we see that for 95% of the centres the prognostic index ratio takes a value between 1.61 and 2.45. This is clinically acceptable as even the lower level of the interval is substantially larger than one. ∎

6.1.2 Frequentist approach using Laplacian integration

The approach proposed by Ripatti and Palmgren (2000) is also based on Laplacian integration, but now in a frequentist rather than in a Bayesian setting.

We start from a more general model specification

$$h_{ij}(t) = h_0(t) \exp\left(\mathbf{x}_{ij}^t \boldsymbol{\beta} + \mathbf{z}_{ij}^t \mathbf{w}\right)$$

with $\mathbf{x}_{ij}$ the fixed effect covariates and $\mathbf{z}_{ij}$ the random effect covariates for the jth subject in cluster i. For the random effects, the following general form for the distribution of the d-dimensional vector $\mathbf{w}$, $f_{\mathbf{w}}(\mathbf{w})$, is assumed

$$\mathbf{w} \sim \mathrm{N}\left(\mathbf{0}, \mathbf{D}(\boldsymbol{\gamma})\right)$$

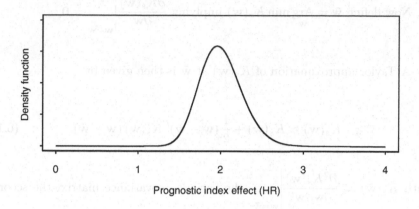

Fig. 6.5. Density of prognostic index effect over centres.

with $\mathbf{D}(\boldsymbol{\gamma})$ the variance–covariance matrix of the random effects vector $\mathbf{w}$ with unknown parameter vector $\boldsymbol{\gamma}$. The marginal likelihood is obtained using ideas similar to the ideas leading to (2.5) but with the gamma distribution replaced by the lognormal distribution resulting in

$$L_{marg}\left(h_0(.),\boldsymbol{\gamma},\boldsymbol{\beta}\right) = \int\limits_{-\infty}^{\infty} \cdots \int\limits_{-\infty}^{\infty} \prod_{i=1}^{s}\prod_{j=1}^{n_i}\left[\left(h_0(y_{ij})\exp\left(\mathbf{x}_{ij}^t\boldsymbol{\beta}+\mathbf{z}_{ij}^t\mathbf{w}\right)\right)^{\delta_{ij}}\right.$$

$$\left.\exp\left(-H_0(y_{ij})\exp\left(\mathbf{x}_{ij}^t\boldsymbol{\beta}+\mathbf{z}_{ij}^t\mathbf{w}\right)\right)\right]f_{\mathbf{W}}(\mathbf{w})d\mathbf{w}$$

$$= c\,|\,\mathbf{D}(\boldsymbol{\gamma})\,|^{-1/2}\int\limits_{-\infty}^{\infty}\cdots\int\limits_{-\infty}^{\infty}\exp\left(-K_s(\mathbf{w})\right)d\mathbf{w}$$

with

$$K_s(\mathbf{w}) = -\sum_{i=1}^{s}\sum_{j=1}^{n_i}\left[\delta_{ij}\left(\log h_0(y_{ij})+\mathbf{x}_{ij}^t\boldsymbol{\beta}+\mathbf{z}_{ij}^t\mathbf{w}\right)\right.$$

$$\left.-H_0(y_{ij})\exp\left(\mathbf{x}_{ij}^t\boldsymbol{\beta}+\mathbf{z}_{ij}^t\mathbf{w}\right)\right]+\frac{1}{2}\mathbf{w}^t\mathbf{D}^{-1}(\boldsymbol{\gamma})\mathbf{w}$$

Now define $\tilde{\mathbf{w}} = \underset{\mathbf{w}}{\text{Arg min}}\, K_s(\mathbf{w})$ implying $\dfrac{\partial K_s(\mathbf{w})}{\partial \mathbf{w}}\bigg|_{\mathbf{w}=\tilde{\mathbf{w}}} = \mathbf{0}.$

A Taylor approximation of $K_s(\mathbf{w})$ at $\tilde{\mathbf{w}}$ is then given by

$$K_s(\mathbf{w}) \approx K_s(\tilde{\mathbf{w}}) + \frac{1}{2}(\mathbf{w} - \tilde{\mathbf{w}})^t \ddot{K}_s(\tilde{\mathbf{w}})(\mathbf{w} - \tilde{\mathbf{w}}) \qquad (6.13)$$

with $\ddot{K}_s(\tilde{\mathbf{w}}) = \dfrac{\partial^2 K_s(\mathbf{w})}{\partial \mathbf{w} \partial \mathbf{w}^t}\bigg|_{\mathbf{w}=\tilde{\mathbf{w}}}$, the variance–covariance matrix, the second-order partial derivatives of $\ddot{K}_s$ with respect to $\mathbf{w}$ and evaluated at $\mathbf{w} = \tilde{\mathbf{w}}$, i.e.,

$$\ddot{K}_s(\tilde{\mathbf{w}}) = \sum_{i=1}^{s}\sum_{j=1}^{n_i} H_0(y_{ij}) \exp\left(\mathbf{x}_{ij}^t \boldsymbol{\beta} + \mathbf{z}_{ij}^t \tilde{\mathbf{w}}\right) \mathbf{z}_{ij} \mathbf{z}_{ij}^t + \mathbf{D}^{-1}(\boldsymbol{\gamma})$$

Therefore,

$$L_{marg}(h_0(.), \boldsymbol{\gamma}, \boldsymbol{\beta}) \approx |\, \mathbf{D}(\boldsymbol{\gamma})\,|^{-1/2} \exp\left(-K_s(\tilde{\mathbf{w}})\right)$$

$$\times \int_{-\infty}^{\infty}\cdots\int_{-\infty}^{\infty} \exp\left(-\frac{1}{2}(\mathbf{w} - \tilde{\mathbf{w}})^t \ddot{K}_s(\tilde{\mathbf{w}})(\mathbf{w} - \tilde{\mathbf{w}})\right) d\mathbf{w}$$

$$= |\, \mathbf{D}(\boldsymbol{\gamma})\,|^{-1/2} \exp\left(-K_s(\tilde{\mathbf{w}})\right)(2\pi)^{d/2}\,|\, \ddot{K}_s(\tilde{\mathbf{w}})\,|^{-1/2}$$

where the last equality follows from the fact that

$$\int_{-\infty}^{\infty}\cdots\int_{-\infty}^{\infty}(2\pi)^{-d/2}\,|\, \ddot{K}_s^{-1}(\tilde{\mathbf{w}})\,|^{1/2}\exp\left(-\frac{1}{2}(\mathbf{w} - \tilde{\mathbf{w}})^t \ddot{K}_s(\tilde{\mathbf{w}})(\mathbf{w} - \tilde{\mathbf{w}})\right) d\mathbf{w} = 1$$

The marginal loglikelihood therefore corresponds to

$$l_{marg}\left(h_0(.), \boldsymbol{\gamma}, \boldsymbol{\beta}\right) \approx -\frac{1}{2}\log \mid \mathbf{D}(\boldsymbol{\gamma}) \mid -\frac{1}{2}\log \mid \ddot{K}_s(\tilde{\mathbf{w}}) \mid -K_s(\tilde{\mathbf{w}})$$

$$= -\frac{1}{2}\log \mid \mathbf{D}(\boldsymbol{\gamma}) \mid$$

$$-\frac{1}{2}\log \left| \sum_{i=1}^{s}\sum_{j=1}^{n_i} H_0(y_{ij})\exp\left(\mathbf{x}_{ij}^t\boldsymbol{\beta}+\mathbf{z}_{ij}^t\tilde{\mathbf{w}}\right)\mathbf{z}_{ij}\mathbf{z}_{ij}^t+\mathbf{D}^{-1}(\boldsymbol{\gamma})\right|$$

$$+l_{pen}\left(h_0(.), \boldsymbol{\gamma}, \boldsymbol{\beta}, \tilde{\mathbf{w}}\right) \qquad (6.14)$$

with

$$l_{pen}\left(h_0(.), \boldsymbol{\gamma}, \boldsymbol{\beta}, \tilde{\mathbf{w}}\right) = -K_s(\tilde{\mathbf{w}})$$

$$= \sum_{i=1}^{s}\sum_{j=1}^{n_i}\left[\delta_{ij}\left(\log h_0(y_{ij}) + \mathbf{x}_{ij}^t\boldsymbol{\beta} + \mathbf{z}_{ij}^t\tilde{\mathbf{w}}\right)\right.$$

$$\left. -H_0(y_{ij})\exp\left(\mathbf{x}_{ij}^t\boldsymbol{\beta} + \mathbf{z}_{ij}^t\tilde{\mathbf{w}}\right)\right] - \frac{1}{2}\tilde{\mathbf{w}}^t\mathbf{D}^{-1}(\boldsymbol{\gamma})\tilde{\mathbf{w}}$$

Assume now that $\boldsymbol{\gamma}$ is known and replace $\tilde{\mathbf{w}}$ by $\mathbf{w}$ in $l_{pen}\left(h_0(.), \boldsymbol{\gamma}, \boldsymbol{\beta}, \tilde{\mathbf{w}}\right)$. Considering now $\mathbf{w}$ as fixed effects parameters we have a penalised Cox full likelihood. In order to convert the penalised full likelihood into a partial likelihood we write

$$l_{pen}\left(h_0(.), \boldsymbol{\gamma}, \boldsymbol{\beta}, \tilde{\mathbf{w}}\right) = l_{ppl}\left(\boldsymbol{\gamma}, \boldsymbol{\beta}, \mathbf{w}\right) + g\left(h_0(.), \boldsymbol{\beta}, \mathbf{w}\right)$$

with

$$l_{ppl}\left(\boldsymbol{\gamma}, \boldsymbol{\beta}, \mathbf{w}\right) = \sum_{i=1}^{s}\sum_{j=1}^{n_i}\left(\delta_{ij}\left(\mathbf{x}_{ij}^t\boldsymbol{\beta} + \mathbf{z}_{ij}^t\mathbf{w}\right) - \log\sum_{qw\in R(y_{ij})}\exp\left(\mathbf{x}_{qw}^t\boldsymbol{\beta} + \mathbf{z}_{qw}^t\mathbf{w}\right)\right)$$

$$-\frac{1}{2}\mathbf{w}^t\mathbf{D}^{-1}(\boldsymbol{\gamma})\mathbf{w}$$

and

$$g\left(h_0(.), \boldsymbol{\beta}, \mathbf{w}\right) = \sum_{i=1}^{s} \sum_{j=1}^{n_i} \Big[\delta_{ij} \left(\log h_0(y_{ij}) + \log \sum_{qw \in R(y_{ij})} \exp\left(\mathbf{x}_{qw}^t \boldsymbol{\beta} + \mathbf{z}_{qw}^t \mathbf{w}\right) \right)$$
$$- H_0(y_{ij}) \exp\left(\mathbf{x}_{ij}^t \boldsymbol{\beta} + \mathbf{z}_{ij}^t \mathbf{w}\right) \Big]$$

Ripatti and Palmgren (2000) show that, for $\boldsymbol{\gamma}$ fixed, the values $\hat{\boldsymbol{\beta}}_{\boldsymbol{\gamma}}$ and $\hat{\mathbf{w}}_{\boldsymbol{\gamma}}$ that maximise $l_{ppl}\left(\boldsymbol{\gamma}, \boldsymbol{\beta}, \mathbf{w}\right)$ also maximise $l_{pen}\left(\hat{h}_0(.), \boldsymbol{\gamma}, \boldsymbol{\beta}, \tilde{\mathbf{w}}\right)$ with $\hat{h}_0(.)$ the discretised baseline hazard estimator that maximises, for $\boldsymbol{\beta}$ and $\mathbf{w}$ fixed, $g\left(h_0(.), \boldsymbol{\beta}, \mathbf{w}\right)$.

Based on the discussion above we can set up an iterative procedure using an inner and an outer loop. In brief the algorithm works as follows:

(i) Inner loop
Fix $\boldsymbol{\gamma}$ and obtain

$$\left(\hat{\boldsymbol{\beta}}_{\boldsymbol{\gamma}}^t, \hat{\mathbf{w}}_{\boldsymbol{\gamma}}^t\right)^t = \operatorname*{Arg\ max}_{(\boldsymbol{\beta}^t, \mathbf{w}^t)^t} l_{ppl}\left(\boldsymbol{\gamma}, \boldsymbol{\beta}, \mathbf{w}\right)$$

(ii) Outer loop
Consider $\hat{\boldsymbol{\beta}}_{\boldsymbol{\gamma}}$ and $\hat{\mathbf{w}}_{\boldsymbol{\gamma}}$ as fixed in $l_{appr}\left(\boldsymbol{\gamma}, \hat{\boldsymbol{\beta}}_{\boldsymbol{\gamma}}, \hat{\mathbf{w}}_{\boldsymbol{\gamma}}\right)$ as defined in (6.17) below and take as updated value for $\boldsymbol{\gamma}$ the value that maximises $l_{appr}\left(\boldsymbol{\gamma}, \hat{\boldsymbol{\beta}}_{\boldsymbol{\gamma}}, \hat{\mathbf{w}}_{\boldsymbol{\gamma}}\right)$. In the further discussion we will show that l_{appr} can be considered as a workable approximation for the marginal loglikelihood l_{marg} given by (6.14).

We now discuss the inner and outer loop in more detail.

In the **inner loop** we consider the maximisation of l_{ppl} given a fixed value for $\boldsymbol{\gamma}$. The estimation equations are given by setting the first derivatives of l_{ppl} with respect to $\boldsymbol{\beta}$ and with respect to $\mathbf{w}$ equal to zero (a vector of dimension p, respectively s), i.e.,

$$\frac{\partial l_{ppl}}{\partial \boldsymbol{\beta}} \equiv \sum_{i=1}^{s} \sum_{j=1}^{n_i} \delta_{ij} \left[\mathbf{x}_{ij} - \frac{\mathbf{x}_{ij} \exp\left(\mathbf{x}_{ij}^t \boldsymbol{\beta} + \mathbf{z}_{ij}^t \mathbf{w}\right)}{\sum\limits_{qw \in R(y_{ij})} \exp\left(\mathbf{x}_{qw}^t \boldsymbol{\beta} + \mathbf{z}_{qw}^t \mathbf{w}\right)} \right] = 0$$

and

$$\frac{\partial l_{ppl}}{\partial \mathbf{w}} \equiv \sum_{i=1}^{s} \sum_{j=1}^{n_i} \delta_{ij} \left[\mathbf{z}_{ij} - \frac{\mathbf{z}_{ij} \exp\left(\mathbf{x}_{ij}^t \boldsymbol{\beta} + \mathbf{z}_{ij}^t \mathbf{w}\right)}{\sum\limits_{qw \in R(y_{ij})} \exp\left(\mathbf{x}_{qw}^t \boldsymbol{\beta} + \mathbf{z}_{qw}^t \mathbf{w}\right)} \right] - \mathbf{D}^{-1}(\boldsymbol{\gamma})\mathbf{w} = \mathbf{0}$$

An approximation to the variance–covariance matrix for $\hat{\boldsymbol{\beta}}$ is given by the inverse of minus the Hessian obtained from l_{ppl}, although it might underestimate the covariances and variances as $\boldsymbol{\gamma}$ is assumed to be known and the uncertainty in the estimation of $\boldsymbol{\gamma}$ (in the outer loop) is not taken into account. Ripatti and Palmgren (2000) demonstrate that the underestimation is small.

In the **outer loop** we first obtain a workable approximation for $l_{marg}\left(h_0(.), \boldsymbol{\gamma}, \boldsymbol{\beta}\right)$.

Replacing in (6.14) $\boldsymbol{\beta}$ by $\hat{\boldsymbol{\beta}}_{\boldsymbol{\gamma}}$ and $\tilde{\mathbf{w}}$ by $\hat{\mathbf{w}}_{\boldsymbol{\gamma}}$ we obtain

$$l_1\left(h_0(.), \boldsymbol{\gamma}, \hat{\boldsymbol{\beta}}_{\boldsymbol{\gamma}}, \hat{\mathbf{w}}_{\boldsymbol{\gamma}}\right)$$

$$= -\frac{1}{2} \log |\mathbf{D}(\boldsymbol{\gamma})|$$

$$- \frac{1}{2} \log \left|\ddot{K}_s\left(\hat{\mathbf{w}}_{\boldsymbol{\gamma}}\right)\right|$$

$$\frac{1}{2}\hat{\mathbf{w}}_{\boldsymbol{\gamma}}^t \mathbf{D}^{-1}(\boldsymbol{\gamma})\hat{\mathbf{w}}_{\boldsymbol{\gamma}}$$

$$+ \sum_{i=1}^{s} \sum_{j=1}^{n_i} \left[\delta_{ij}\left(\log h_0(y_{ij}) + \mathbf{x}_{ij}^t\hat{\boldsymbol{\beta}}_{\boldsymbol{\gamma}} + \mathbf{z}_{ij}^t\hat{\mathbf{w}}_{\boldsymbol{\gamma}}\right)\right.$$

$$\left. - H_0(y_{ij}) \exp\left(\mathbf{x}_{ij}^t\hat{\boldsymbol{\beta}}_{\boldsymbol{\gamma}} + \mathbf{z}_{ij}^t\hat{\mathbf{w}}_{\boldsymbol{\gamma}}\right)\right] \qquad (6.15)$$

Ignoring the dependence on $\boldsymbol{\gamma}$ of $\hat{\boldsymbol{\beta}}_{\boldsymbol{\gamma}}$ and $\hat{\mathbf{w}}_{\boldsymbol{\gamma}}$ in the fourth term on the right-hand side of (6.15) we can further replace $l_1\left(h_0(.), \boldsymbol{\gamma}, \hat{\boldsymbol{\beta}}_{\boldsymbol{\gamma}}, \hat{\mathbf{w}}_{\boldsymbol{\gamma}}\right)$ by

$$l_2\left(h_0(.), \boldsymbol{\gamma}, \hat{\boldsymbol{\beta}}_{\boldsymbol{\gamma}}, \hat{\mathbf{w}}_{\boldsymbol{\gamma}}\right) = -\frac{1}{2} \log |\mathbf{D}(\boldsymbol{\gamma})|$$

$$- \frac{1}{2} \log \left|\ddot{K}_s\left(\hat{\mathbf{w}}_{\boldsymbol{\gamma}}\right)\right| - \frac{1}{2}\hat{\mathbf{w}}_{\boldsymbol{\gamma}}^t \mathbf{D}^{-1}(\boldsymbol{\gamma})\hat{\mathbf{w}}_{\boldsymbol{\gamma}} \qquad (6.16)$$

since, in the outer loop, our interest is maximisation with respect to γ. In (6.16) the matrix $\ddot{K}_s(\hat{\mathbf{w}}_\gamma)$ also contains $\hat{\mathbf{w}}_\gamma$ and the baseline hazard.

From the discussion on the likelihoods given above recall that, to get rid of the baseline hazard, $l_{pen}(h_0(.), \gamma, \beta, \tilde{\mathbf{w}}) \equiv -K_s(\tilde{\mathbf{w}})$ in $l_{marg}(h_0(.), \gamma, \beta)$ given by (6.14) has been replaced by $l_{ppl}(\gamma, \beta, \mathbf{w})$. We repeat this idea here and replace $\ddot{K}_s(\hat{\mathbf{w}}_\gamma)$ by

$$\ddot{l}_{ppl}\left(\gamma, \hat{\beta}_\gamma, \hat{\mathbf{w}}_\gamma\right) = \left.\frac{\partial^2 l_{ppl}(\beta, \mathbf{w}, \gamma)}{\partial \mathbf{w} \partial \mathbf{w}^t}\right|_{\beta=\hat{\beta}_\gamma, \mathbf{w}=\hat{\mathbf{w}}_\gamma}$$

For the outer loop, we therefore propose an approximation for the marginal loglikelihood:

$$l_{appr}\left(\gamma, \hat{\beta}_\gamma, \hat{\mathbf{w}}_\gamma\right) = -\frac{1}{2}\log|\mathbf{D}(\gamma)|$$

$$-\frac{1}{2}\log\left|\ddot{l}_{ppl}\left(\gamma, \hat{\beta}_\gamma, \hat{\mathbf{w}}_\gamma\right)\right| - \frac{1}{2}\hat{\mathbf{w}}_\gamma^t \mathbf{D}^{-1}(\gamma)\hat{\mathbf{w}}_\gamma \quad (6.17)$$

In the outer loop we obtain, for $\hat{\beta}_\gamma$ and $\hat{\mathbf{w}}_\gamma$ fixed,

$$\hat{\gamma} = \underset{\gamma}{\text{Arg max}}\, l_{appr}\left(\gamma, \hat{\beta}_\gamma, \hat{\mathbf{w}}_\gamma\right)$$

To obtain the estimating equation for γ, note that (see Section 12.10 in Searle (1982) for details)

$$\frac{d}{d\gamma}\log|\mathbf{D}(\gamma)| = \text{tr}\left(\mathbf{D}^{-1}(\gamma)\frac{d\mathbf{D}(\gamma)}{d\gamma}\right) \quad (6.18)$$

$$\frac{d}{d\gamma}\hat{\mathbf{w}}_\gamma^t \mathbf{D}^{-1}(\gamma)\hat{\mathbf{w}}_\gamma = -\hat{\mathbf{w}}_\gamma^t \mathbf{D}^{-1}(\gamma)\frac{d\mathbf{D}(\gamma)}{d\gamma}\mathbf{D}^{-1}(\gamma)\hat{\mathbf{w}}_\gamma \quad (6.19)$$

$$\frac{d}{d\gamma}\log\left|\ddot{l}_{ppl}\left(\gamma, \hat{\beta}_\gamma, \hat{\mathbf{w}}_\gamma\right)\right| = \text{tr}\left[\left(\ddot{l}_{ppl}\left(\gamma, \hat{\beta}_\gamma, \hat{\mathbf{w}}_\gamma\right)\right)^{-1}\right.$$

$$\left.\times \mathbf{D}^{-1}(\gamma)\frac{d\mathbf{D}(\gamma)}{d\gamma}\mathbf{D}^{-1}(\gamma)\right] \quad (6.20)$$

where we use that $\mathbf{D}^{-1}(\gamma)$ is the only term in $\ddot{l}_{ppl}(\beta, \mathbf{w}, \gamma)$ that depends on

γ and that

$$-\frac{d}{d\gamma}\mathbf{D}^{-1}(\gamma) = \mathbf{D}^{-1}(\gamma)\frac{d\mathbf{D}(\gamma)}{d\gamma}\mathbf{D}^{-1}(\gamma)$$

From (6.17)–(6.20) we easily obtain that the estimating equation for γ is

$$-\frac{1}{2}\ \mathrm{tr}\left(\mathbf{D}^{-1}(\gamma)\frac{d\mathbf{D}(\gamma)}{d\gamma}\right)$$

$$-\frac{1}{2}\mathrm{tr}\left[\left(\ddot{l}_{ppl}\left(\gamma,\hat{\beta}_\gamma,\hat{\mathbf{w}}_\gamma\right)\right)^{-1}\mathbf{D}^{-1}(\gamma)\frac{d\mathbf{D}(\gamma)}{d\gamma}\mathbf{D}^{-1}(\gamma)\right]$$

$$+\frac{1}{2}\hat{\mathbf{w}}_\gamma^t\mathbf{D}^{-1}(\gamma)\frac{d\mathbf{D}(\gamma)}{d\gamma}\mathbf{D}^{-1}(\gamma)\hat{\mathbf{w}}_\gamma = 0 \qquad\qquad (6.21)$$

Finally, for the Fisher information matrix, we differentiate with respect to γ the terms on the right-hand side of (6.21) and we take the expectation with respect to $\mathbf{w}$ (using that $\mathrm{E}\left(\hat{\mathbf{w}}_\gamma\right) \approx \mathbf{0}$ since $\mathrm{E}\left(\mathbf{w}\right) = \mathbf{0}$). This gives

$$-\frac{1}{2}\ \mathrm{tr}\left(-\mathbf{D}^{-1}(\gamma)\frac{d\mathbf{D}(\gamma)}{d\gamma}\mathbf{D}^{-1}(\gamma)\frac{d\mathbf{D}(\gamma)}{d\gamma} + \mathbf{D}^{-1}(\gamma)\frac{d^2\mathbf{D}(\gamma)}{d\gamma d\gamma^t}\right)$$

$$+\frac{1}{2}\mathrm{tr}\left[\left(\ddot{l}_{ppl}\left(\gamma,\hat{\beta}_\gamma,\hat{\mathbf{w}}_\gamma\right)\right)^{-1}\frac{d\mathbf{D}^{-1}(\gamma)}{d\gamma}\left(\ddot{l}_{ppl}\left(\gamma,\hat{\beta}_\gamma,\hat{\mathbf{w}}_\gamma\right)\right)^{-1}\frac{d\mathbf{D}^{-1}(\gamma)}{d\gamma}\right.$$

$$\left.+\ddot{l}_{ppl}\left(\gamma,\hat{\beta}_\gamma,\hat{\mathbf{w}}_\gamma\right)\frac{d^2\mathbf{D}^{-1}(\gamma)}{d\gamma d\gamma^t}\right] \qquad\qquad (6.22)$$

Example 6.2 Prognostic index heterogeneity for a bladder cancer multicentre trial: a frequentist analysis

As in Example 6.1 we fit model (6.1) for the bladder cancer data (Example 1.10) assuming uncorrelated random effects, i.e., we assume that $\mathbf{D}(\mathbf{w})$ the variance–covariance matrix of $\mathbf{w}^t = (w_{01},\dots,w_{0s},w_{11},\dots,w_{1s})$ takes form

$$\mathbf{D}(\mathbf{w}) = \mathbf{D}(\gamma) = \begin{pmatrix} \gamma_0\mathbf{I}_s & \mathbf{0} \\ \mathbf{0} & \gamma_1\mathbf{I}_s \end{pmatrix}$$

In this example, the prognostic index is a binary covariate: $x_{ij} = 1$ (poor prognosis) or $x_{ij} = 0$ (good prognosis).

The corresponding $\mathbf{z}_{ij}$ is vector

$$\mathbf{z}_{ij}^t = (0,\ldots,1,\ldots,0 \mid 0,\ldots,x_{ij},\ldots,0)$$

with one in position i and x_{ij} in position $s+i$. A different way to write $\mathbf{z}_{ij}^t\mathbf{w}$ is as follows: for

$$\mathbf{c}^t = (w_{01}, w_{01} + w_{11}, w_{02}, w_{02} + w_{12}, \ldots, w_{0s}, w_{0s} + w_{1s})$$

and

$$\tilde{\mathbf{z}}_{ij}^t = (0,\ldots,0,1 - x_{ij}, x_{ij}, 0, \ldots, 0)$$

with $1 - x_{ij}$ in position $2i - 1$ and x_{ij} in position $2i$, we have (note that $x_{ij} = 0$ or $x_{ij} = 1$)

$$\mathbf{z}_{ij}^t\mathbf{w} = \tilde{\mathbf{z}}_{ij}^t\mathbf{c}$$

Note that, with $\otimes$ the Kronecker product,

$$\mathbf{D}(\mathbf{c}) = \mathbf{I}_s \otimes \begin{pmatrix} \gamma_0 & \gamma_0 \\ \gamma_0 & \gamma_0 + \gamma_1 \end{pmatrix} \tag{6.23}$$

We can fit the Ripatti and Palmgren method (Ripatti and Palmgren, 2000) in Splus using the coxme function. This function uses the variance–covariance specification given in (6.23). The estimated hazard ratio $\exp(\hat{\beta}_1)$ equals 1.987 and the 95% confidence interval is $[1.63; 2.42]$, the variance component estimates are $\hat{\gamma}_0 = 0.09411$ and $\hat{\gamma}_1 = 0.01375$. These results are similar to the results obtained in Example 6.1.

The coxme function can also handle the more general variance–covariance matrix for $\mathbf{c}$ of form

$$\mathbf{D}(\mathbf{c}) = \mathbf{I}_s \otimes \begin{pmatrix} \gamma_0 & \gamma_0 + \gamma_{01} \\ \gamma_0 + \gamma_{01} & \gamma_0 + \gamma_1 + \gamma_{01} \end{pmatrix}$$

with γ_{01} the covariance of w_{0i} and w_{1i}. For the current example the covariance is estimated to be zero.

To have an example where the covariance γ_{01} is not zero we analyse the bladder cancer data set with treatment as covariate instead of prognostic index. Fitting the model with uncorrelated random effects, we obtain as estimate for the hazard ratio 0.94 and the 95% confidence interval is $[0.802; 1.104]$. The estimates for the variance components are $\hat{\gamma}_0 = 0.107$ and $\hat{\gamma}_1 = 0.083$. Introducing covariance between the two random effects gives $\hat{\gamma}_{01} = 0.041$ as estimate for the covariance and $\hat{\gamma}_0 = 0.086$ and $\hat{\gamma}_1 = 0.093$ as estimates for the variance components. The estimate of the hazard ratio in this extended model is 0.95 and the 95% confidence interval is $[0.82; 1.09]$. ■

6.2 Multilevel frailty models

In this section, we study techniques to fit models with nested clusters. Consider for instance Example 1.11 where data are collected on child mortality in Ethiopia. Two cluster levels are present in these data: children are clustered in villages and villages are clustered in districts. The model is given by

$$h_{ijk}(t) = h_0(t)u_i z_{ij} \exp\left(\mathbf{x}_{ijk}^t \boldsymbol{\beta}\right)$$

with $h_{ijk}(t)$ the hazard at time t of subject k, $k = 1, \ldots, n_{ij}$ clustered in the jth subcluster, $j = 1, \ldots, s_i$, of cluster i, $i = 1, \ldots, s$; u_i is the frailty term for cluster i and z_{ij} is the frailty term for subcluster j nested in cluster i. Different distributional assumptions will be made regarding these frailty terms. In Section 6.2.1, we assume that the frailty terms are independent and gamma distributed, and maximise the marginal likelihood using penalised splines for the baseline hazard. In Section 6.2.2, a Weibull baseline hazard with independent normal distributed random effects will be fitted.

6.2.1 Maximising the marginal likelihood with penalised splines for the baseline hazard

In the maximum marginal likelihood approach, proposed by Rondeau et al. (2003, 2006), the frailty terms are assumed to be independent and one-parameter gamma distributed, i.e., $U_i \sim \text{Gamma}(1/\theta, 1/\theta)$ and also $Z_{ij} \sim \text{Gamma}(1/\eta, 1/\eta)$. For this choice of the two frailty densities, the frailty density at the subcluster level can still be integrated out analytically. The conditional likelihood (conditional on the frailty terms) for cluster i is given by

$$L_i\left(h_0(.), \boldsymbol{\beta} \mid u_i, z_{i1}, \ldots, z_{is_i}\right) = \prod_{j=1}^{s_i} \prod_{k=1}^{n_{ij}} (h_0(y_{ijk})u_i z_{ij} \exp(\mathbf{x}_{ijk}^t \boldsymbol{\beta}))^{\delta_{ijk}}$$
$$\times \exp(-H_0(y_{ijk})u_i z_{ij} \exp(\mathbf{x}_{ijk}^t \boldsymbol{\beta}))$$

with y_{ijk}, δ_{ijk}, and $\mathbf{x}_{ijk}$ respectively the observed time (either event or censoring time), the censoring indicator, and the covariate information vector for subject k in subcluster j nested in cluster i. The marginal likelihood for cluster i then corresponds to

$$
L_{marg,i}(h_0(.),\theta,\eta,\boldsymbol{\beta}) = \int_0^\infty \int_0^\infty \cdots \int_0^\infty \prod_{j=1}^{s_i} \prod_{k=1}^{n_{ij}} \left[(h_0(y_{ijk})u_i z_{ij}\exp(\mathbf{x}_{ijk}^t\boldsymbol{\beta}))^{\delta_{ijk}}\right.
$$

$$
\times \left. \exp(-H_0(y_{ijk})u_i z_{ij}\exp(\mathbf{x}_{ijk}^t\boldsymbol{\beta}))\right]
$$

$$
\times \left(\frac{1}{\eta^{1/\eta}\Gamma(1/\eta)}\right)^{s_i} \prod_{j=1}^{s_i} z_{ij}^{1/\eta-1}\exp\left(-z_{ij}/\eta\right)
$$

$$
\times \frac{1}{\theta^{1/\theta}\Gamma(1/\theta)} u_i^{1/\theta-1}\exp\left(-u_i/\theta\right) dz_{i1}\ldots dz_{is_i} du_i \quad (6.24)
$$

Integrating out the frailty terms $z_{i1},\ldots,z_{is_i}$ analytically we obtain

$$
L_{marg,i}(h_0(.),\theta,\eta,\boldsymbol{\beta}) =
$$

$$
\prod_{j=1}^{s_i}\prod_{k=1}^{n_{ij}}\left(h_0(y_{ijk})\exp(\mathbf{x}_{ijk}^t\boldsymbol{\beta})\right)^{\delta_{ijk}} \frac{1}{\theta^{1/\theta}\Gamma(1/\theta)} \prod_{j=1}^{s_i} \frac{\Gamma(1/\eta+d_{ij})}{(1/\eta)^{d_{ij}}\Gamma(1/\eta)}
$$

$$
\times \int_0^\infty \frac{u_i^{1/\theta-1+d_i}\exp\left(-u_i/\theta\right)}{\prod_{j=1}^{s_i}\left(1+\eta u_i \sum_{k=1}^{n_{ij}} H_0(y_{ijk})\exp(\mathbf{x}_{ijk}^t\boldsymbol{\beta})\right)^{1/\eta+d_{ij}}}du_i \quad (6.25)
$$

with d_{ij} the number of events in subcluster j nested in cluster i and d_i the total number of events in cluster i. By taking the logarithm of (6.25) and summing over the s clusters we obtain the marginal loglikelihood $l_{marg}(h_0(.),\theta,\eta,\boldsymbol{\beta})$. The marginal loglikelihood still contains the baseline and cumulative baseline hazard $h_0(.)$ and $H_0(.)$. A flexible approach is to use splines to model the baseline hazard. Splines are piecewise polynomial functions that are combined in a linear and smooth way (using constraints at the interval boundaries). Rondeau et al. (2006) use cubic M-splines for the baseline hazard function and I-splines (integrated M-splines) for the baseline cumulative hazard function. To control the degree of smoothness, a penalty term for the roughness of the baseline hazard is added to the marginal loglikelihood. The penalty is the product of a smoothing factor κ and the integral of the squared second derivative of the baseline hazard which is a global measure for the curvature of the baseline hazard

$$l_{pmarg}(h_0(.), \theta, \eta, \boldsymbol{\beta}, \kappa) = l_{marg}(h_0(.), \theta, \eta, \boldsymbol{\beta}) - \kappa \int_0^\infty \left(h_0^{(2)}(t)\right)^2 dt \quad (6.26)$$

The smoothing parameter κ can be chosen by visual inspection of the penalising effect for a set of particular κ values or by fixing the number of degrees of freedom to estimate the baseline hazard (Gray, 1992). Another way to choose the smoothing parameter is by maximising a likelihood cross-validation criterion (Joly et al., 1998).

The algorithm thus consists of maximisation of the penalised marginal log-likelihood $l_{pmarg}(h_0(.), \theta, \eta, \boldsymbol{\beta}, \kappa)$ for which the robust Marquardt algorithm (Marquardt, 1963) is used. The penalised marginal loglikelihood expression $l_{pmarg}(h_0(.), \theta, \eta, \boldsymbol{\beta}, \kappa)$ still contains integrals, one for each frailty term at the higher cluster level. Gaussian quadrature is used to evaluate these integrals in a numerical way. The first and second derivatives of $l_{pmarg}(h_0(.), \theta, \eta, \boldsymbol{\beta}, \kappa)$, from which the Hessian and therefore the asymptotic variance–covariance matrix is obtained, are also calculated numerically using finite differences.

To fit this multilevel frailty model on concrete data, the software package "frailtypack", developed in R by Rondeau and Gonzalez (2005), can be used.

Example 6.3 Modelling multilevel child mortality data through maximising the marginal loglikelihood with penalised splines for the baseline hazard

A frailty model is fitted to the child mortality data presented in Example 1.11. Two cluster levels occur in this example. The district (woreda) is the cluster at the highest level. A district contains different villages (kebele), the low level of clustering. Within each village all infants are followed up. The estimate of the variance related to the villages is 0.045 (s.e. = 0.028); the estimate of the variance related to the districts is 0.0073 (s.e. = 0.00007). The estimate of the gender effect is $\hat{\beta} = -0.137$ (s.e. = 0.071) resulting in a hazard ratio of death of female versus male of 0.87, the 95% confidence interval is $[0.76; 1.00]$, i.e., the gender effect is marginally significant. ∎

6.2.2 The Bayesian approach for multilevel frailty models using Gibbs sampling

The Bayesian approach using MCMC techniques, proposed in Section 5.3.4 for the semiparametric frailty model with one frailty term, becomes even more interesting for multilevel frailty models. In this section we give a number of examples with increasing complexity and we demonstrate how easily the Bayesian MCMC approach adapts to the increased model complexity.

In this section, we use Gibbs sampling and we consider the frailties as parameters that need to be sampled. We start from the model discussed in Section 2.4; we assume a Weibull baseline hazard and one (one-parameter) gamma frailty term, but replace the Metropolis algorithm used in Section 2.4 by Gibbs sampling. The assumption of a gamma frailty density leads to rather simple expressions for the conditional posterior densities of some of the parameters.

The more common choice for frailty distributions in multilevel models, however, is the normal distribution for the random effects (or equivalently the lognormal distribution for the frailties). It leads typically to more complex expressions for the conditional posterior densities, but it has the advantage that more complex hierarchical structures can be easily described by the multivariate normal distribution. We first discuss the frailty model with one normal distributed random effect. Next, we extend this model to contain two hierarchical random effects. Finally, we demonstrate that the Bayesian approach can be used to fit models for interval-censored data; the proposed models are straightforward extensions of the models considered for right-censored data.

Fiting the parametric frailty model with one frailty term using Gibbs sampling

Consider the following frailty model:

$$h_{ij}(t) = h_0(t)u_i \exp\left(\mathbf{x}_{ij}^t \boldsymbol{\beta}\right) \tag{6.27}$$

and assume that the frailties are Gamma$(1/\theta, 1/\theta)$ distributed. For a Weibull baseline hazard, model (6.27) can be written as

$$h_{ij}(t) = \lambda u_i \rho t^{\rho-1} \exp\left(\mathbf{x}_{ij}^t \boldsymbol{\beta}\right) \tag{6.28}$$

To use Gibbs sampling based on the posterior conditional densities of the parameters of interest, we need to specify the conditional data likelihood and the prior densities of the parameters. Denote the prior densities by $f(\lambda)$, $f(\rho)$, $f(u_i)$, and $f(\beta_a)$, $a = 1, \ldots, p$. Additionally, a prior density $f(\theta_R)$ is put on $\theta_R = 1/\theta$, which is the precision of the frailties (the inverse of the variance). To ensure logconcavity of all conditional posterior densities, the following prior distributions are chosen:

$$f(\rho) = \text{Gamma}(a_1, a_2)$$

$$f(\lambda) = \text{Gamma}(b_1, b_2)$$

The conditional data likelihood, $f(\mathbf{y} \mid \lambda, \rho, \boldsymbol{\beta}, \mathbf{u})$, is given by

$$\prod_{i=1}^{s} \prod_{j=1}^{n_i} \left(\lambda u_i \exp(\mathbf{x}_{ij}^t \boldsymbol{\beta}) \rho y_{ij}^{\rho-1} \right)^{\delta_{ij}} \exp(-\lambda u_i \exp(\mathbf{x}_{ij}^t \boldsymbol{\beta}) y_{ij}^{\rho}) \quad (6.29)$$

For U_i and λ we obtain the following conditional posterior densities:

$$f(u_i \mid \mathbf{y}, \mathbf{d}, \boldsymbol{\beta}, \lambda, \rho, \theta_R) = \text{Gamma}\left(1/\theta + d_i, 1/\theta + \lambda \sum_{j=1}^{n_i} \exp(\mathbf{x}_{ij}^t \boldsymbol{\beta}) y_{ij}^{\rho} \right)$$
$$(6.30)$$

and

$$f(\lambda \mid \mathbf{y}, \mathbf{d}, \boldsymbol{\beta}, \rho, \mathbf{u}) = \text{Gamma}\left(b_1 + d, b_2 + \sum_{i=1}^{s} \sum_{j=1}^{n_i} u_i \exp(\mathbf{x}_{ij}^t \boldsymbol{\beta}) y_{ij}^{\rho} \right) \quad (6.31)$$

with $\mathbf{d}^t = (d_1, \ldots, d_s)$ and $d = \sum_{i=1}^{s} d_i$. For the other parameters, the following proportionality relationships hold for the conditional posterior densities:

$$f(\rho \mid \mathbf{y}, \mathbf{d}, \boldsymbol{\beta}, \lambda, \mathbf{u}) \propto \left(\prod_{i=1}^{s} \prod_{j=1}^{n_i} y_{ij}^{\delta_{ij}} \right)^{\rho-1} \rho^{d+a_1-1}$$

$$\times \exp\left(-\lambda \sum_{i=1}^{s} \sum_{j=1}^{n_i} u_i \exp(\mathbf{x}_{ij}^t \boldsymbol{\beta}) y_{ij}^{\rho} - \rho a_2 \right)$$

$$f(\beta_a \mid \mathbf{y}, \mathbf{d}, \rho, \lambda, \boldsymbol{\beta}_{(-a)}, \mathbf{u}) \propto \exp\left(\boldsymbol{\beta}^t \sum_{i=1}^{s} \sum_{j=1}^{n_i} \delta_{ij} \mathbf{x}_{ij} - \lambda \sum_{i=1}^{s} \sum_{j=1}^{n_i} u_i \exp(\mathbf{x}_{ij}^t \boldsymbol{\beta}) y_{ij}^{\rho} \right)$$

$$\times f(\beta_a)$$

and

$$f(\theta_R \mid \mathbf{y}, \mathbf{d}, \mathbf{u}) \propto \prod_{i=1}^{s} \left(\frac{u_i^{\theta_R-1} \exp(-\theta_R u_i)}{\theta_R^{-\theta_R} \Gamma(\theta_R)} \right) f(\theta_R)$$

All these conditional posterior distributions are logconcave, hence, adaptive rejection sampling can be used (see Section 4.1.1 in Ibrahim et al. (2001) for more details).

Within this Bayesian context, a common choice for the frailty is the lognormal distribution resulting in the following model:

$$h_{ij}(t) = h_0(t) \exp\left(\mathbf{x}_{ij}^t \boldsymbol{\beta} + w_i\right) \tag{6.32}$$

with the assumption that the random effects w_i are $N(0, \gamma)$ distributed. For a Weibull baseline hazard the model (6.32) can be written as

$$h_{ij}(t) = \lambda \rho t^{\rho-1} \exp\left(\mathbf{x}_{ij}^t \boldsymbol{\beta} + w_i\right)$$

$$= \rho t^{\rho-1} \exp\left(\alpha + \mathbf{x}_{ij}^t \boldsymbol{\beta} + w_i\right) \tag{6.33}$$

with $\alpha = \log \lambda$. A common choice (and the default used in WinBUGS) for the prior densities is as follows:

$$f(\beta_a) = N(0, \kappa), \quad a = 1, \ldots, p$$

$$f(\alpha) = N(0, \kappa)$$

$$f(\rho) = \text{Gamma}(a_1, a_2)$$

Finally, a uniform prior for the hyperparameter $\sqrt{\gamma}$, the standard deviation of the random effects, is assumed, i.e., $f(\sqrt{\gamma}) \propto 1$. With this choice for the prior distributions, Gibbs sampling can be performed, although the required resampling techniques are more complex than the ones used in the gamma frailty model (Gray, 1994; Matsuyama et al., 1998).

Example 6.4 The parametric frailty model with normal random cow effects for the udder quarter infection data

We fit a frailty model with Weibull baseline hazard to the udder quarter infection data (Example 1.4) using Gibbs sampling techniques available in WinBUGS (Spiegelhalter et al., 2003). We consider cow as a normal distributed random effect and heifer as a covariate in the model. We generate four independent chains using 2500 iterations as burn-in period and 2500 iterations as sample to construct the posterior density. The obtained $\hat{R}$ statistic given by (2.37) is very close to one, indicating convergence of the chains. The summary statistics of the posterior densities of the parameters of interest are given in

Table 6.1. The results obtained here are similar to the results obtained in Example 4.16 using Gaussian quadrature to integrate out the normal distributed random effects numerically. The medians for β and λ are the same as in Example 4.16, whereas the median for ρ corresponds to 2.53 and is slightly higher than 2.49, the estimate obtained from the Gaussian quadrature approach. Finally, the median for the variance is substantially higher than the estimate for γ obtained from Gaussian quadrature. ∎

Table 6.1. Summary statistics of the univariate posterior density functions based on the parametric survival model with Weibull baseline hazard and normal distributed random cow effects for the udder quarter infection data set.

Parameter	Mean	s.e.	Quantiles				
			2.5%	25%	50%	75%	97.5%
λ	0.33	0.10	0.16	0.26	0.32	0.38	0.55
ρ	2.53	0.13	2.26	2.44	2.53	2.62	2.79
β	0.46	0.40	-0.32	0.20	0.46	0.73	1.22
γ	3.31	0.70	2.14	2.81	3.24	3.72	4.85

Fitting the parametric frailty model with two nested normal distributed random effects using Gibbs sampling

We further extend the frailty model (6.32) and include as extra random effect the farm to which the cow belongs:

$$h_{ijk}(t) = \rho t^{\rho-1} \exp\left(\alpha + \mathbf{x}_{ijk}^t \boldsymbol{\beta} + f_i + w_{ij}\right) \tag{6.34}$$

with $h_{ijk}(t)$ the hazard function of udder quarter k from cow j belonging to farm i and f_i the $N(0, \gamma_f)$ distributed random effect of farm i. All the other parameter characteristics remain the same as in the previous section. We only have to add the prior density of the hyperparameter $\sqrt{\gamma_f}$, the standard deviation of the random farm effects, to the model assumptions. We assume a uniform prior, i.e., $f(\sqrt{\gamma_f}) \propto 1$.

The conditional data likelihood, $f(\mathbf{y} \mid \lambda, \rho, \boldsymbol{\beta}, \mathbf{w}, \mathbf{f})$, is given by

$$\prod_{i=1}^{s} \prod_{j=1}^{n_i} \prod_{k=1}^{n_{ij}} \left(\phi_{ijk} \rho y_{ijk}^{\rho-1}\right)^{\delta_{ijk}} \exp(-\phi_{ijk} y_{ijk}^{\rho}) \tag{6.35}$$

with $\phi_{ijk} = \exp\left(\alpha + \mathbf{x}_{ijk}^t \boldsymbol{\beta} + f_i + w_{ij}\right)$. Posterior densities can be obtained and Gibbs sampling can be used to obtain a sample from each of the conditional posterior densities, on which statistical inference can be based.

Example 6.5 The parametric frailty model with normal distributed random farm and cow effects for the udder quarter infection data

We again fit a frailty model with Weibull baseline hazard to the udder quarter infection data (Example 1.4) using Gibbs sampling techniques available in WinBUGS (Spiegelhalter et al., 2003). Note that we use the midpoint imputation here: we only know that the infection time lies in a certain interval, and we use the midpoint of that interval as the infection time. We introduce both farm and cow as normal distributed random effects and heifer as a covariate in the model. We generate four independent chains using 2500 iterations as burn-in period and 2500 iterations as sample to construct the posterior density. The $\hat{R}$ statistic given by (2.37) is very close to one.

The summary statistics of the posterior densities of the parameters of interest are given in Table 6.2. The conditional posterior densities of α, ρ, and β of model (6.32) and this model (6.34) are similar. The median of the variance of the random cow effect is 2.37 for model (6.34) versus 3.24 for model (6.32). The median of the variance of the random farm effects is 0.78 and is substantially smaller than that of the cow effects. ■

Table 6.2. Summary statistics of posterior density functions based on the parametric frailty model with Weibull baseline hazard and normal distributed random farm and cow effects for the udder quarter infection data set.

			Quantiles				
Parameter	Mean	s.e.	2.5%	25%	50%	75%	97.5%
λ	0.33	0.12	0.15	0.25	0.31	0.40	0.63
ρ	2.50	0.13	2.25	2.41	2.50	2.59	2.78
β	0.46	0.40	-0.32	0.20	0.46	0.73	1.22
γ	2.43	0.59	1.49	2.01	2.37	2.77	3.79
γ_f	0.90	0.63	0.05	0.48	0.78	1.19	2.46

Fitting the parametric frailty model for interval-censored data with two nested normal distributed random effects

It is straightforward to fit a version of model (6.34) for a data set with interval-censored and right-censored data. The only change we need to make is the specification of the conditional data likelihood. The likelihood now takes form

$$\prod_{i=1}^{s} \prod_{j=1}^{n_i} \prod_{k=1}^{n_{ij}} \left[\exp\left(-\phi_{ijk}\left(l_{ijk}\right)^{\rho}\right) - \exp\left(-\phi_{ijk}\left(r_{ijk}\right)^{\rho}\right) \right]^{\delta_{ijk}}$$

$$\left(\exp\left(-\phi_{ijk} r_{ijk}^{\rho}\right)\right)^{1-\delta_{ijk}} \tag{6.36}$$

with r_{ijk} the censoring time for right-censored subjects ($\delta_{ijk} = 0$) and l_{ijk} and r_{ijk} the start and the end of the interval in which the event takes place for interval-censored subjects ($\delta_{ijk} = 1$).

Example 6.6 The parametric frailty model with normal distributed random farm and cow effects for the interval-censored udder quarter data

We again fit a frailty model with Weibull baseline hazard to the interval-censored udder quarter infection data (Example 1.4) using Gibbs sampling techniques with both farm and cow as normal distributed random effects and heifer as a covariate in the model. Compared to Example 6.5 we now take the interval-censored nature of the data in consideration and use the likelihood expression (6.36). We generate four independent chains using 2500 iterations as burn-in period and 2500 iterations as sample to construct the posterior density. The $\hat{R}$ statistic given by (2.37) is very close to one. The summary statistics of the posterior densities of the parameters of interest are given in Table 6.3.

The main differences with the results presented in Table 6.2 are observed for the parameters λ and ρ and to a lesser extent for γ_f, with a smaller median value for ρ and a higher median value for λ for the model based on interval-censored data. This is due to the fact that for midpoint imputation the first event is only observed after a certain time; therefore the hazard function must start from a lower value (smaller λ) and increase faster (higher ρ) in the case of midpoint imputation. ∎

Table 6.3. Summary statistics of posterior density functions based on the parametric frailty model with Weibull baseline hazard and normal distributed random farm and cow effects for the interval-censored infection times of the udder quarter infection data set.

Parameter	Mean	s.e.	Quantiles				
			2.5%	25%	50%	75%	97.5%
λ	0.47	0.15	0.24	0.36	0.45	0.55	0.83
ρ	2.02	0.11	1.80	1.94	2.01	2.09	2.25
β	0.46	0.40	−0.32	0.2	0.46	0.73	1.22
γ	2.42	0.61	1.44	1.98	2.35	2.78	3.82
γ_f	0.74	0.59	0.01	0.32	0.63	1.02	2.16

6.3 Further extensions and references

To fit multilevel frailty models we can use maximum penalised likelihood techniques (Section 6.2.1) or Bayesian techniques (Section 6.2.2). Also EM algorithms have been proposed to fit multilevel frailty models (Sastry, 1997). Manda (2001) compares the EM algorithm with Gibbs sampling for the analysis of a nested frailty model with two levels of clustering. Manda (2000) further describes the use of Gibbs sampling for the semiparametric model with three levels of clustering. Yau (2001) also proposes methods for the analysis of multivariate survival data with three levels of clustering using Cox partial likelihood in the context of the generalised linear mixed model. Finally, for multifrailty data, Vaida and Xu (2000) use the EM algorithm in combination with Markov Chain Monte Carlo methods to obtain expected values of the frailties in the E-step of the EM algorithm.

7

Extensions of the frailty model

7.1 Censoring and truncation

In this section we discuss, for multivariate survival data, a number of censoring schemes that are more complex than right censoring. A variety of inferential techniques have been proposed to analyse such complex data sets. For some of the censoring schemes frailty models have been studied. Based on examples we explain how one arrives at different censoring schemes and we give references for further reading.

Consider the following dental caries data. For tooth j of subject i time at risk starts from the emergence time a_{ij} of the tooth. The tooth is followed up until time c_{ij}. We first consider the situation where for each tooth j of subject i, we have the exact emergence time a_{ij}. Whenever the caries event time t_{ij} (i.e., the time from emergence to the time of observed caries) is smaller than c_{ij}, the event time is observed. If t_{ij} is larger than c_{ij}, the event time is not observed and the observation for that particular tooth is right-censored.

When the subject is only examined on preset visit times rather than daily, the caries event time is not known exactly: the available information is that t_{ij} is in the interval $]l_{ij}, r_{ij}]$ with l_{ij} the last visit time without observed caries and r_{ij} the first visit time with observed caries, obviously for subjects having $r_{ij} \leq c_{ij}$. This type of censoring, interval censoring, is discussed in Sections 2.3 and 6.2.2. Interval censoring for multivariate survival data has been studied by different authors (Goggins and Finkelstein, 2000; Bogaerts et al., 2002; Kim and Xue, 2002; Bellamy et al., 2004; Glynn and Rosner, 2004). We have doubly interval censoring if the interval censoring occurs for both the emergence time a_{ij} and the event time t_{ij} (Komárek et al., 2005b).

Now assume that a particular tooth was not followed up from its emergence time, but rather from time o_{ij} ($o_{ij} > a_{ij}$). Caries might have been observed already for such a tooth at the first visit to the dentist, i.e., for tooth j of subject i caries already developed before the first visit to the dentist ($t_{ij} < o_{ij}$). This is a left-censored observation; we only know that the caries event happened before a particular time but not exactly when. Obviously this type of information should not be discarded. Applications of left-censored data in the context of frailty models have been considered by Vu (2004).

Survival data that contain both left- and right-censored observations are called doubly-censored data. For examples of doubly-censored multivariate survival data see Jones and Rocke (2002) and Kim (2006).

Apart from censoring also data truncation can occur in survival data. Left truncation occurs when the tooth was not followed up from its emergence time a_{ij}, but from a later time o_{ij}, at which time the tooth does not have caries yet and is therefore still at risk. Left truncation in the context of multivariate survival data has been studied by Salter and Solomon (1997), Williamson et al. (2002), Jiang et al. (2005a), and Petersen et al. (2006).

Throughout the book we assumed independence between the event time and the censoring time, as explained in Section 1.4. This assumption has been relaxed by several authors in the context of multivariate survival data. Informative and nonignorable drop-out is discussed in Matsuyama (2003), Jiang et al. (2005b), and Lee et al. (2005). Informative censoring is studied in Wang et al. (2001), Dunson and Dinse (2002), Huang and Wolfe (2002), and Huang et al. (2004). Kosorok et al. (2002) considered dependent censoring.

7.2 Correlated frailty models

The shared frailty model is a common model for clustered survival data. In the shared frailty model all subjects belonging to the same cluster share the same frailty term, i.e., the frailty terms of any two subjects j and j' in cluster i are identical: $U_{ij} = U_{ij'} = U_i$. Therefore $\rho_u = \text{Corr}(U_{ij}, U_{ij'}) = \text{Corr}(U_i, U_i) = 1$.

Yashin et al. (1993, 1995) introduced the correlated frailty model model to model bivariate survival data. In the (bivariate) correlated frailty model the frailties for the individuals or components within a pair are not identical, as they are in the shared frailty model, but they are still correlated. The correlated frailty model is given by

$$h_{ij}(t) = h_0(t)u_{ij}\exp\left(\mathbf{x}_{ij}^t\boldsymbol{\beta}\right)$$

with U_{i1} and U_{i2} correlated, but with (U_{i1}, U_{i2}), $i = 1, \ldots, s$, independent between clusters. Different distributional assumptions have been proposed for the U_{ij}'s. As an example, we will discuss the gamma distribution assumption which is studied by several authors (Pickles et al., 1994; Yashin and Iachine, 1995, 1997; Petersen, 1998; Wienke et al., 2001, 2002, 2003).

Using gamma distributions the dependence structure between the frailty terms can be constructed as follows. Let $Q_{il}, l = 0, 1, 2$ be three independent gamma distributed random variables, i.e., $Q_{il} \sim \text{Gamma}(k_l, \lambda)$ and α a positive real number.

The frailty terms are then given by

$$U_{i1} = Q_{i0} + Q_{i1}$$

$$U_{i2} = \alpha \left(Q_{i0} + Q_{i2} \right)$$

from which follows

$$U_{i1} \sim \text{Gamma}(k_0 + k_1, \lambda)$$

$$U_{i2} \sim \text{Gamma}(k_0 + k_2, \lambda/\alpha)$$

We further restrict U_{i1} and U_{i2} to have mean equal to one and denote their variances by σ_1^2 and σ_2^2 and their correlation by ρ_u. It follows that

$$\frac{k_0 + k_1}{\lambda} = 1 \text{ and } \alpha \frac{k_0 + k_2}{\lambda} = 1$$

and

$$\frac{k_0 + k_1}{\lambda^2} = \sigma_1^2 \text{ and } \alpha^2 \frac{k_0 + k_2}{\lambda^2} = \sigma_2^2$$

The covariance between U_{i1} and U_{i2} is given by

$$\text{Cov}\left(U_{i1}, U_{i2} \right) = \text{E}\left(U_{i1} U_{i2} \right) - \text{E}\left(U_{i1} \right) \text{E}\left(U_{i2} \right) \qquad (7.1)$$

In order to derive an expression for the first term on the right-hand side of (7.1) we require

$$\text{E}\left(Q_{i0}^2 \right) = \text{Var}\left(Q_{i0} \right) + \left(\text{E}\left(Q_{i0} \right) \right)^2$$

$$= \frac{k_0}{\lambda^2} + \left(\frac{k_0}{\lambda} \right)^2 = \frac{k_0^2 + k_0}{\lambda^2}$$

We then have for the first term on the right-hand side of (7.1)

$$\text{E}\left(U_{i1} U_{i2} \right) = \text{E}\left(\left(Q_{i0} + Q_{i1} \right) \alpha \left(Q_{i0} + Q_{i2} \right) \right)$$

$$= \alpha \text{E}\left(Q_{i0}^2 + Q_{i0} Q_{i1} + Q_{i0} Q_{i2} + Q_{i1} Q_{i2} \right)$$

$$= \frac{\alpha}{\lambda^2} \left(k_0^2 + k_0 + k_0 k_1 + k_0 k_2 + k_1 k_2 \right)$$

Therefore, the correlation between U_{i1} and U_{i2} is given by

$$\rho_u = \frac{\text{Cov}\,(U_{i1}, U_{i2})}{\sqrt{\text{Var}\,(U_{i1})\,\text{Var}\,(U_{i2})}}$$

$$= \frac{\alpha\lambda^{-2}\left(k_0^2 + k_0 + k_0 k_1 + k_0 k_2 + k_1 k_2\right) - 1}{\sigma_1 \sigma_2}$$

$$= \frac{\alpha k_0}{\lambda^2 \sigma_1 \sigma_2}$$

The parameters related to the Q_{il}'s are therefore given by

$$\lambda = \frac{1}{\sigma_1^2}, \quad k_0 = \frac{\rho_u}{\sigma_1 \sigma_2}, \quad k_1 = \frac{1}{\sigma_1^2} - \frac{\rho_u}{\sigma_1 \sigma_2}, \text{ and } k_2 = \frac{1}{\sigma_2^2} - \frac{\rho_u}{\sigma_1 \sigma_2}$$

and finally

$$\alpha = \left(\frac{\sigma_2}{\sigma_1}\right)^2$$

Using $k_1 \geq 0$ and $k_2 \geq 0$, we easily obtain that

$$0 \leq \rho_u \leq \min\left(\frac{\sigma_1}{\sigma_2}, \frac{\sigma_2}{\sigma_1}\right) \tag{7.2}$$

Similar techniques as for the shared frailty model can be applied to fit correlated frailty models. Other distributions have been used for the frailty terms of the correlated frailty model, such as the power variance function (Yashin and Iachine, 1999) and the lognormal distribution (Xue and Brookmeyer, 1996; Yau, 2001). Aalen and Hjort (2002) introduced general correlated frailty models using frailties generated by nonnegative Lévy processes.

7.3 Joint modelling

The main focus in the book is on the analysis of clustered event times considering only one event type, e.g., death, infection, or insemination. In this section we consider clustered event times where the observable events within a cluster are not of the same type. We furthermore discuss the joint modelling of longitudinally obtained measurements (not time to event) together with an event time. We briefly mention some settings that have been studied and give some references for further reading.

A first setting is competing risks. In the competing risk setting each subject is at risk for a number of events, e.g., death due to different causes. A subject is either right-censored or experiences one of the events. Upon experiencing an event, the subject is no longer at risk for the other events. Incorporating dependence between the event times of the different event types leads to unidentifiability (Peterson, 1976; Prentice et al., 1978; Crowder, 2000). It is therefore required to assume independence between the event times. Naskar et al. (2005) introduce a frailty term for subjects within a cluster, but conditional on the frailty term the competing risk event times are assumed to be independent.

With some restrictions on the competing risk model, dependence between the event times of the different event types can, however, be modelled. One such restriction, considered by Faraggi and Korn (1996), is to assume that the treatment affects only one event type and not the others. Another restriction corresponds to the case of semicompeting risks (Fine et al., 2001). In semicompeting risks, one event type can still be observed after having observed the other event type, but not the other way around. A typical case arises in clinical cancer trials, where the death event can still be observed after the patient has experienced the cancer progression event, but not the other way around.

A second setting of joint modelling occurs for multivariate survival data consisting of both recurrent events and a terminal event; the terminal event precludes any further occurrence of the recurrent event. This setting has been studied in the context of the frailty model by Liu et al. (2004), whereas Mahé and Chevret (1999b) and Chen and Cook (2004) model this setting in terms of marginal proportional hazards models.

In a third setting both longitudinal covariate information and an event time are available. In such cases, the hazard function is important but also the longitudinal covariate information process is of interest. Including the longitudinal data as time-varying covariates has some major drawbacks. First, the information should be available in a continuous way, which is not often the case. Furthermore, the uncertainty in the measurements of the longitudinal data is not taken into account.

A two-stage modelling approach was proposed by Tsiatis et al. (1995): first a model is constructed for the evolution of the longitudinal data. Next the estimates from that model are used as covariate information in the survival model. Some drawbacks of this approach are discussed by Wulfsohn and Tsiatis (1997). A better approach is to model the longitudinal data and the event time information jointly (Henderson et al., 2000). Using a latent zero-mean bivariate Gaussian process one jointly models the repeated measurements of the time-dependent covariates and the hazard process. The details are as follows. Let $W_i(t) = (W_{i1}(t), W_{i2}(t))$ denote the bivariate Gaussian process and let subject i have longitudinal measurements at time $t_{i1}, t_{i2}, \ldots$ given by $Z_{i1}, Z_{i2}, \ldots$.

The model for the longitudinal covariates is then given by

$$Z_{ij} = \mathbf{x}_{i1}^t(t_{ij})\boldsymbol{\beta}_1 + W_{i1}(t_{ij}) + e_{ij} \tag{7.3}$$

with $\mathbf{x}_{i1}^t(t_{ij})$ and $\boldsymbol{\beta}_1$ the, possibly time-varying, covariates with corresponding regression coefficients and $e_{ij} \sim \mathrm{N}(0, \sigma^2)$ the random error term. The hazard function is

$$\lambda_i(t) = \lambda_0(t) \exp\left(\mathbf{x}_{i2}^t(t)\boldsymbol{\beta}_2 + W_{i2}(t)\right) \tag{7.4}$$

It is further assumed that conditional on the covariate information and $W_i(t)$ the longitudinal covariates and event time data are independent. The zero-mean bivariate Gaussian process $W_i(t) = (W_{i1}(t), W_{i2}(t))$ is general and needs to be specified in more detail. An often-used model is based on the assumption of a linear random effects model with random intercept and random slope, $W_{i1}(t) = U_{i1} + U_{i2}t$, where (U_{i1}, U_{i2}) are zero-mean bivariate Gaussian variables with variances σ_1^2 and σ_2^2 and correlation ρ. Furthermore, we have the proportionality assumption $W_{i2}(t) = \gamma W_{i1}(t)$.

A more complex model described by Henderson et al. (2000) has the same model specification for $W_{i1}(t)$ but for $W_{i2}(t)$ we have

$$W_{i2}(t) = \gamma_1 U_{i1} + \gamma_2 U_{i2} + \gamma_3 (U_{i1} + U_{i2}t) + U_{i3} \tag{7.5}$$

where $U_{i3} \sim \mathrm{N}(0, \sigma_3^2)$ and independent of (U_{i1}, U_{i2}). The model parameters γ_1, γ_2, and γ_3 describe the association induced through the random intercept, the random slope, and the random effects model $W_{i1}(t)$.

More flexible distributional assumptions have been proposed by Brown and Ibrahim (2003) based on Dirichlet process priors in a Bayesian context.

7.4 The accelerated failure time model

The vast majority of techniques developed for frailty models is based on the proportional hazards model. An alternative model is the accelerated failure time model. The basics of the accelerated failure time model for independent survival data are given in Section 1.4.3.

Furthermore we demonstrated in Example 2.2 how the proportional hazards frailty model can be rewritten in terms of an accelerated failure time model. The parameter estimates obtained for the parametric proportional hazards frailty model can be easily translated into parameter estimates in terms of the accelerated failure time model. More elaborate extensions of the accelerated failure time model for multivariate survival data are available. The accelerated failure time model with random effect can be obtained by extending model (1.15)

$$\log T_{ij} = \mu + \mathbf{x}_{ij}^t \boldsymbol{\alpha} + w_i + \sigma E_{ij}$$

with T_{ij} the event time for subject j from cluster i, μ the intercept, $\mathbf{x}_{ij}$ the vector of covariates for subject j from cluster i, $\boldsymbol{\alpha}$ the vector containing the covariate effects, w_i the random effect for cluster i, σ the scale parameter, and finally E_{ij} the random error term for subject j from cluster i. The random error term is assumed to have a fully specified distribution. Different assumptions have been proposed leading to event time distributions other than the Weibull (e.g., gamma, inverse Gaussian, lognormal, and loglogistic). Lambert et al. (2004) propose to integrate out the random effects through numerical integration routines. Pan (2001) bases the parameter estimation on the EM algorithm whereas Chang (2004) proposes rank-based techniques to estimate the marginal fixed effects in the accelerated failure time model. Komárek et al. (2005a) and Komárek and Lesaffre (2006) discuss the analysis of multivariate survival data based on the accelerated failure time model in a Bayesian context, modelling the error term by a classical normal mixture or penalised normal mixture, and the random effects by a multivariate normal distribution. Accelerated failure time models with random effect can also be fitted through the hierarchical likelihood approach suggested by Lee and Nelder (1996) and making use of the pseudo-response variable of Buckley and James (1979) to take into account the censoring (Ha et al., 2002).

References

Aalen, O.O. (1988). Heterogeneity in survival analysis. *Stat. Med.* **7**, 1121-1137.

Aalen, O.O. (1992). Modelling heterogeneity in survival analysis by the compound Poisson distribution. *Ann. Appl. Probab.* **2**, 951-972.

Aalen, O.O. (1994). Effects of frailty in survival analysis. *Stat. Methods Med. Res.* **3**, 227-243.

Aalen, O.O. and Hjort, N.L. (2002). Frailty models that yield proportional hazards. *Stat. Probab. Lett.* **58**, 335-342.

Adkinson, R.W., Ingawa, K.H., Blouin, D.C. and Nickerson, S.C. (1993). Distribution of clinical mastitis among quarters of the bovine udder. *J. Dairy Sci.* **76**, 3453-3459.

Allard, P., Bernard, P., Fradet, Y. and Tetu, B. (1998). The early clinical course of primary Ta and T1 bladder cancer: a proposed prognostic index. *Brit. J. Urol.* **81**, 692-698.

Andersen, E.W. (2005). Two-stage estimation in copula models used in family studies. *Lifetime Data Anal.* **11**, 333-350.

Andersen, P.K., Borgan, O., Gill, R.D. and Keiding, N. (1993). *Statistical models based on counting processes.* Springer Verlag, New York.

Andersen, P.K., Klein, J.P. and Zhang, M. (1999). Testing for centres effects in multicentre survival studies: a Monte Carlo comparison of fixed and random effects. *Stat. Med.* **18**, 1489-1500.

Andersen, P.K., Ekstrom, C.T., Klein, J.P., Shu, Y.Y. and Zhang, M.J. (2005). A class of goodness of fit tests for copula based on bivariate right-censored data. *Biom. J.* **47**, 815-824.

Anderson, J.E., Louis, T.A., Holm, N.V. and Harvald, B. (1992). Time-dependent association measures for bivariate survival distributions. *J. Am. Stat. Assoc.* **87**, 641-650.

Asefa, M., Drewett, R. and Hewison, J. (1996). An Ethiopian birth cohort study: the study design. *Paediatr. Perinat. Epidemiol.* **10**, 443-462.

Asefa, M., Drewett, R. and Tessema, F. (2000). A birth cohort study in South-West Ethiopia to identify factors associated with infant mortality that are amenable for intervention. *Ethiop. J. Health Dev.* **14**, 161-168.

Balakrishnan, N. and Peng, Y.W. (2006). Generalized gamma frailty model. *Stat. Med.* **25**, 2797-2816.

Barlow, R. and Proschan, F. (1975). *Statistical theory of reliability and lifetesting.* Holt, Rinehart & Winston, New York.

Barnard, G.A. (1963). Some logical aspects of the fiducial argument. *J. R. Stat. Soc. Ser. B-Stat. Methodol.* **25**, 111-114.

Beard, R.E. (1959). Note on some mathematical mortality models. In: *The lifespan of animals. Ciba colloquium on Aging,* G.E.W. Wolstenholme and M. O'Connor (eds). Little, Brown, Boston, 302-311.

Bellamy, S.L., Li, Y., Ryan, L.M., Lipsitz, S., Canner, M.J. and Wright, R. (2004). Analysis of clustered and interval-censored data from a community-based study in asthma. *Stat. Med.* **23**, 3607-3621.

Bjarnason, H. and Hougaard, P. (2000). Fisher information for two gamma frailty bivariate Weibull models. *Lifetime Data Anal.* **6**, 59-71.

Bogaerts, K., Leroy, R., Lesaffre, E. and Declerck, D. (2002). Modelling tooth emergence data based on multivariate interval-censored data. *Stat. Med.* **21**, 3775-3787.

Brown, E.R. and Ibrahim, J.G. (2003). A Bayesian semiparametric joint hierarchical model for longitudinal and survival data. *Biometrics* **59**, 221-228.

Buckley, J. and James, I. (1979). Linear regression with censored data. *Biometrika* **66**, 429-436.

Carlin, B.P. and Louis, T.A. (1996). *Bayes and empirical Bayes methods for data analysis.* Chapman and Hall, London.

Chang, S. (2004). Estimating marginal effects in accelerated failure time models for serial sojourn times among repeated events. *Lifetime Data Anal.* **10**, 175-190.

Chen, B.E. and Cook, R.J. (2004). Tests for multivariate recurrent events in the presence of a terminal event. *Biostatistics* **5**, 129-143.

Chen, M.C. and Bandeen-Roche, K. (2005). A diagnostic for association in bivariate survival models. *Lifetime Data Anal.* **11**, 245-264.

Chen, M.H., Ibrahim, J.G. and Sinha, D. (2002). Bayesian inference for multivariate survival data with a cure fraction. *J. Multivar. Anal.* **80**, 101-126.

Claeskens, G., Nguti, R. and Janssen, P. (2007). One-sided tests in shared frailty models. *Test* (to appear).

Clayton, D.G. (1978). A model for association in bivariate life tables and its application in epidemiological studies of family tendency in chronic disease incidence. *Biometrika* **65**, 141-151.

Clayton, D.G. (1991). A Monte Carlo method for Bayesian inference in frailty models. *Biometrics* **47**, 467-485.

Collett, D. (2003). *Modelling survival data in medical research.* Second edition. Chapman and Hall, London.

Cox, D.R. (1972). Regression models and life tables (with discussion). *J. R. Stat. Soc. Ser. B-Stat. Methodol.* **34**, 187-220.

Crowder, M. (2000). Characterizations of competing risks in terms of independent-risks proxy models. *Scand. J. Stat.* **27**, 57-64.

Cui, S.F. and Sun, Y.Q. (2004). Checking for the gamma frailty distribution under the marginal proportional hazards frailty model. *Stat. Sin.* **14**, 249-267.

Dabrowska, D.M. (1988). Kaplan-Meier estimate on the plane. *Ann. Stat.* **16**, 1475-1489.

Dempster, A.P., Laird, N.M. and Rubin, D.B. (1977). Maximum likelihood from incomplete data via the EM algorithm (with discussion). *J. R. Stat. Soc. Ser. B-Stat. Methodol.* **39**, 1-38.

De Vliegher, S., Barkema, H.W., Opsomer, G., de Kruif, A. and Duchateau, L. (2005). Association between somatic cell count in early lactation and culling of dairy heifers using Cox frailty models. *J. Dairy Sci.* **88**, 560-568.

Doksum, K.A. (1974). Tailfree and neutral random probabilities and their posterior distributions. *Ann. Probab.* **2**, 209-230.

Duchateau, L. and Janssen, P. (2004). Penalized partial likelihood for frailties and smoothing splines in time to first insemination models for dairy cows. *Biometrics* **60**, 608-614.

Duchateau, L. and Janssen, P. (2005). Understanding heterogeneity in generalized mixed and frailty models. *Am. Stat.* **59**, 143-146.

Duchateau, L., Janssen, P., Kezic, I. and Fortpied, C. (2003). Evolution of recurrent asthma event rate over time in frailty models. *J. R. Stat. Soc. Ser. C-Appl. Stat.* **52**, 355-363.

Duchateau, L., Opsomer, G., Dewulf, J. and Janssen, P. (2005). The nonlinear effect (determined by the penalised partial-likelihood approach) of milk-protein concentration on time to first insemination in Belgian dairy cows. *Prev. Vet. Med.* **68**, 81-90.

Ducrocq, V. and Casella, G. (1996). A Bayesian analysis of mixed survival models. *Genet. Sel. Evol.* **28**, 505-529.

Ducrocq, V. and Sölkner, J. (1994). "The survival kit", a Fortran package for the analysis of survival data. In: *5th World Congress on Genetics Applied to Livestock Production, Vol. 22, pp. 51-52*, University of Guelph, Guelph, Ontario, Canada.

Dunson, D.B. and Dinse, G.E. (2002). Bayesian models for multivariate current status data with informative censoring. *Biometrics* **58**, 79-88.

Durrleman, V., Nikeghbali, A. and Roncalli, T. (2000). Which copula is the right one? *Technical Report.* Groupe de Recherche Opérationnelle, Crédit Lyonnais, France.

Economou, P. and Caroni, C. (2005). Graphical tests for the assumption of gamma and inverse Gaussian frailty distributions. *Lifetime Data Anal.* **11**, 565-582.

Fandamu, P., Duchateau, L., Speybroeck, N., Marcotty, T., Mbao, V., Mtambo, J., Mulumba, M. and Berkvens, D. (2005a). Theileria parva seroprevalence in traditionally kept cattle in southern Zambia and El Niño. *Int. J. Parasitol.* **35**, 391-396.

Fandamu, P., Duchateau, L., Speybroeck, N., Mulumba, M. and Berkvens, D. (2005b). East Coast Fever and multiple El Niño Southern oscillation ranks. *Vet. Parasitol.* **135**, 147-152.

Faraggi, D. and Korn, E.L. (1996). Competing risks with frailty models when treatment affects only one failure type. *Biometrika* **83**, 467-471.

Feller, W. (1971). *An introduction to probability theory and its applications, Volume 2.* Wiley, New York.

Fine, J.P., Jiang, H. and Chappell, R. (2001). On semi-competing risks data. *Biometrika* **88**, 907-919.

Fine, J.P., Glidden, D.V. and Lee, K.E. (2003). A simple estimator for a shared frailty regression model. *J. R. Stat. Soc. Ser. B-Stat. Methodol.* **65**, 317-329.

Fleming, T.R. and Harrington, D.P. (1991). *Counting processes and survival analysis.* Wiley, New York.

Fong, D.Y.T., Lam, K.F., Lawless, J.F. and Lee, J.W. (2001). Dynamic random effects models for times between repeated events. *Lifetime Data Anal.* **7**, 345-362.

Freedman, L.S. (1982). Tables of the number of patients required in clinical trials using the logrank test. *Stat. Med.* **1**, 121-129.

Frees, E.W., Carriere, J. and Valdez, E. (1996). Annuity valuation with dependent mortality. *J. Risk Insur.* **63**, 229-261.

Gamerman, D. (1997). *Markov Chain Monte Carlo.* Chapman and Hall, London.

Gelman, A. (2003). Prior distributions for variance parameters in hierarchical models. *Bayesian Anal.* **1**, 515-533.

Gelman, A. and Rubin, D.B. (1992). Inference from iterative simulation using multiple sequences (with discussion). *Stat. Sci.* **7**, 457-511.

Gelman, A., Roberts, G. and Gilks, W. (1995). Efficient metropolis jumping rules. In *Bayesian statistics*, J.M. Bernardo, J.O. Berger, A.P. Dawid and A.F.M. Smith (eds). Oxford University Press, New York.

Gelman, A., Carlin, J.B., Stern, H.S. and Rubin, D.B. (2004). *Bayesian data analysis.* Second edition. Chapman and Hall, London.

Genest, C. and MacKay, J. (1986). The joy of copulas: bivariate distributions with uniform marginals. *Am. Stat.* **40**, 280-283.

Gilks, W.R. and Wild, P. (1992). Adaptive rejection sampling for Gibbs sampling. *J. R. Stat. Soc. Ser. C-Appl. Stat.* **41**, 337-348.

Gill, R.D. (1984). Understanding Cox's regression model: a martingale approach. *J. Am. Stat. Assoc.* **79**, 441-447.

Gill, J. (2002). *Bayesian methods. A social and behavioral sciences approach.* Chapman and Hall, London.

Gillick, M. (2001). Pinning down frailty. *J. Gerontol. Ser. A-Biol. Sci. Med. Sci.* **56**, M134-M135.

Gjessing, H.K., Aalen, O.O. and Hjort, N.L. (2003). Frailty models based on Levy processes. *Adv. Appl. Probab.* **35**, 532-550.

Glidden, D.V. (1999). Checking the adequacy of the gamma frailty model for multivariate failure times. *Biometrika* **86**, 381-393.

Glidden, D.V. (2000). A two-stage estimator of the dependence parameter for the Clayton-Oakes model. *Lifetime Data Anal.* **6**, 141-156.

Glidden, D.V. and Vittinghoff, E. (2004). Modelling clustered survival data from multicentre clinical trials. *Stat. Med.* **23**, 369-388.

Glynn, R.J. and Rosner, B. (2004). Multiple imputation to estimate the association between eyes in disease progression with interval-censored data. *Stat. Med.* **23**, 3307-3318.

Goethals, K., Ampe, B., Berkvens, D., Laevens, H., Janssen, P. and Duchateau, L. (2007). Modelling interval-censored, clustered cow udder quarter infection times through the shared gamma frailty model. *Technical report*.

Goggins, W.B. and Finkelstein, D.M. (2000). A proportional hazards model for multivariate interval-censored failure time data. *Biometrics* **56**, 940-943.

Gray, R.J. (1992). Flexible methods for analyzing survival data using splines, with applications to breast cancer prognosis. *J. Am. Stat. Assoc.* **87**, 942-951.

Gray, R.J. (1994). A bayesian analysis of institutional effects in a multicenter cancer clinical trial. *Biometrics* **50**, 244-253.

Gupta, R.C. and Kirmani, S.N.U.A. (2006). Stochastic comparisons in frailty models. *J. Stat. Plan. Infer.* **10**, 3647-3658.

Ha, I.D., Lee, Y. and Song, J. (2002). Hierarchical-likelihood approach for mixed linear models with censored data. *Lifetime Data Anal.* **8**, 163-176.

Harkanen, T., Hausen, H., Virtanen, J.I. and Arjas, E. (2003). A non-parametric frailty model for temporally clustered multivariate failure times. *Scand. J. Stat.* **30**, 523-533.

He, W.Q. and Lawless, J.F. (2003). Flexible maximum likelihood methods for bivariate proportional hazards models. *Biometrics* **59**, 837-848.

Henderson, C.R. (1975). Best linear unbiased estimation and prediction under a selection model. *Biometrics* **31**, 423-447.

Henderson, R., Diggle, P. and Dobson, A. (2000). Joint modelling of longitudinal measurements and event time data. *Biostatistics* **1**, 465-480.

Hjort, N.L. (1990). Nonparametric Bayes estimators based on Beta processses in models of life history data. *Ann. Stat.* **18**, 1259-1294.

Hougaard, P. (1986a). A class of multivariate failure time distributions. *Biometrika* **73**, 671-678.

Hougaard, P. (1986b). Survival models for heterogeneous populations derived from stable distributions. *Biometrika* **73**, 387-396.

Hougaard, P. (2000). *Analysis of multivariate survival data*. Springer Verlag, New York.

Huang, X.L. and Wolfe, R.A. (2002). A frailty model for informative censoring. *Biometrics* **58**, 510-520.

Huang, X.L., Wolfe, R.A. and Hu, C.C. (2004). A test for informative censoring in clustered survival data. *Stat. Med.* **23**, 2089-2107.

Huang, Y.J. and Chen, Y.Q. (2003). Marginal regression of gaps between recurrent events. *Lifetime Data Anal.* **9**, 293-303.

Huster, W.J., Brookmeyer, R. and Self, S.G. (1989). Modelling paired survival data with covariates. *Biometrics* **45**, 145-156.

Ibrahim, J.G., Chen, M. and Sinha, D. (2001). *Bayesian survival analysis.* Springer Verlag, New York.

Jeffreys, H. (1961). *Theory of probability.* Third edition. Oxford University Press, New York.

Jeong, J.H. and Jung, S.H. (2006). Rank tests for clustered survival data when dependent subunits are randomized. *Stat. Med.* **25**, 361-373.

Jeong, J.H., Jung, S.H. and Wieand, S. (2003). A parametric model for long-term follow-up data from phase III breast cancer clinical trials. *Stat. Med.* **22**, 339-352.

Jiang, H.Y., Fine, J.P. and Chappell, R. (2005a). Semiparametric analysis of survival data with left truncation and dependent right censoring. *Biometrics* **61**, 567-575.

Jiang, H.Y., Fine, J.P., Kosorok, M.R. and Chappell, R. (2005b). Pseudo self-consistent estimation of a copula model with informative censoring. *Scand. J. Stat.* **32**, 1-20.

Johnson, N.L., Kotz, S. and Balakrishnan, N. (1994). *Continuous univariate distributions, Volume 2.* Second edition. John Wiley & Sons, New York.

Joly, P., Commenges, D. and Letenneur, L. (1998). A penalized likelihood approach for arbitrarily censored and truncated data: application to age-specific incidence of dementia. *Biometrics* **54**, 185-194.

Jones, G. and Rocke, D.M. (2002). Multivariate survival analysis with doubly-censored data: application to the assessment of Accutane treatment for fibrodysplasia ossificans progressiva. *Stat. Med.* **21**, 2547-2562.

Julien, J.P., Bijker, N., Fentiman, I.S., Peterse, J.L., Delledonne, V., Rouanet, P., Avril, A., Sylvester, R., Mignolet, F., Bartelink, H. and Van Dongen, J.A. (2000). Radiotherapy in breast-conserving treatment for ductal carcinoma in situ: first results of the EORTC randomised phase III trial 10853. *Lancet* **355**, 528-533.

Kalbfleisch, J.D. (1978). Nonparametric Bayesian analysis of survival time data. *J. R. Stat. Soc. Ser. B-Stat. Methodol.* **40**, 214-221.

Kendall, M.G. (1938). A new measure of rank correlation. *Biometrika* **30**, 81-93.

Kim, M.Y. and Xue, X.N. (2002). The analysis of multivariate interval-censored survival data. *Stat. Med.* **21**, 3715-3726.

Kim, Y.J. (2006). Regression analysis of doubly-censored failure time data with frailty. *Biometrics* **62**, 458-464.

Klein, J.P. (1992). Semiparametric estimation of random effects using the Cox model based on the EM algorithm. *Biometrics* **48**, 795-806.

Klein, J.P. and Moeschberger, M.L. (1997). *Survival analysis. Techniques for censored and truncated data.* Springer Verlag, New York.

Komárek, A. and Lesaffre, E. (2006). Bayesian semi-parametric accelerated failure time model for paired doubly interval-censored data. *Stat. Model.* **6**, 3-22.

Komárek, A., Lesaffre, E. and Hilton, J.F. (2005a). Accelerated failure time model for arbitrarily censored data with smoothed error distribution. *J. Comput. Graph. Stat.* **14**, 726-745.

Komárek, A., Lesaffre, E., Harkanen, T., Declerck, D. and Virtanen, J.I. (2005b). A Bayesian analysis of multivariate doubly-interval-censored dental data. *Biostatistics* **6**, 145-155.

Kosorok, M.R. and Gangnon, R.E. (2006). Resolving the tail instability in weighted log-rank statistics for clustered survival data. *Stat. Probab. Lett.* **76**, 304-309.

Kosorok, M.R., Fine, J.P., Jiang, H.Y. and Chappell, R. (2002). Asymptotic theory for the gamma frailty model with dependent censoring. *Ann. Inst. Stat. Math.* **54**, 476-499.

Lambert, P., Collett, D., Kimber, A. and Johnson, R. (2004). Parametric accelerated failure time models with random effects and an application to kidney transplant survival. *Stat. Med.* **23**, 3177-3192.

Lee, Y. and Nelder, J.A. (1996). Hierarchical generalised linear models (with discussion). *J. R. Stat. Soc. Ser. B-Stat. Methodol.* **58**, 619-678.

Lee, Y.J., Noh, M. and Ryu, K.K. (2005). HGLM modelling of dropout process using a frailty model. *Comput. Stat.* **20**, 295-309.

Legrand, C., Sylvester, R., Duchateau, L., Janssen, P. and Therasse, P. (2002). Treatment outcome studies; pitfalls in current methods and practice. *Eur. J. Cancer* **38**, 1173-1180.

Legrand, C., Ducrocq, V., Janssen, P., Sylvester, R. and Duchateau, L. (2005). A Bayesian approach to jointly estimate center and treatment by center interaction heterogeneity in a proportional hazards model. *Stat. Med.* **24**, 3789-3804.

Legrand, C., Duchateau, L., Janssen, P., Ducrocq, V. and Sylvester, R. (2007). Validation of prognostic indices using the frailty model. *Technical report.*

Li, Q.H. and Lagakos, S.W. (2004). Comparisons of test statistics arising from marginal analysis of multivariate survival data. *Lifetime Data Anal.* **10**, 389-405.

Li, Y., Betensky, R.A., Louis, D.N. and Cairncross, J.G. (2002). The use of frailty hazard models for unrecognized heterogeneity that interacts with treatment: considerations of efficiency and power. *Biometrics* **58**, 232-236.

Liang, K.Y., Self, S.G. and Chang, Y.C. (1993). Modeling marginal hazards in multivariate failure time data. *J. R. Stat. Soc. Ser. B-Stat. Methodol.* **55**, 441-453.

Liang, K.Y., Self, S.G., Bandeen-Roche, K. and Zeger, S. (1995). Some recent developments for regression analysis of multivariate failure time data. *Lifetime Data Anal.* **1**, 403-415.

Lin, D.Y. (1994). Cox regression-analysis of multivariate failure time data —
the marginal approach. *Stat. Med.* **13**, 2233-2247.

Lipsitz, S.R. and Parzen, M. (1996). A jackknife estimator of variance for Cox
regression for correlated survival data. *Biometrics* **52**, 291-298.

Lipsitz, S.R., Dear, K.B.G. and Zhao, L. (1994). Jackknife estimators of variance for parameter estimates from estimating equations with applications
to clustered survival data. *Biometrics* **50**, 842-846.

Liu, D.C. and Nocedal, J. (1989). On the limited memory BFGS method for
large scale optimization. *Math. Program.* **45**, 503-528.

Liu, L., Wolfe, R.A. and Huang, X.L. (2004). Shared frailty models for recurrent events and a terminal event. *Biometrics* **60**, 747-756.

Longini, I.M. and Halloran, M.E. (1996). A frailty mixture model for estimating vaccine efficacy. *J. R. Stat. Soc. Ser. B-Appl. Stat.* **45**, 165-173.

Lundin-Olsson, L., Nyberg, L. and Gustafson, Y. (1998). Attention, frailty
and falls: the effect of a manual task on basic mobility. *J. Am. Geriatr.
Soc.* **46**, 758-761.

Machin, D., Cheung, Y.B. and Parmar, M.K.B. (2006). *Survival analysis.
A practical approach.* Second edition. John Wiley & Sons, West Sussex,
England.

Mahé, C. and Chevret, S. (1999a). Estimating regression parameters and degree of dependence for multivariate failure time data. *Biometrics* **55**, 1078-
1084.

Mahé, C. and Chevret, S. (1999b). Estimation of the treatment effect in a
clinical trial when recurrent events define the endpoint. *Stat. Med.* **18**, 1821-
1829.

Makeham, W.M. (1867). On the law of mortality. *J. Inst. Act.* **13**, 325.

Maller, R.A. and Zhou, X. (2003). Testing for individual heterogeneity in
parameteric models for event-history data. *Math. Methods Stat.* **12**, 276-
304.

Manatunga, A.K. and Oakes, D. (1999). Parametric analysis for matched pair
survival data. *Lifetime Data Anal.* **5**, 371-387.

Manda, S.O.M. (2000). A Bayesian analysis of multivariate survival data from
multi-stage cluster sampling. *Commun. Stat.-Theory Methods* **29**, 769-782.

Manda, S.O.M. (2001). A comparison of methods for analysing a nested frailty
model to child survival in Malawi. *Aust. N. Z. J. Stat.* **43**, 7-16.

Manda, S.O.M. and Meyer, R. (2005). Bayesian inference for recurrent events
data using time-dependent frailty. *Stat. Med.* **24**, 1263-1274.

Marquardt, D. (1963). An algorithm for least-squares estimation of nonlinear
parameters. *SIAM J. Appl. Math.* **11**, 431-441.

Martinussen, T. and Pipper, C.B. (2005). Estimation in the positive stable
shared frailty Cox proportional hazards model. *Lifetime Data Anal.* **11**,
99-115.

Matsuyama, Y. (2003). Sensitivity analysis for the estimation of rates of
change with non-ignorable drop-out: an application to a randomized clinical
trial of the vitamin D-3. *Stat. Med.* **22**, 811-827.

Matsuyama, Y., Sakamoto, J. and Ohashi, Y. (1998). A Bayesian hierarchical survival model for the institutional effect in a multi-centre cancer clinical trial. *Stat. Med.* **17**, 1893-1908.

McGilchrist, C.A. (1993). REML estimation for survival models with frailty. *Biometrics* **49**, 221-225.

McGilchrist, C.A. and Aisbett, C.W. (1991). Regression with frailty in survival analysis. *Biometrics* **47**, 461-466.

McLachlan, G.J. and McGiffin, D.C. (1994). On the role of finite mixture models in survival analysis. *Stat. Methods Med. Res.* **3**, 211-226.

Moger, T.A. and Aalen, O.O. (2005). A distribution for multivariate frailty based on the compound Poisson distribution with random scale. *Lifetime Data Anal.* **11**, 41-59.

Moger, T.A., Aalen, O.O., Halvorsen, T.O., Storm, H.H. and Tretli, S. (2004). Frailty modelling of testicular cancer incidence using Scandinavian data. *Biostatistics* **5**, 1-14.

Morgan, B.J.T. (1992). *Analysis of quantal response data*. Chapman and Hall, London.

Morley, J.E., Perry, H. and Miller, D.K. (2002). Something about frailty. *J. Gerontol. Ser. A-Biol. Sci. Med. Sci.* **57**, M698-M704.

Murphy, S.A. (1995). Asymptotic theory for the frailty model. *Ann. Stat.* **23**, 182-198.

Naskar, M., Das, K. and Ibrahim, J.G. (2005). A semiparametric mixture model for analyzing clustered competing risks data. *Biometrics* **61**, 729-737.

Neal, R.M. (2003). Slice sampling (with discussion). *Ann. Stat.* **31**, 705-767.

Neijenhuis, F., Barkema, H.W., Hogeveen, H. and Noordhuizen, J.P.T.M. (2001). Relationship between teat-end callosity and occurrence of clinical mastitis. *J. Dairy Sci.* **84**, 2664-2672.

Nelsen, R.B. (1997). Dependence and order in families of Archimedean copulas. *J. Multivar. Anal.* **60**, 111-122.

Nelsen, R.B. (2006). *An introduction to copulas*. Second edition. Springer Verlag, New York.

Ng, S.K., McLachlan, G.J., Yau, K.K.W. and Lee, A.H. (2004). Modelling the distribution of ischaemic stroke-specific survival time using an EM-based mixture approach with random effects adjustment. *Stat. Med.* **23**, 2729-2744.

Nielsen, G.G., Gill, R.D., Andersen, P.K. and Sorensen, T.I.A.A. (1992). A counting process approach to maximum likelihood estimation in frailty models. *Scand. J. Stat.* **19**, 25-43.

Oakes, D. (1982). A model for association in bivariate survival data. *J. R. Stat. Soc. Ser. B-Stat. Methodol.* **44**, 414-422.

Oakes, D. (1989). Bivariate survival models induced by frailties. *J. Am. Stat. Assoc.* **84**, 487-493.

Pan, W. (2001). Using frailties in the accelerated failure time model. *Lifetime Data Anal.* **7**, 55-64.

Parner, E. (1998). Asymptotic theory for the correlated gamma-frailty model. *Ann. Stat.* **26**, 183-214.

Patterson, H.D. and Thompson, R. (1971). Recovery of interblock information when block sizes are unequal. *Biometrika* **58**, 545-554.

Perks, W. (1932). On some experiments in the graduation of mortality statistics. *J. Inst. Act.* **63**, 12.

Petersen, J.H. (1998). An additive frailty model for correlated lifetimes. *Biometrics* **54**, 646-661.

Petersen, L., Sorensen, T.I.A., Nielsen, G.G. and Andersen, P.K. (2006). Inference methods for correlated left truncated lifetimes: parent and offspring relations in an adoption study. *Lifetime Data Anal.* **12**, 5-20.

Peterson, A.V. (1976). Bounds for a joint distribution function with fixed subdistribution functions: Applications to competing risks. *Proc. Natl. Acad. Sci. U. S. A.* **73**, 11-13.

Phelps, A.L. and Weissfeld, L.A. (1997). A comparison of dependence estimators in bivariate copula models. *Commun. Stat.-Simul. Comput.* **26**, 1583-1597.

Pickles, A., Crouchley, R., Simonoff, E., Eaves, L., Meyer, J., Rutter, M., Hewitt, J. and Silberg, J. (1994). Survival models for developmental genetic data: age of onset of puberty and antisocial behavior in twins. *Genet. Epidemiol.* **11**, 155-170.

Pipper, C.B. and Martinussen, T. (2003). A likelihood based estimation equation for the Clayton-Oakes model with marginal proportional hazards. *Scand. J. Stat.* **30**, 509-521.

Podsiadlo, D. and Richardson, S. (1991). The timed up and go — a test of basic functional mobility for frail elderly persons. *J. Am. Geriatr. Soc.* **39**, 142-148.

Prentice, R.L., Kalbfleisch, J.D., Peterson, A.V., Flournoy, N., Farewell, V.T. and Breslow, N.E. (1978). The analysis of failure times in the presence of competing risks. *Biometrics* **34**, 541-554.

Price, D.L. and Manatunga, A.K. (2001). Modelling survival data with a cured fraction using frailty models. *Stat. Med.* **20**, 1515-1527.

Ripatti, S. and Palmgren, J. (2000). Estimation of multivariate frailty models using penalized partial likelihood. *Biometrics* **56**, 1016-1022.

Risselada, M., van Bree, H., Kramer, M., Chiers, K., Duchateau, L. and Verleyen, P. (2006). Evaluation of nonunion fractures in dogs by use of B-mode ultrasonography, power Doppler ultrasonography, radiography, and histologic examination. *Am. J. Vet. Res.* **67**, 1354-1361.

Rockwood, K. (2005). Frailty and its definition: a worthy challenge. *J. Am. Geriatr. Soc.* **53**, 1069-1070.

Rondeau, V., Commenges, D. and Joly, P. (2003). Maximum penalized likelihood estimation in frailty models. *Lifetime Data Anal.* **9**, 139-153.

Rondeau, V. and Gonzalez, J.R. (2005). Frailtypack: A computer program for the analysis of correlated failure time data using penalized likelihood estimation. *Comput. Meth. Programs Biomed.* **80**, 154-164.

Rondeau, V., Filleul, L. and Joly, P. (2006). Nested frailty models using maximum penalized likelihood estimation. *Stat. Med.* **25**, 4036-4052.

Roy, D. and Mukherjee, S.P. (1998). Multivariate extensions of univariate lifetime distributions. *J. Multivar. Anal.* **67**, 72-79.

Salter, A. and Solomon, P.J. (1997). Truncated recurrent event survival models for methadone data. *Biometrics* **53**, 1293-1303.

Sastry, N. (1997). A nested frailty model for survival data, with an application to the study of child survival in northeast Brazil. *J. Am. Stat. Assoc.* **92**, 426-435.

Schall, R. (1991). Estimation in generalised linear models with random effects. *Biometrika* **78**, 719-727.

Searle, S.R. (1982). *Matrix algebra useful for statistics.* John Wiley & Sons, New York.

Self, S.G. and Liang, K.L. (1987). Asymptotic properties of maximum likelihood estimators and likelihood ratio tests under nonstandard conditions. *J. Am. Stat. Assoc.* **82**, 605-610.

Shih, J.H. and Louis, T.A. (1995a). Inferences on the association parameter in copula models for bivariate survival data. *Biometrics* **51**, 1384-1399.

Shih, J.H. and Louis, T.A. (1995b). Assessing gamma frailty models for clustered failure time data. *Lifetime Data Anal.* **1**, 205-220.

Silverman, B.W. (1986). *Density estimation for statistics and data analysis.* Chapman and Hall, London.

Sinha, D., Ibrahim, J.G. and Chen, M.H. (2003). A Bayesian justification of Cox's partial likelihood. *Biometrika* **90**, 629-641.

Sklar, A. (1959). Fonctions de répartition á n dimensions et leurs marges. *Publ. Inst. Stat. Univ. Paris* **8**, 229-231.

Spiegelhalter, D., Thomas, A., Best, N. and Lunn, D. (2003). *WinBUGS User Manual.* Available from http://www.mrc-bsu.cam.ac.uk/bugs.

Spiekerman, C.F. and Lin, D.Y. (1998). Marginal regression models for multivariate failure time data. *J. Am. Stat. Assoc.* **93**, 1164-1175.

Stram, D.O. and Lee, J.W. (1994). Variance components testing in longitudinal mixed effects models. *Biometrics* **50**, 1171-1177.

Sylvester, R.J., van der Meijden, A.P.M., Oosterlinck, W., Witjes, A., Bouffioux, C., Denis, L., Newling, D.W.W. and Kurth, K. (2006). Predicting recurrence and progression in individual patients with stage TaT1 bladder cancer using EORTC risk tables: a combined analysis of 2596 patients. *Eur. Urol.* **49**, 466-477.

Therneau, T.M. and Grambsch, P.M. (2000). *Modeling survival data. Extending the Cox model.* Springer Verlag, New York.

Therneau, T.M., Grambsch, P.M. and Pankratz, V.S. (2003). Penalized survival models and frailty. *J. Comput. Graph. Stat.* **12**, 156-175.

Tierney, L. and Kadane, J.B. (1986). Accurate approximations for posterior moments and marginal densities. *J. Am. Stat. Assoc.* **81**, 82-86.

Tsiatis, A.A., Degruttola, V. and Wulfsohn, M.S. (1995). Modelling the relationship of survival to longitudinal data measured with error. Applications to survival and CD4 counts in patients with AIDS. *J. Am. Stat. Assoc.* **90**, 27-37.

Tweedy, M. (1984). An index which distinguishes between some important exponential families. Statistics: applications and new directions. In *Proceedings of the Indian Statistical Institute Golden Jubilee International Conference*, J. Ghosh and J. Roy (Eds), 579-604.

Vaida, F. and Xu, R. (2000). Proportional hazards model with random effects. *Stat. Med.* **19**, 3309-3324.

Vangroenweghe, F., Duchateau, L., Boutet, P., Rainard, P., Paape, M.J., Lekeux, P. and Burvenich, C. (2005). Effect of Carprofen treatment following experimentally induced Escherichia coli mastitis in primiparous cows. *J. Dairy Sci.* **88**, 2361-2376.

Vaupel, J.W. and Yashin, A.I. (1985). Heterogeneity's ruses: some surprising effects of selection on population dynamics. *Am. Stat.* **39**, 176-185.

Vaupel, J.W., Manton, K.G. and Stallard, E. (1979). The impact of heterogeneity in individual frailty on the dynamics of mortality. *Demography* **16**, 439-454.

Viswanathan, B. and Manatunga, A.K. (2001). Diagnostic plots for assessing the frailty distribution in multivariate survival data. *Lifetime Data Anal.* **7**, 143-155.

Vu, H.T.V. (2004). Estimation in semiparametric conditional shared frailty models with events before study entry. *Comput. Stat. Data Anal.* **45**, 621-637.

Wang, M.C., Qin, J. and Chiang, C.T. (2001). Analyzing recurrent event data with informative censoring. *J. Am. Stat. Assoc.* **96**, 1057-1065.

Weller, J.I., Saran, A. and Zeliger, Y. (1992). Genetic and environmental relationships among somatic cell count, bacterial infection, and clinical mastitis. *J. Dairy Sci.* **75**, 2532-2540.

White, H. (1982). Maximum likelihood estimation under mis-specified models. *Econometrica* **50**, 1-26.

Wienke, A., Holm, N.V., Skytthe, A. and Yashin, A.I. (2001). The heritability of mortality due to heart diseases: a correlated frailty model applied to Danish twins. *Twin Res.* **4**, 407-411.

Wienke, A., Christensen, K., Skytthe, A. and Yashin, A.I. (2002). Genetic analysis of cause of death in a mixture model with bivariate lifetime data. *Stat. Model.* **2**, 89-102.

Wienke, A., Holm, N.V., Christensen, K., Skytthe, A., Vaupel, J.W. and Yashin, A.I. (2003). The heritability of cause-specific mortality: a correlated gamma-frailty model applied to mortality due to respiratory diseases in Danish twins born 1870–1930. *Stat. Med.* **22**, 3873-3887.

Wild, C.J. (1983). Failure time models with matched data. *Biometrika* **70**, 633-641.

Williamson, J.M., Lin, H.M. and Bush, T.J. (2002). A simple two-sample rank test for multivariate survival outcomes with left truncation and right censoring. *Biom. J.* **44**, 213-225.

Wintrebert, C.M.A., Putter, H., Zwinderman, A.H. and van Houwelingen, J.C. (2004). Centre-effect on survival after bone marrow transplantation: application of time dependent frailty models. *Biom. J.* **46**, 512-525.

Wu, C.F.J. (1986). Jackknife, bootstrap and other resampling methods in regression analysis — discussion. *Ann. Stat.* **14**, 1261-1295.

Wulfsohn, M.S. and Tsiatis, A.A. (1997). A joint model for survival and longitudinal data measured with error. *Biometrics* **53**, 330-339.

Xue, X. and Brookmeyer, R. (1996). Bivariate frailty model for the analysis of multivariate survival data. *Lifetime Data Anal.* **2**, 277-290.

Yashin, A.I. and Iachine, I.A. (1995). Genetic analysis of durations: correlated frailty model applied to survival of Danish twins. *Genet. Epidemiol.* **12**, 529-538.

Yashin, A.I. and Iachine, I.A. (1997). How frailty models can be used for evaluating longevity limits: taking advantage of an interdisciplinary approach. *Demography* **34**, 31-48.

Yashin, A.I. and Iachine, I.A. (1999). Dependent hazards in multivariate survival problems. *J. Multivar. Anal.* **71**, 241-261.

Yashin, A.I., Vaupel, J.W. and Iachine, I.A. (1993). Correlated individual frailty: an advantageous approach to survival analysis of bivariate data. *Working paper series: Population Studies of Aging 7*, CHS, Odense University.

Yashin, A.I., Vaupel, J.W. and Iachine, I.A. (1995). Correlated individual frailty: an advantageous approach to survival analysis of bivariate data. *Math. Popul. Stud.* **5**, 145-159.

Yau, K.K.W. (2001). Multilevel models for survival analysis with random effects. *Biometrics* **57**, 96-102.

Yau, K.K.W. and McGilchrist, C.A. (1997). Use of generalised linear mixed models for the analysis of clustered survival data. *Biom. J.* **39**, 3-11.

Yau, K.K.W. and McGilchrist, C.A. (1998). ML and REML estimation in survival analysis with time dependent correlated frailty. *Stat. Med.* **17**, 1201-1213.

Yin, G.S. and Ibrahim, J.G. (2005). A class of Bayesian shared gamma frailty models with multivariate failure time data. *Biometrics* **61**, 208-216.

Applications and Examples Index

Author Index

Subject Index

Accelerated failure time model, vii, 1, 3, 26, 27, 30, 31, 53, 54, 196, 292, 293

Adaptive rejection sampling, 241, 250, 251, 254, 282

Akaike's information criterion, 60, 61

Asymptotic efficiency, 84, 109

Bayes theorem, 66, 142, 203, 240

Bayesian analysis, viii, 1–3, 43, 65, 66, 68, 74, 199, 233, 246, 255, 259–261, 279, 280, 286, 292, 293

Best linear unbiased predictor, 211

Bivariate Gaussian process, 291, 292

Bivariate survival data, 3, 77, 95–98, 100, 104, 111, 116, 123, 138, 141, 144, 145, 159, 171, 185, 288

Censoring
  distribution, 19
  doubly, 288
  informative, 288
  interval, 8, 17, 19, 20, 43, 61, 63, 64, 280, 284, 285, 287
  left, 287, 288
  right, 5, 8, 17, 19, 20, 24, 43, 61, 62, 153, 167, 280, 284, 285, 287, 288, 291

Competing risks, 291

Confounding, 82, 86

Copula, vii, 2, 77, 93–104, 116, 121, 158, 159, 172
  Archimedean, 95, 97, 104, 106, 107, 138
  Clayton, 77, 97, 99–101, 103, 138, 172
  inverse Gaussian, 160, 172

positive stable, 171–173

power variance function family, 185

Correlated frailty model, 3, 288, 290

Credible set, 65

Cross ratio function, 117, 126–129, 141, 144–147, 163–165, 175, 176, 188, 189

Delta method, 31, 64

EM algorithm, vii, 1, 3, 199–204, 207–210, 214, 215, 218, 246, 247, 286, 293

Fisher information matrix, 46, 47, 84, 85, 116, 275

Fixed effects model, 2, 77–87

Frailty distribution
  compound Poisson, 2, 117, 118, 190, 191, 193, 196, 258
  gamma, 2, 35, 37, 43, 44, 54, 61–63, 65, 66, 79, 100–102, 105, 111, 113–115, 117, 118, 130, 131, 134, 136, 138, 140–145, 147, 163, 164, 174, 176, 177, 180, 191, 196, 199, 200, 203, 207, 210, 213–215, 221, 222, 224, 228, 230, 232–234, 238, 245, 247, 258, 259, 269, 277, 280, 282, 288
  inverse Gaussian, 2, 54, 117, 118, 150, 152, 155, 156, 158, 160–164, 167, 170, 174, 176, 177, 179, 187
  lognormal, 2, 117, 118, 195, 196, 210–215, 221, 222, 224, 228, 230, 232, 234, 244, 245, 247, 249, 258, 265, 269, 277, 280, 282, 284, 290

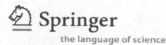
springer.com

The Statistical Analysis of Recurrent Events

Richard J. Cook and Jerald F. Lawless

The purpose of this book is to present models and statistical methods for the analysis of recurrent event data. No single comprehensive treatment of these areas currently exists. The authors provide broad but detailed coverage of the major approaches to analysis, while also emphasizing the modeling assumptions that they are based on. Thus, they consider important models such as Poisson and renewal processes, with extensions to incorporate covariates or random effects.

2007. 416 pp. (Statistics for Biology and Health) Hardcover
ISBN 978-0-387-69809-0

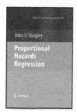

Proportional Hazards Regression

John O'Quigley

This book focuses on the theory and applications of a very broad class of models—proportional hazards and non-proportional hazards models, the former being viewed as a special case of the latter—which underlie modern survival analysis. Unlike other books in this area the emphasis is not on measure theoretic arguments for stochastic integrals and martingales. Instead, while inference based on counting processes and the theory of martingales is covered, much greater weight is placed on more traditional results such as the functional central limit theorem.

2007. 480 pp. (Statistics for Biology and Health) Hardcover
ISBN 978-0-387-25148-6

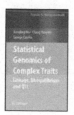

Statistical Genomics of Complex Traits

Rongling Wu, Changxing Ma, and George Casella

The book introduces the basic concepts and methods that are useful in the statistical analysis and modeling of DNA-based marker and phenotypic data that arise in agriculture, forrestry, experimental biology, and other fields. It concentrates on the linkage analysis of markers, map construction and quantitative trait locus (QTL) mapping and assumes a background in regression analysis and maximum likelihood approaches.

2007. 365 pp. (Statistics for Biology and Health) Hardcover
ISBN 978-0-387-20334-8